BEFORE YOU PUT THAT ON

Other style books by Lloyd Boston

Men of Color: Fashion, History, Fundamentals (Artisan)

Make Over Your Man: The Woman's Guide to Dressing Any Man in Her Life (Broadway)

BEFORE YOU PUT THAT ON

365 DAILY STYLE TIPS FOR HER

Written and Illustrated by

LLOYD BOSTON

ATRIA BOOKS

NEW YORK LONDON TORONTO SYDNEY

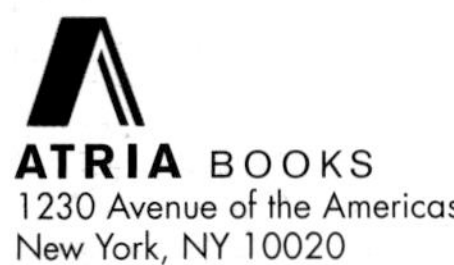
ATRIA BOOKS
1230 Avenue of the Americas
New York, NY 10020

Photographs by Keith Major

ISBN-13: 978-0-7432-8169-0
ISBN-10: 0-7432-8169-1

First Atria Books hardcover edition September 2005

10 9 8 7 6 5 4 3 2 1

Manufactured in the United States of America

All illustrations in this book were created by Lloyd Boston with Windsor & Newton Designers Gouache and Berol Prismacolor thick lead art pencils.

For my mother, Lynell, and "Uncle Jake" and "Aunt Jean," thanks for keeping me safe

CONTENTS

PREFACE

I love my job! Yes, I am probably one of the few who can honestly say that I truly love my job. As an author, television host, and fashion editor, I basically go clothing shopping for a living. And with the help of television I can assist millions of real women in looking and feeling better each and every day using what I find. A blessing.

Before You Put That On is a book for real women of all shapes, sizes, and lifestyles in search of better style year-round. Not just for special occasions or job interviews, but every time you leave the house.

First, I'd like to thank real women everywhere for almost writing my latest book for me! That may sound strange, but it is true. Between the days that I am serving as the on-air fashion editor for America's number-one morning show, NBC's *Today*, I have had the privilege to travel America as spokesperson for numerous fashion designers, mass brands, and labels, spreading the gospel of high style and easy tips on looking great—from intimate fashion shows in boutiques and department stores, to local morning television makeover spots at the crack of dawn, to special appearances for women's organizations and national conventions. Style has fast become the new motivational genre for women and men.

While getting on and off airplanes and trains and in and out of automobiles, I have witnessed so many real women (not fashion models) going about their day in the most unflattering clothing. And it makes me so sad. Mostly because on each of these women there was at least one redeeming outfit area that could have been played up, but they consciously or unconsciously chose to play it down. Many times I just wanted to reach out and politely whisper a tiny little anonymous tip: "Go one size larger on your bra, miss." Or, "Add a cuff to those pants for maximum glamour." I would have been slapped or security would have been called. So I chose to keep my mouth shut.

Instead of looking and sounding like an insane fashion stalker, I decided to take all of the wrongs I have witnessed and "right" them for every woman to benefit from, each day of any given year. Enter *Before You Put That On*.

A tip a day? 365 of them? It may sound intimidating to absorb, but I mean, really, why care about how you look every day? No one else does. Your kids love it when you show up to parent/teacher night dressed like you've been plowing the farm all day. Your husband really doesn't care because he gets his eyeful of the women at work who actually still take the time to do their nails and hair regularly. And your boss, why bother? Looking at you in the cramped cubicle year after year from her corner office suits her just fine. Not anymore.

Although every tip in this book won't speak to every woman, much of the style advice that is offered each day are fashion solutions using what you may very well already own. Some tips you may already know, so this is just confirmation that you are doing the right style thing.

You will notice somewhat generic clothing descriptions, and that I deal with "big picture" style (your top, your bottom, your shoes) often devoid of designer names, specific accessories, prints and patterns, etcetera. This was intentional to allow women of all bodies, budgets, and lifestyles to read the style ideas, interpret them to suit their needs, and most of all empower a personal style power without them having to run out and find a specific floral skirt with lace trim and beading. Who has time?

An artist for as long as I can remember, I have always been fascinated with the way women dress—from images of celebrities on the big and small screens, to real women who would never imagine that a young man was noticing their shoes and lipstick. I think it began with my second-grade teacher—Miss Sanders had the most beautiful lip color that stuck together just in the corners of her mouth when she spoke. You never saw her reapply as the day went on; it was just always perfectly in place atop her full lips.

My mom was a walking supermodel to me as I was growing up. I distinctly remember feeling so secure holding her hand on the way to preschool—yes, that early—and noticing the jingle of the stacks of thin sterling-silver bracelets on her wrists, and the sound her slim frame made as she walked across the gravel parking lot in her stacked wedge shoes. I would always try to walk harder to make the same noise, but my tiny body just wasn't heavy enough pull it off.

This spark led to well over fifteen years in the fashion and television industries, and nothing pleases me more than helping real women get dressed, and seeing them look and feel their absolute best afterward. I'm always amazed by how much pain women put up with when there are so many more comfortable solutions that are just as stylish. From shoes to undergarments, there is a world of possibilities so many women rush by to get to their old standbys. *Before You Put That On* unearths many of them.

Kind of like sleeping on the remote, you usually wake up on some channel that scares you in the middle of the night. This is what happens when you just start getting dressed each day and not dressing well. To do this, sometimes all you need is a little pearl of inspiration to set you on your way. And note that although each day has a specific tip, they are very universal and can be used whenever you need a boost. Go ahead and use the tip from January 13 on May 23!

Whether they realize it or not, when most women give a thumbs-up to a red carpet star or magazine page, they are saying that they'd love to look like that one day, one night. It may seem like an insurmountable task, though. This is why a little growth each day is the best way to get there. Hopefully, with the help of my book, and within the course of a calendar year, you will be on track to a stylish New Year and newer style!

I hope to show you how one key piece can give you a multitude of looks. As you turn the pages you will see how to go from your desk to dinner in no time. And finally figure out what really needs to be retired without hesitation from your packed closet.

Sometimes life can seem like one big to-do list, and most women forget to put themselves at the very top. This is where *Before You Put That On* comes in, boasting daily tips for low-maintenance high fashion.

My sincere hope is that this book will be a continuum to my TV work of helping real women everywhere to look and, most important, feel their absolute best. One woman, one day, one outfit at a time.

You have to invest in your appearance to shine, not only monetarily through clothing and accessories, but also with a little time and thought. This book asks you for just a few short minutes each day. For some this may be over coffee in the morning as you plan your outfit, whereas for others it will be a bedtime read that allows you to dream up a better outfit for tomorrow than you wore today. Make it a private ritual that gives you a little time to look within yourself and exceed your own style expectations. This is all that really matters.

You will come to find that having style is like riding a bike. You will know it when you have it, and so will every woman who passes you by. You've witnessed this before, and know it right away. And just like you respond to other women with great style, you'll begin to get the same reactions. Sometimes it is as simple as a locked glance, but those who know, will know.

JANUARY

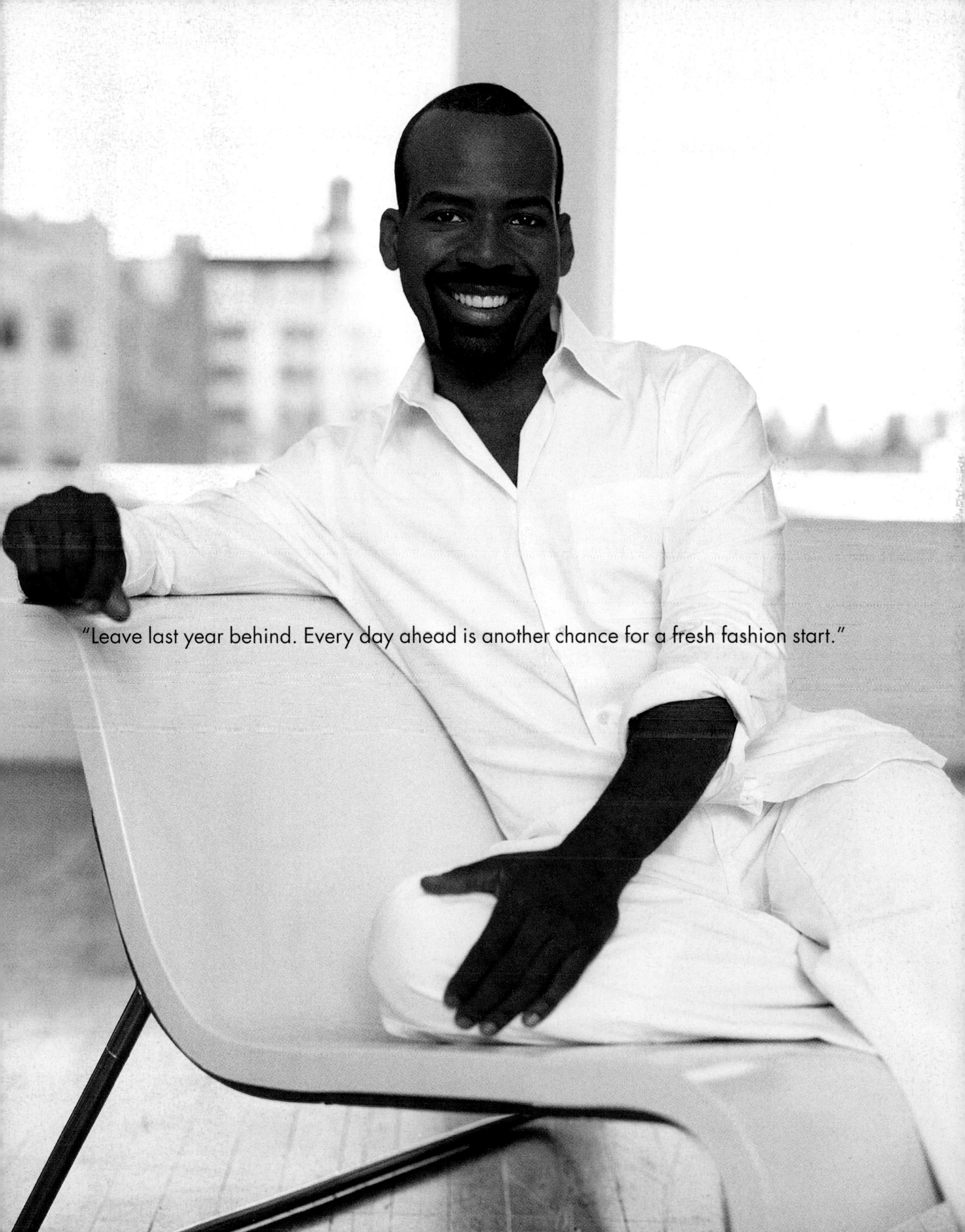
"Leave last year behind. Every day ahead is another chance for a fresh fashion start."

JANUARY 1 | CLAIM THIS YEAR AS YOUR MOST STYLISH EVER. MAKE A PACT WITH YOURSELF TO EXPLORE NEW IDEAS, BREAK BAD HABITS, AND BE OPEN TO CHANGE.

To have style is to give shape to the way you carry yourself. Our focus here is primarily on the way you dress, but the truth is that every way in which you present yourself to the world is important.

Set a tone for the new year rather than commit yourself to resolutions—which most of us break in ninety days' time. Think of adding or practicing good habits, as opposed to denying yourself. If you're in the habit of wearing black, commit to adding some color. If you're accustomed to loose garments, try more tailored or form-fitting ones. Start one item at a time.

Don't claim New Year's resolutions, embrace a positive evolution.

Affirmation:
Before I put anything on, I will take two minutes each day to focus on ways to a more stylish me.

JANUARY 2 | WEAR WORKOUT CLOTHES THAT WILL INSPIRE YOU TO KEEP IT MOVING.

Motivating yourself to exercise is tough whether you're working out to a program on DVD in the privacy of your home or in a public or co-ed space. You know the scene at the gym. Some members—the gym bunnies—are in better shape than others and hop around letting everyone know it. Others—maybe you—slink around trying to draw as little attention as possible.

Give yourself a self-esteem boost. Wear workout clothes that make you look and *feel* good—own two or three outfits that are simple, comfortable, and fit well. Try a tank in a bright color, paired with a darker drawstring yoga pant and your cleanest sneakers, athletic shoes, or even ballet slippers, depending on the activity. Or, invest in a supple velour sweat suit in a dark neutral with a bright-colored shoe.

The cut of your workout gear should cover enough of you so that you never feel exposed, yet not large enough to make you feel like you are under a tarp. For instance, swap the XXL giveaway T-shirts for lightweight, zip-front track jackets that can be opened to reveal more, as your body takes on the new shape. And instead of oversized men's sweatpants, opt for ultrathin, drawstring lounge pants that offer the full coverage of a pajama pant without the thick, visual-pound-adding bulk of traditional sweats.

No need to go to great expense by buying brand-named athletic gear, and definitely avoid working out in heavy makeup or high-maintenance coiffed hair (though a subtle energizing scent could be nice). The idea is that when you look good, you feel better about doing anything—even if it's an activity you dread. High style can inspire you to high performance and results that stick.

JANUARY 3 | ADD PRINTS AND PATTERNS TO THE BEST EFFECT.

Prints, plaids, and stripes are a stylish option for all women no matter what your size. So why, you might be asking yourself, has it been such a long-held belief that patterns only flatter tall and/or slender women and take fashion points away from fuller or shorter figures?

The key to looking fabulous in that floral-patterned garment or checked jacket is balanced proportions and an overall look that doesn't overshadow your personality. Leave the solids in the drawer for a change.

Try a horizontal striped T-shirt under a tailored blazer with your favorite jeans. Try a muted-plaid skirt with a knee boot to give your look some energy in the dead of winter. If you are larger or smaller than the average woman, avoid extremes such as teeny prints, microflorals, or, on the opposite end, large checks or patterns in bright colors. Moderation applies well here. When in doubt, go for the medium-size prints that make a chic style statement without screaming for attention.

JANUARY 4

TAKE AN EXPERT STYLE CUE FROM TOP NEW YORK STYLE-MAKER ADAM GLASSMAN, CREATIVE DIRECTOR OF *O, THE OPRAH MAGAZINE.*

What is your best-kept personal style secret?

Buy good-quality, well-tailored clothing, mostly in natural fabrics like cashmere, wool, and cotton. Think of fabrics that are good for three seasons a year. It's better to spend extra money on pieces that last a long time.

What are the three fashion essentials every well-dressed woman should own?

1. Crisp white shirts. You can never have enough. They are great for work, weekend, or evening for a casual evening look, paired with a dressy skirt, pants, or suits.
2. Great-fitting wool gabardine pants with some stretch in them. They travel great, wear well, and don't have to be dry-cleaned as often. Get them in navy, khaki, medium gray, tan, or black.
3. Four styles of shoes . . .
   - A low-heel sling-back in black
   - A flat for work and comfort
   - An evening shoe—a high heel, mule, or flat
   - A casual shoe like a moccasin or deck shoe, for traveling or weekends

What are the biggest mistakes women make when getting dressed?

Not thinking about their outfit. It's important to spend time on creating a look. Some people have an innate sense of style and it comes easily to them. For those who don't have this, it is important to learn how to dress just as we learn how to do other things in our lives that we are not as great at. First impressions are a factor in life whether we like it or not, so keep that in mind when you go out the door. If you are not comfortable in trendy clothes stick with classics and simple lines. It is important that people see you first and your clothes second. You should wear the clothes, not let the clothes wear you!

Who is the most stylish woman in existence, in your opinion? And what do you appreciate about her look?

Supermodel Linda Evangelista—no matter what she puts on she looks amazing. And Naomi Campbell looks great in vintage or runway looks.

If you could whisper a fail-safe style tip into the ears of women everywhere, without them feeling bad by hearing it, what would it be?

Think before you shop. Take stock of what you own, what you need, and how to replenish your wardrobe. Do not shop just because it's a "buy or steal," or looks good on someone else. Know your body and work with, not against, it.

JANUARY 5 | WOODEN HANGERS, PLEASE.

I had to go there. Who can forget those infamous words forever linked with Joan Crawford: no wire hangers. The idea here is not to remind you of a nightmare, but rather to fulfill your desire for a dream closet to store your elements of style.

True style isn't just about the clothes, after all. It's also about how the clothes are organized, stored, and maintained. Most of us are not able to dial up a closet design company and have them gut-renovate and then install custom shelving and cabinetry. But we can afford to treat our clothes better—even with the standard too-small closets most apartment and house dwellers have—by investing in quality wooden hangers. You'll need two basic types: those that are tapered for dresses, blouses, and jackets, and those that have clips for pants and skirts.

The average cost for basic blond wood hangers is around $5 new, in most stores. You can choose the more expensive versions made of mahogany, walnut, or cedar, but any wood will serve the purpose. Look for them at flea markets for a bargain price. Whatever the price, they extend the life of your clothes because they are sturdy. They hold their shape (better than wire or plastic), and allow the garment to hold its shape and prevent wrinkles and creases.

Buy ten at a time, and before you know it, you'll have a closet that not only better serves your clothes, but is more pleasing to your eye.

JANUARY 6

GET A LITTLE HELP FROM YOUR FRIENDS. ASK A FEW GOOD FRIENDS TO COMMIT TO TOTAL HONESTY IN GIVING YOU FEEDBACK ON HOW YOU LOOK.

Give the woman in your mirror some support. You can't possibly expect her to make sure you're perfect in your presentation all by herself. She can't see you the way others see you because, among other reasons, she's too close.

Choose a few friends who have a taste and style that has always impressed you. Ask them to form an honesty alliance. Think The Supremes. The Go-Go's. Destiny's Child. I bet they all used this tip to keep one another looking ready for the world stage.

JANUARY 7

DO A SHOE-HEEL INVENTORY. MAKE SURE WHAT YOU OWN MEETS THE STANDARD: FIT, FLATTERY, AND TIMELESSNESS.

The right shoes can not only complete your look, they can increase your confidence and add polish to your posture as well. Here's a checklist:

Nude-colored high heels
Black closed-toe work pumps in solid leather
Work sling-back
Black evening pumps in satin, embellished leather, patent leather, or a fun skin
1–1½-inch kitten heel with a slightly pointed toe
High-heeled sandal
Real or faux skin heels, simply the best you can afford
Barely there strappy heel
Metallic high heel
Ankle strap pumps
Peep-toe pumps

JANUARY 8 | TAKE AN EXPERT STYLE CUE FROM MICHAEL KORS, A TOP AMERICAN DESIGNER.

What is your best-kept personal style secret?
Dark colors on top, light colors on the bottom.

What are the three fashion essentials every well-dressed woman should own?
A perfect khaki trench coat to wear over everything from jeans to a gown; a knee-length, fitted, black sheath dress that can go from the office to a black-tie party depending on accessories; and a pair of oversized black sunglasses to give you instant glamour no matter how tired you are.

What are the biggest mistakes women make when getting dressed?
Not looking in a three-way mirror—everyone else is seeing you from the back, why shouldn't you? Thinking that things will look perfect off the rack—even jeans and a T-shirt can be made more fabulous and flattering with tailoring.

Who is the most stylish woman in existence, in your opinion? And what do you appreciate about her look?
Jackie O. She had an editor's eye and was able to filter the look of each decade into her own style. She never forgot that the right clothes and accessories are all about framing your personality.

If you could whisper a fail-safe style tip into the ears of women everywhere, without them feeling bad by hearing it, what would it be?
Never think in terms of quantity, always in terms of quality. Given the choice between cutting edge and classic, always steer to the classic—you can't go wrong.

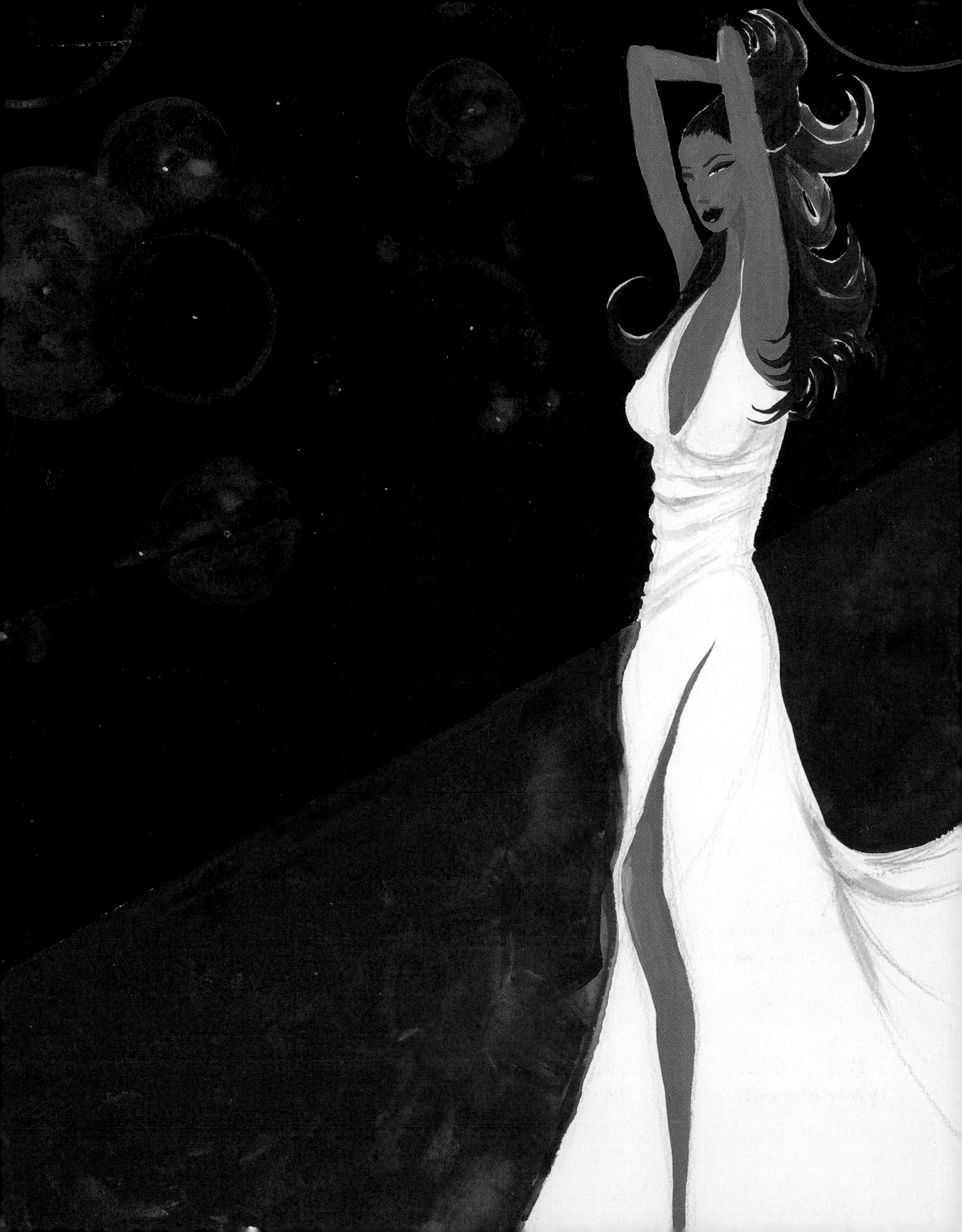

JANUARY 9 | BE A BETTER SHOPPER. LEARN A NEW FASHION TERM.

Ruching (roo-shing) • *Trimming made by pleating a strip of lace, ribbon, net, fine muslin, or silk so that it ruffles on both sides. Made by stitching through the center of pleating. Also spelled* rouche, ruche.

Women who want their midsection to look svelte should know the power of ruching, a trimming effect that creates a visual tension, almost as if gathered fabric is being obviously pulled to one direction. You will find ruching on everything from swimsuits to evening gowns. The look of a tensely ruched garment can create a slimming illusion to the eye and actually minimize a "questionable" area.

When shopping for the perfect top that is both elegant and functional, be sure to ask the most seasoned sales representative you can find if there are any tops that have ruched details. If they aren't certain what you mean, simply say "the gathered sections of fabric on a top."

The look can also bring to mind the 1940s, when women delighted in a sexy fit that was still sophisticated and left something to the imagination. Think of Betty Grable, the original bombshell swimsuit pinup girl who regularly offered curves yet revealed little to nothing, thanks to the power of ruching.

JANUARY 10 | TAKE AN EXPERT BEAUTY CUE FROM MALLY RONCAL, A TOP CELEBRITY MAKEUP ARTIST AND FOUNDER OF MALLY BEAUTY.

What is your best-kept personal beauty secret?
I use a facial mask that I make in my own kitchen. Take one egg white and some cornmeal, mix it together, and put it on your face. When it dries, wash it off and your skin will glow! Also, I put olive oil on my hair as a deep conditioner. Works wonders.

What are the three beauty essentials every woman should own?
1. An eyelash curler is an instant pick-me-up that immediately makes you look gorgeous and wide-awake.
2. Black eyeliner can be used for a soft polished look just on the upper lashes or for an instant smoky eye by lining all around and smudging with a Q-tip or your finger. It's a perfect way to define your eyes.

(CONTINUED)

3. A swipe of a beautiful, natural-looking blush like juicy coral, fresh apricot, or youthful pink instantly wakes up the face and makes you look alive.

What are the biggest mistakes women make when applying makeup?
Wearing too much base or using the wrong color base. Remember that base is meant to be invisible! I see lots of women out there covering up their beautiful skin with loads of heavy base.

Heavy, dark lip liner is another. Women think that by overdrawing their lips in a dark liner that they are making their lips look bigger. In actuality it makes the lips look smaller. Opt for a nude lip liner that matches your lip tone exactly. You will achieve the fullest lip-look possible.

Who is the most stylish woman in existence, in your opinion?
Jacqueline Kennedy Onassis, who exuded timeless, effortless glamour.

If you could whisper a fail-safe beauty tip into the ears of women everywhere, without them feeling bad by hearing it, what would it be?
Take care of your skin. It is the number-one beauty tip. When you have beautiful skin you hardly need any makeup!

JANUARY 11 | THINK OF THE PEN YOU PULL OUT AS A REFLECTION OF YOUR STYLE.

Your fifty-nine-cent writing pen might be stealing your fashion edge in the moments that really count. Sure, it probably makes no difference to you when writing a check behind closed doors, since the recipient will never know. But when you have a stylish, quality pen in your hand out in the open, even the most mundane use gets a first-class upgrade.

It wasn't until the 1940s that a woman would pull out a ballpoint pen to write with in private or in public. A proper lady used a fountain pen, as did just about everyone else for that matter. The heavy and sometimes messy metal fountain pens that most of us see as special or fancy were standard in the handbag of a woman, with or without notable style. Today, choosing to write with a quality, design-forward writing pen, be it fountain or not, versus a disposable, plastic ballpoint, is a decision that can punctuate your entire look.

Think about it. Your every commonplace action leading up to your pen has your attention; why stop? Your blouse of silk is a favorite and fits perfectly, your watch or bracelet says a bit about who you are. Your gorgeous ring is a symbol of something important. You spent $30 on that perfect manicure and lotion that leave your hands supple. And out comes a chewed-up, plastic pen with clotted ink in the tube's chamber.

Use this moment to look at what you are pulling out to write with. Maybe you have a few pens. Discard the weakest and keep the one that looks the best. If that pen is still not commensurate with your taste level when it is time to seal the deal, or just write a monthly bill, it's time to treat yourself to one that is. No need to send me a handwritten thank-you either, although with a new pen I'm sure you will want to.

JANUARY 12 | IDENTIFY YOUR "LIFE PALETTE" AND BEGIN TO TRUST IT.

Most people have a favorite color or several colors that they prefer and viscerally respond to. I refer to those colors as a "life palette."

Take a close look at your closet, your bedroom, your makeup drawer, or shelf of nail polish. You will no doubt see that you probably have a particular color pattern within each. It might be mostly neutrals in your closet, with bold pastel accents throughout. Your makeup might be all warm tones with dusty, burnished finishes. And your nail colors might be all sheer pastels with a hint of shimmer.

We sometimes unconsciously select the colors we like and create a continuum of this grouping in all that we do, yet often we do not trust it to guide us—especially when shopping. Sometimes we look at a mannequin and want to purchase the entire outfit—or wonder if we should instead just buy the red skirt we adore. Trusting the latter choice allows you to lean on the palette of what you already own, knowing that this new addition (in a color from your life palette) will undoubtedly complement many of the items already in your closet—thus saving you money and space.

Embrace the colors you instinctively love, and your wardrobe will eventually fall into place as if a designer dressed you.

JANUARY 13 | MAKE YOUR OWN TIME-SAVING STYLE FILE.

Actresses do it. Professional stylists do it. Even your favorite top designers do it. They all call it "inspiration." I call it a "style file." A style file is the way to better style in less time and with less stress. It is simple, eliminates clutter (you'll be tossing out magazine pages upon pages that will never matter again), and keeps you feeling new.

The next time you flip through a magazine and see a look that really makes you swoon, look a little closer at what the women in the images are wearing and break the outfits down into pieces. You can glean a fashion idea from just about any image if you take the time to really see the clothing elements and not get distracted by who is wearing it, her size, hair, and the exotic location—we call this the fantasy. It is what sells the clothes, but it can also give you the road map to a great outfit. You will wonder why you hadn't done this sooner since it is virtually free when you stop to think about the time you save versus the cost of a fashion magazine.

Tear out what you like, even if it is just a shot of a belt buckle. Keep the pages in a binder or folder and divide them by season, daytime, nighttime, intimates, shoes—whatever works for you. There's just one rule: Run to it if you are ever short on time or new outfit ideas, which happens to even the most stylish women. But not you, right after the very first rrrrrrip!

JANUARY 14 | LOOK FOR FALL/WINTER CLEARANCE SALES.

The middle of January is when most larger department stores and retail chains begin to drastically cut prices on the many items you have been swooning over for months. What a great time to stock up on finds for next winter, or for the rest of this one. Call a salesperson to get a feel for what the reductions are before bursting into the store. Many times, if you know what is ahead, you can plan accordingly, or go at a later time when reductions really meet your pocketbook right where they should.

Be sure to get on your favorite store's mailing list, for select stores will cut prices in small reductions from now through the end of the month, and hold a massive two-day clearance event—usually over a weekend or holiday weekend. You will know about it first. And whatever does not sell is sometimes shipped off to an outlet store owned by the same brand—so all is not lost. Find out where it is located, and get on its mailing list as well.

JANUARY 15 | SEAMLESS BRAS RULE.

Do you own a nude seamless bra? If your answer is no, please close this book immediately and get yourself to the nearest lingerie or department store. Find the manager, not just a salesperson, and tell them that I sent you to purchase one.

Unlike the push-up, racerback, no-wire, or even the strapless bra, the nude seamless bra is, by far, the most versatile bra a woman can own whether worn to the office or for a weekend brunch with friends. The undergarment lines will virtually disappear, working ingeniously beneath a myriad of fabrics, from your best wool sweaters and cashmere tops, to simple cotton shirts and tees.

When selecting a nude version, remember that the standard nude may not be your nude. For some women, nude is a deep chocolate brown; for others, a flesh tone similar to a Band-Aid. Take the time to find one that is near invisible, like that of a quality makeup foundation for the face.

In general, seamless or not, always opt for bra fabrics that have clean and smooth surfaces, not the bras with lots of frilly straps, sweet ribbons, or chunky topstitched seam lines.

JANUARY 16 | WEAR A HAT FOR STYLE, NOT JUST FOR WARMTH.

When Faye Dunaway's portrayal of the infamous Bonnie Parker in the 1967 movie *Bonnie and Clyde* had her wearing a sleek, simple beret, hat sales of the same style shot up almost instantly around the globe. Primarily because she looked just as powerful as her male counterparts—even in her fitted pencil skirts and bold lipstick. And as the 1970s approached, what woman didn't want a little more power? So female fans of the now-classic style flick sat up and took notice.

As we look around at women on the street today, the business of hats as stylish accessories is virtually dead, when, in fact, wearing a hat is one of the simplest ways to add a smidge of verve to a basic coat, cool-weather pantsuit, or your favorite jeans and turtleneck sweater. Especially if you want to look more original than the next woman on the street.

Whether a beret, a fedora, a floppy brim, or a newsboy, build your entire outfit around how it makes you feel. Take a wool newsboy or beret and give a menswear twist to a blazer and trouser combo. Hark back to the 1970s with a felt floppy-brimmed hat à la Diana Ross in *Mahogany*, which can bring a shirtdress up to runway standards. Or go "gangster" with a stingy-brimmed fedora tilted to one side—just like one of the many signature looks of the ultrafeminine Sophia Loren in the 1960s.

Wouldn't you just love to feel the joy today that Mary Tyler Moore did as she flung up her beret in the opening sequence of her legendary hit television show? Well, you've got to toss one on before you can toss it up!

JANUARY 17 | PROTECT YOUR DRESS SHOES WITH RUBBER SOLES AND CEDAR SHOE TREES.

Telling a woman's station in life is easy. Look at her shoes and you will instantly know her whole story—or at least the story she wants you to know.

Is she a pampered princess who travels by car and driver? Is she someone who is on her feet all day long, and then runs for the bus home? Maybe she's the CEO of a Fortune 500 company who trots from her carpeted corner office to fancy lunch meetings all week. One look at her shoes will give you a clue as to which road she's been traveling—or one day hopes to travel.

While most women tend to worry more about the style of their shoes or how they match a particular outfit, the actual condition and appearance of their shoe of choice gets kicked to the curb. The visuals are at once sad and funny: puppy-nibbled heels, "witchy" curled toes, cat-scratched leather surfaces, and the classic super-stretched opening à la Minnie Mouse. These attributes can make even the most expensive pair of designer shoes look like a hand-me-down.

Take a moment and commit to caring for new shoes and revitalizing your existing shoe collection in a way that will make you shine from the bottom up. Here are two simple things you can do to ensure that your shoes remain ready for their close-up for years to come:

THE GOOD WOOD

When looking at the price of new shoes, automatically add an additional $20 to the price tag. This will get you in the habit of factoring in the cost of cedar shoe trees for each and every pair of dress shoes. Choose cedar over plastic for their ability to absorb moisture, maintain the shoes' original shape, and naturally iron out creases caused by walking and toe-flexing.

WHERE THE RUBBER MEETS THE ROAD

Have rubber soles applied to the bottoms of your new and old shoes. You can even find ultrathin versions to keep your stilettos looking sleek, while adding a layer of protection between you and hard-paved surfaces. When they wear down, you simply replace them—not your shoes.

JANUARY 18

LOOK BACK AT WOMEN'S HISTORY AND USE THE STRENGTH AND STYLE OF YOUR FOREMOTHERS TO INSPIRE TOTAL CONFIDENCE IN YOUR CLOTHES—AND IN YOUR CHARACTER.

January 18, 1777: Baltimore newspaper publisher and postmaster Mary Katherine Goddard produced the first printed copy of the Declaration of Independence.

The image that most people connect with the signing of the Declaration of Independence is one of fancifully coiffed powdered wigs and pronounced hosiery gracing well-shaped legs, but not on women. It is refreshing to know that a Maryland woman, Mary Katherine Goddard, was at the center of this historic event. Goddard produced the very first printed copy of this document that would forever change the way Americans would lead their lives—a document that would inspire democracy around the globe.

Make history in your own way on this day by kicking off the year in winning outfits that speak of importance and character. This simply means a more conscious approach to pulling the best you together each day so that you won't be rendered invisible—or worse, forgotten.

And although you are a few weeks into the year, it is not too late to add a small amendment to your New Year's evolution to pick your clothes with a greater consciousness. In the spirit of Mary Katherine Goddard, try claiming this one today so that you won't be forgotten:

What I choose to wear from tip-to-toe will reflect the fact that I am a woman in the know.
Every piece that I wear, be it a blouse or a dress, will inspire, flatter, and more than impress.

JANUARY 19 | GET "MODEL CONFIDENCE" BY PUTTING FITNESS, NOT JUST FASHION, IN THE FOREFRONT OF YOUR MIND.

One trick of the fashion industry is the use of the fashion model: a woman who generally (and subliminally) represents the ideal of what every woman wishes to be. I also learned this is not always the case, for one woman can never be all things to all women. Thankfully, the term *model* now applies to a more diverse profile of professional women ranging from stick thin to curvy and plus-size, blond with Nordic blue eyes, to chocolate brown with thick, curly hair, and they are working alone and alongside one another. Beautiful! How their function serves the industry is obvious: When you look through a magazine and see a garment worn by such a model, you may buy it. Perfect business.

But I also think women can be *personally* inspired by models, even beyond the clothes. And the reason is their fit bodies, slim or curvy, that allows them to jump into anything and make it look amazing! The way every woman wishes she could.

And although many of these working gals are naturally fit, many have to work at it—as should you, so you can have the same unbridled joy of jumping into any garment you fancy.

Use this as a reminder to keep fitness ahead of fashion as the year passes. Take these women as your role model: With a fit body you feel great about, at any size, you can toss on jeans and a T-shirt and look just as good, if not better, than the out-of-shape woman dressed in thousands of dollars worth of designer clothing.

JANUARY 20 | HAPPY BIRTHDAY, AQUARIUS GIRL.

An earth sign with next to no limits, you reach for style where others dare not go. Off-the-beaten-path boutiques, thrift stores, consignment shops, and the good old Goodwill if you are really in the spirit to hunt down a find.

This never means that you'll be seen in some old ragtag dress scurrying about town. Shopping thrifty is about finding items with character and original details that excite you (and others). You'll mix in with these cost-effective finds a piece of estate jewelry, a crafts fair necklace from Santa Barbara, and new stiletto boots from a luxury department store and blow the minds of the entire room.

Eartha Kitt and Sarah McLachlan are cross-generational Aquarians who rely on the power of style freedom to fuel their on-stage images. And, just like you, if that spotlight dimmed tomorrow, the world will remain a style stage for them. Sometimes even a fashion runway!

JANUARY 21 | PACK A SCENTED CANDLE ON YOUR NEXT TRIP.

Getting away this or any time of the year is all about truly escaping from the dullness of your day-to-day life. Leaving behind the daily to-do list, the waking up on time and rushing to deadlines, and the nights of leftovers. By escaping to another place, your body and mind have a chance to refresh and restore themselves. Your personal style benefits from taking a break to another atmosphere, too, for it allows you to turn off (within reason) the need to feel put together.

One thing that always ties the mood of a getaway together is a signature scent. Whether intentional or by happenstance, the smell of your surroundings can leave a clear mark in your memory to the sights, feelings, sounds, and textures of wherever you are. It may be a cabin in the mountains, a Caribbean villa, or something as basic as a cute roadside motel in America's heartland. A change is a change. Scent is, in fact, the strongest sense tied to one memory.

A really inexpensive way to keep an escape alive is to pack a scented candle along with your clothes and toiletries. Choose a scent that is new to you, with a very distinct aroma. For you it may be intense lavender, eucalyptus, or even a mix of ginger and honeysuckle. Light your candle as you get dressed for a fun evening, burn it when you are in between showering from the beach and taking that rare midday nap, or let it waft you through breakfast in bed from a distance.

When you face your real world back home, and the glow of vacation leaves your skin and mind, remember that you always have an inexpensive way back without packing a bag. It works like a charm. Simply take out your candle and light it up to be instantly transported back, if only for an hour before the family gets home or you have to rush off to work.

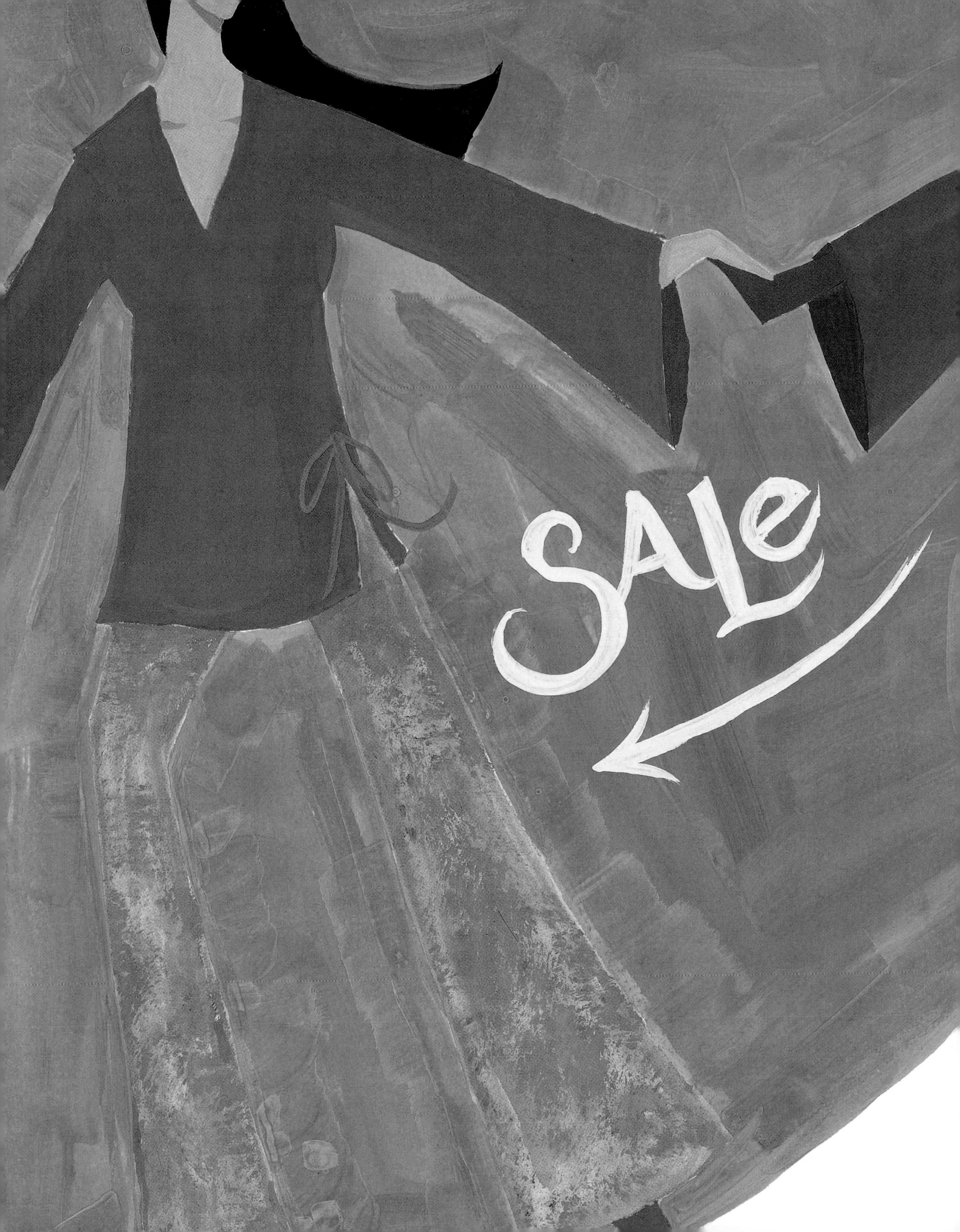
SALE

JANUARY 22 | TRY FEATURING A CAFTAN AND DRAWSTRING LOUNGE PANTS FOR COMFORT AND STYLE.

Instead of the oversized vacation souvenir T-shirt-and-stretch-pant combo, wear a caftan and drawstring pants. An exotic caftan and a pair of drawstring lounge pants will give you the same loose, free-spirited feel. Buy a men's pair of lounge pants if you need more room! You can find these at any East Indian clothing or fabric store for around $30 at the most.

Instead of sneakers, wear a new pair of backless slides to complete the Eastern look. They're probably even more comfy, and are more befitting the look.

JANUARY 23 | ADD AN ASIAN PRINT TO YOUR LOOK WHILE POLICING YOURSELF ON THE PERFECT WAY TO DO IT.

The lull of the midwinter blahs is chilly enough on its own—why not keep the sparkle of the season going, starting right now? While the year is still relatively new (at least in Western culture) keep the holiday festivities alive in your wardrobe for as long as you can. Wearing dashes of intense color, texture, and lively prints makes the holidays linger on sweetly—instead of rushing that "unplugged" feeling that happens just after the champagne goes flat, and the big clean-up on January 1.

Asian prints seem to patiently wait their turn to come "in" and "out" of fashion with a Zenlike confidence, knowing that, for the most stylish women, they are always "in" heavy wardrobe rotation. Whether opting for signature Chinese prints that take cues from the country's traditional paintings and interior design embroideries, often featuring swirly dragons, artful lanterns, and soothing clouds atop scenic mountains, or heading to Japanese prints where majestic pagodas, flora, and foliage dance around peaking mountains, your visual journey is almost limitless. Silk fabrics with black or dark grounds are probably the most recognizable, but brighter colors like lime and coral look just as good, even this time of year.

A Chinese cheongsam, the simple, straight-lined dress with a mandarin collar closing diagonally at the side (and daringly high side slits) is an amazing party dress. Or consider just a pair of embroidered Chinese slippers for nights entertaining at home. And how about a Japanese kimono with your white jeans instead of that expected blazer?

THREE WAYS TO ALWAYS LOOK STYLISH IN ASIAN PRINTS

• Pair bolder Asian prints with casual Western separates. Embroidered silk tops with fun jeans or tailored trousers give the look of a confident world traveler—not a wannabe.

• Avoid adding stereotypical accessories with Asian prints. For instance, lacquered chopsticks in the hair are a no-no, unless that is the only reference to the East you are featuring.

• Be sure the fit is roomy and forgiving. Many Eastern silhouettes are cut narrow. There's nothing worse than a skintight scene of a babbling brook and birds across an ample bustline.

JANUARY 24 | TAKE AN EXPERT STYLE CUE FROM KENNETH COLE, A TOP NEW YORK DESIGNER.

What is your best-kept personal style secret?
Style needs to appear innate and effortless. To the degree that it looks forced or overplanned, then your outfit looks contrived.

What are the three fashion essentials every well-dressed woman should own?
1. Comfortable and stylish shoes that you can wear to work and wear out that evening.
2. A blazer that works with jeans *and* with a skirt.
3. Self-confidence—the most important essential.

What are the biggest mistakes women make when getting dressed?
Women must always do a last-minute mirror check before leaving the house. Look at yourself and examine your outfit from all angles.

Who is the most stylish woman in existence, in your opinion? And what do you appreciate about her look?
I have three daughters and a beautiful wife. All are distinctly stylish.

If you could whisper a fail-safe style tip into the ears of women everywhere, without them feeling bad by hearing it, what would it be?
Always smile. If you think you look great, then you do. It's a self-fulfilling prophecy.

JANUARY 25 | POP STYLE QUIZ.

1. Which fashion designer was most identified with first lady Jacqueline Kennedy during her White House years?

A. Oleg Cassini
B. Karl Lagerfeld
C. Bonnie Cashin
D. Halston

2. Which pants silhouette should petite women avoid?

A. Jodhpur pants
B. Cigarette pants
C. Drawstring pants
D. Capri pants

3. The statement "A fashion is nothing but an induced epidemic" was made by which of the following scholars?

A. George Bernard Shaw
B. Oscar Wilde
C. Diana Vreeland
D. None of the above

4. Knee boots and knee-length skirts look best with . . .

A. No skin showing from hem to boot
B. Some skin showing from hem to boot
C. A receipt from the Salvation Army
D. A meter maid's badge

(Answers: 1-A, 2-D, 3-A, 4-B)

JANUARY 26 | TAKE AN EXPERT STYLE CUE FROM MARC BOUWER, A TOP NEW YORK DESIGNER.

What is your best-kept personal style secret?

What is important about dressing is wearing the right undergarments or no undergarments at all. Some body types need to be reshaped by corsetry before you put on the gown or outfit. It is the shape that is the most important thing. Some you want to show, some you want to hide. A G-string can show a bulge, so you may need to wear nothing. Start with the inside first.

What are the three fashion essentials every well-dressed woman should own?

I believe in four: a basic black pencil skirt, a wrinkle-proof white button-down blouse, a cashmere wrap, and a great pair of strappy black stilettos.

What are the biggest mistakes women make when getting dressed?

They get too used to themselves in one particular proportion or silhouette as they age, or as fashion changes. You need to look objectively and be very much aware of what's going on in the world of fashion. Otherwise you can get stuck in a time warp. Coloring changes, fashion changes. If you don't want to grow old with your audience, reinvention is the key to looking young and fashionable. Simple things like a new haircut or color and silhouette will do the trick.

Who is the most stylish woman, in your opinion? And what do you appreciate about her look?

My favorite is Angelina Jolie! The new Angelina has let her own beauty shine through. The clothes are never too much. They are sexy and simple—for example, the white dress that we did for her for the Academy Awards. Let your own beauty shine through and don't be afraid to be sexy.

Women should keep it simple, not tacky. If you are covered, make sure that there is interest in fabrication or added detail. The more open you are, the less detail you need. The more covered, the more detail.

Like a canvas, let the beauty shine through. Not fussy! If you wear a black turtleneck sweater, wear a fantastic pair of earrings or chain belt. The simpler the silhouette, the more you can add to it and be chic.

One last fail-safe tip for every woman?

Grooming is important. Hair should be beautifully styled or a great haircut. Makeup should be applied properly. It doesn't matter how much you wear as long as it's blended properly. Again, grooming is essential!

JANUARY 27 | GET TEN-MINUTE STYLE FOR AN IMPORTANT MEETING THAT LOOKS LIKE YOU SPENT HOURS PULLING IT TOGETHER.

Sometimes all you have is ten minutes to create a look that speaks of all you wish to represent. You've got to think fast, on your feet, pray you have the right clothing and accessories, and that they are clean, wrinkle-free, and within reach. So every minute counts.

Here is a great ten-minute style solution for an important business meeting:

Minutes 1:00–2:00:
Before anything, grab your smartest skirt or pantsuit in a solid color and place it in the bathroom while you shower for a free steaming to remove any wrinkles.

Minutes 3:00–4:00:
Pull out an ultrathin blouse and a fine-gauge sweater to layer atop it—or toss over your shoulders if you remove your jacket. Add color or pattern on one, not both.

Minutes 5:00–6:00:
Add a sharp side part to your hair, and put it back or up. Even a simple chignon looks smarter, more feminine, and more thought-out with a defined side part.

Minutes 7:00–8:00:
Choose sling-back heels over chunky heels or sensible flats, especially if you are presenting in front of a room. Keep comfy shoes on standby for afterward.

Minutes 9:00–10:00:
Keep makeup minimal. Focus on undereye darkness using concealer, plus all-in-one foundation/powder, a whish of clear mascara on brows and lashes, a lip color that reads like your own natural tone—but with shine—and go!

JANUARY 28 | SHOP SMARTER AND SAFER.

Some of the little-known perks provided by stores and malls can make your shopping day easier and give you more time and energy to nab an even better outfit. Keep the following short list in mind whenever your shopping mall experience begins to change from a nice day out to a nightmare:

•Many department stores, such as Nordstrom, offer a coat and bag check to help you take the load off of long shopping trips. It can make a huge difference in your energy and focus.

•Most department stores have personal shopping services that, at no cost, will preselect options for just about anything you're shopping for before you arrive. There is no obligation to buy, or silent pressure, just an array of options waiting for you, like you're a celebrity.

•Take advantage of the charge/send payment option at most mall stores. The establishment will ship your goods to your front door for current standard mail rates and save you the hassle of toting goods from store to store. Some U.S. residents can actually save tax fees when shipping to their home state.

•Department and specialty store gift registries make for great hints to friends, even if you are not getting married. Why not use it as a birthday, housewarming, or graduation registry?

•In the heightened state of worldwide security, mall security has really stepped up its game, and some malls now offer escorts to your car after dark, as well as jumper cables for harried shoppers who have left their lights on. Request services like these to make your shopping experience hassle-free.

JANUARY 29

TAKE AN EXPERT STYLE CUE FROM SUZE YALOF SCHWARTZ, A TOP NEW YORK STYLE-MAKER, EXECUTIVE FASHION AND BEAUTY EDITOR AT LARGE OF *GLAMOUR* MAGAZINE.

What is your best-kept personal style secret?
Skin-tone high-heeled sling-backs. They make me look taller and are invisible.

What female celebrity (dead or alive) has kept global style moving forward? What is it about her that makes it happen?
Jackie O—her look is timeless and appears in some form or another on every runway every season.

Why do so many women love your magazine? And what should they expect month to month to help them lead more stylish lives?
It doesn't matter whether you are a size 2 or 22. Women love to look and feel glamorous, and we show them how to do it effortlessly and affordably.

Why is it so easy for real women to look just as good as the stars on the red carpet today?
Because magazines like *Glamour* show them how to find their clothes, makeup, and hairstyles on our pages.

As a busy person, what one style tip—that always gets you by and looking fabulous—would you love other busy people to know?
Concealer and bronzing gel. You can put makeup on in less than sixty seconds—you can't be too busy for that.

What are the three fashion essentials every well-dressed woman should own?
A chic, black, fitted coat; a tan pencil skirt; and white jeans.

What are the biggest mistakes women make when getting dressed?
They forget to care and then they spend the whole day feeling bad and insecure—taking a little time and pride in your outfits can make your day.

If you could whisper a fail-safe style tip into the ears of women everywhere, without them feeling bad by hearing it, what would it be?
Dark denim makes everyone look skinnier.

JANUARY 30 | LET ME COUNT THE WAYS.

Before walking out of any store with your next clothing purchase, test yourself on how many ways you can wear what you are planning to buy.

Skirts are a great example for this challenge. They're one of the few items that, if chosen properly, can go from sporty to sexy to serious with the change of accessories and tops. Think of anything you select as a three-in-one possibility, and then you know you are getting your money's worth.

This may not hold true for supercasual items like trendy jeans or very dressy, tailored clothing such as satin eveningwear. But certainly apply it to midlevel apparel that can swing up or down.

Here are some questions that will help. If you answer yes to three of them, then off to the register you go with no hesitation:

Can I wear this with my sexiest heels?
Will this look appropriate with dressy flats?
Would I love this on a date with a sexy top (or bottom)?
Is this appropriate as a separate for a business presentation or interview?
Might this transition from day to night with the help of accessories?
Will this work for a total day of fun?
Is this office-appropriate?

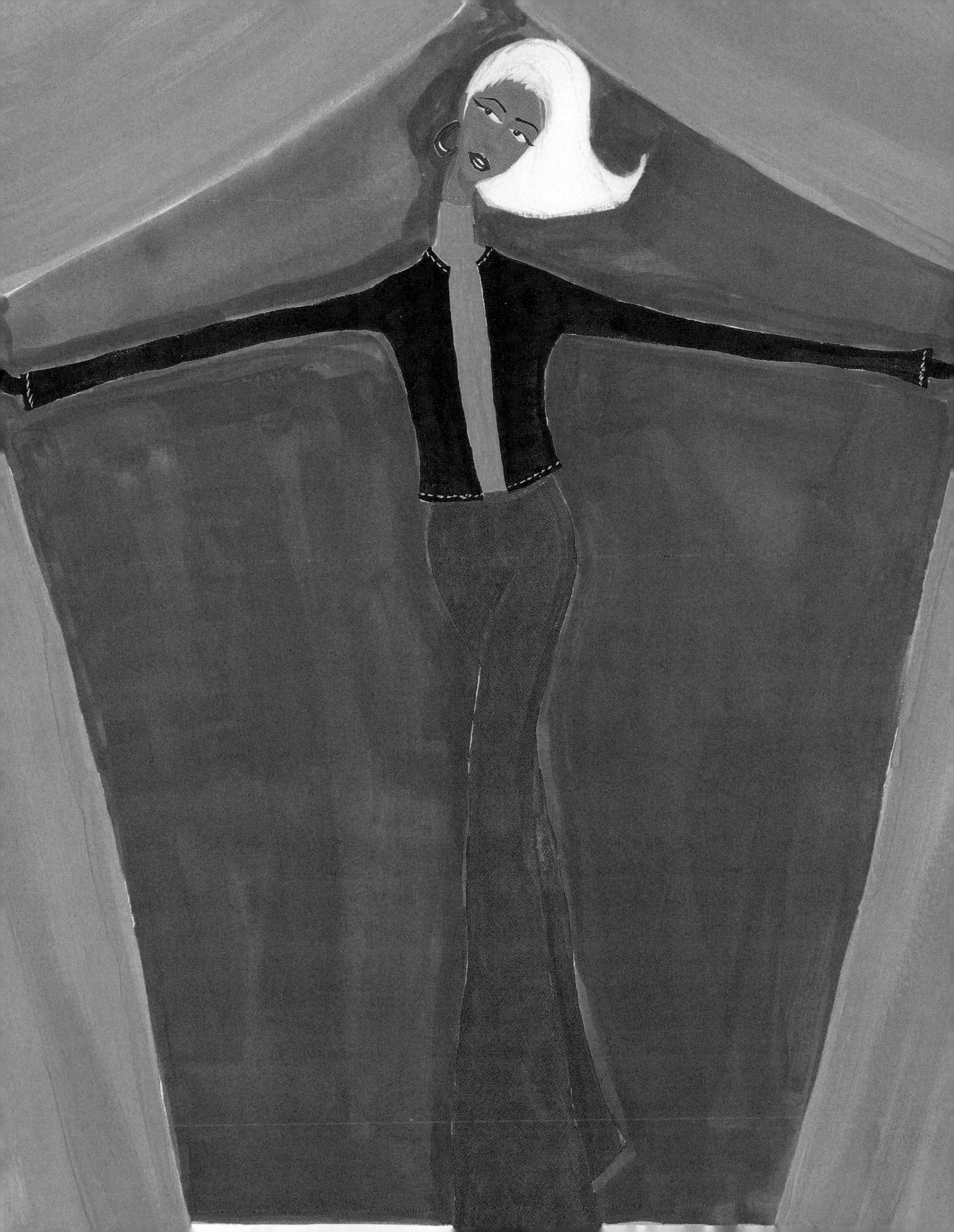

JANUARY 31

IF YOU ARE SHORT ON TIME, AND IF ALL ELSE FAILS, CREATE YOUR OWN VERSION OF THIS SUREFIRE, STYLISH OUTFIT COMBINATION AND RUN WITH IT!

If this is one of those days when it seems the clock is jumping ahead ten minutes at a time, and you can't seem to dream up another original outfit, here is a fast solution that can get you back on real time.

For most women, this time of year calls for clothing and accessories to do triple duty—providing major warmth, spirit-lifting style, and layered protection—without being bulky and adding visual poundage.

By looking at some women, you would think that this perfect style trifecta was unachievable. Wrong. The trick lies in combining convertible layers that morph as your day does, providing options for quick changes, added insulation, or just a release from having too much on in heated spaces.

Get a block of time back right now. Look in your closet and try to mirror this style equation as best as you can with what you have. Don't worry if the items you own aren't an exact match. Within this template, choose your own colors and details. Getting the look not so letter perfect gives it your hint of personal style, which is always better than an exact copy.

Top: thin solid turtleneck sweater
Bottom: tweed pants
Feet: three-quarter-length boots
Accessories: hoop earrings; leather or suede gloves
Flex piece: leather or suede blazer or zip-front cropped jacket

FEBRUARY

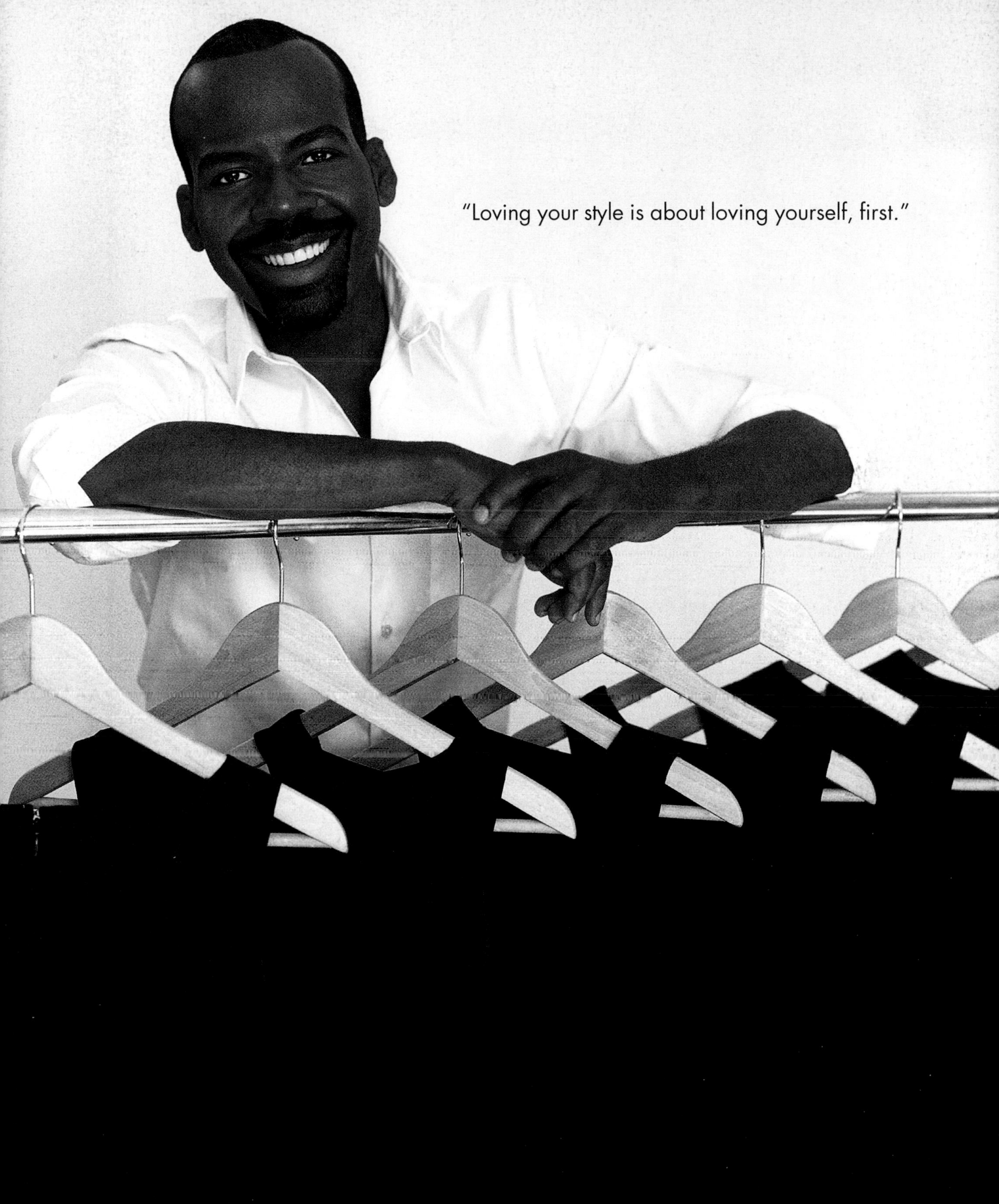
"Loving your style is about loving yourself, first."

FEBRUARY 1 | SHOW YOURSELF SOME LOVE BEFORE ANY VALENTINE GREETING ARRIVES.

Use this month to love yourself. Don't wait for it to come from another.

Make a list of what you love about yourself. Appreciate your every curve and smile knowing that they are yours and yours alone. Peer at your nose and think of the character it brings to your face, making you the woman you are. Pay yourself a compliment as you check yourself in the mirror. A simple one that anyone can remember: "Damn, I look good!"

Affirmation:
The month of love is about showing affection to myself before anyone else.
I will dress myself as if I were taking the gorgeous "me" out to dinner, dancing, and a night on the town.

FEBRUARY 2 | GROUNDHOG DAY COULDN'T BE A LESS SEXY CELEBRATION. BUT YOU CAN STILL USE IT AS A COUNTDOWN TO *GET* SEXY.

Groundhog Day celebrates the rise of Punxsutawney Phil from his hole. As legend has it, if he sees his shadow, he'll retreat, and we are in for six more weeks of winter. If he doesn't, he remains aboveground and spring is nearby.

If you get the news that he has ducked back in and six more weeks of cold weather are upon us, that's a reason to rejoice. Why? You now have six near-guaranteed weeks of prep time before you show more skin and lighten up your clothing. You can accomplish a lot toward becoming a more beautiful you in six weeks! Here is a quick week-by-week countdown of style and beauty steps you can take:

Week six: Start drinking eight glasses of water daily for your skin and overall body tone.
Week five: Round up spring shoes and drop them off for tune-ups at the local shoe repair.
Week four: Schedule four pedicures through to week one and beat the open-toe rush.
Week three: Buy a bright spring trench coat before they all disappear.
Week two: Grab that jump rope to burn as many calories in ten minutes as you would running for thirty.
Week one: Focus on eight hours of sleep nightly, so you can ease up on the heavier winter makeup.

FEBRUARY 3 | GO FOR OPEN-TOE SHOES.

Think of your best evening events in the cooler months. You arrive on the red carpet, if only in your mind, stepping straight from a fabulous car into a heated venue. Is a sometimes heavy, close-toe pump really necessary? Especially with that flowing gown that is just screaming for an elegant set of perfectly polished toes to peek out and complete the look.

I wouldn't recommend open-toe shoes for any other time but glamorous evening events in the cooler months. This applies to women who actually live in environments where winter really means *winter*. L.A. and Miami divas need not adhere, for your toes can feel the breeze almost year-round, day or night.

Wearing shoes that expose the feet, whether a peep-toe pump or a strappy sandal that bares all, is a way to increase an outfit's softness and femininity. And unlike closing off the foot once the weather goes south, it is now okay to reveal the lady in you, if only by night, all year long. You may have to stand by the fireplace for a few moments upon entry to your winter evening event, but you'll look far more fashionable in the process!

FEBRUARY 4 | CELEBRATE BLACK HISTORY MONTH BY TAKING A STYLE CUE FROM BIRTHDAY GIRL ROSA PARKS, BORN ON THIS DAY IN 1913.

Parks was a gentle woman who sparked a freedom movement by standing her ground and keeping her seat. She held fast in a quiet storm of confidence that sent one of the loudest messages of protest in American history.

Parks was a seamstress; dressing people well was her source of income. Thanks to great women such as Rosa Parks, you can choose to be a seamstress or the CEO of a corporation manufacturing clothes. What principles do you stand for? Consider whether you look the part of a woman with the courage of her convictions.

FEBRUARY 5 | THERE IS A CURE FOR THE WINTERTIME BLUES.

Do you have a case of cabin fever? And even if you are getting out of the house each day to head to work, or a day of errands, you are probably running into yet another heated indoor space. Midwinter days such as this can be uninspiring for women who aren't living in some tranquil paradise—think Hawaii. Before you jump into what is cozy and comfy, such as a sweatshirt and the same old jeans, consider something that is rather bright, flirty, and flattering.

CONSIDER WEARING THIS

•Instead of jeans, pull out a pair of cotton twill chinos (a fabric cousin to denim) in white! Yes, bright white! Pale khaki will do in a pinch.

•Instead of the sweatshirt you cleaned the basement in last week, opt for two T-shirts worn together! One short or cap-sleeve, and one long sleeve in a contrasting color to be worn beneath. Try one in aqua, the other in mango—or whatever combination inspires you. Together they will be as warm as most sweatshirts.

•Ditch the snow boots, especially if there is no snow to drudge through, and step into a pair of sneaker/shoe hybrids. Think bowling shoes—very cool again!

FEBRUARY 6 | BAGGY CLOTHES DO NOT MAKE FOR A SLIMMER-LOOKING YOU.

Remember this: When you add extra fabric, you add visual pounds. Tentlike trapeze jackets, shapeless dresses, and oversized tops, contrary to popular beliefs, do not minimize figures.

Drapey clothes only make you *feel* more comfortable. Drop-waist dresses, triangularly shaped swing coats, and prairie skirts instantly put your style out to pasture.

Clothes that fit your body, not squeeze you in, are the correct choice. Look for waisted jackets, scoop necklines, and fitted tops that gently release below the bustline—not balloon out. Also, darting on blouses add taper without smashing you in.

FEBRUARY 7 | REMEMBER TO INVEST IN DUPLICATES WHEN YOU'RE SHOPPING A GREAT SALE.

This is the time of year when most retailers are practically giving away their fall and winter merchandise. If you find an amazing deal (60 percent or more off), leave with two of the same item. If you have two pairs of those killer classic high-heeled shoes that feel as comfortable as slippers, you can keep one pair fresh for special occasions while the other becomes the "workhorse" pair that you wear more often.

I learned this trick from my years working in front of television cameras, where everything you wear looks best if it's new. Also, whether or not they realize it, television viewers expect personalities to never be seen in the same outfit twice. This inspired me to find ways to keep *everything* looking new!

FEBRUARY 8 | SCHEDULE A *PROFESSIONAL* BRA FITTING.

Studies conducted by bra manufacturers show that over half of adult American women are wearing the wrong size bra on a daily basis.

Even the most stylish outfit can be visually destroyed when worn atop an ill-fitting bra. Undergarments are the true foundation for consistent and solid style.

Women have more choices than ever before when it comes to bras. Some enhance, others minimize, and some simply add support. The perfect fit is the key to making you look great in the clothes you wear over it.

Your best bet is to visit an independent shop that only deals in bras, since often salespeople in bra departments of more general stores aren't specialists and can't really give you expert advice.

When fitted, give yourself the stick-and-move test to make certain you are walking out with everything up where it belongs!

THE QUICK "STICK AND MOVE" BRA FIT TEST

A foolproof way to test true fit is by slipping your finger beneath the strip of fabric that connects your bra cups. This part should rest flat to the skin. If you feel a sticking sensation, graduate to a larger cup size. If it is loose, wrinkles, or creases, drop down a size.

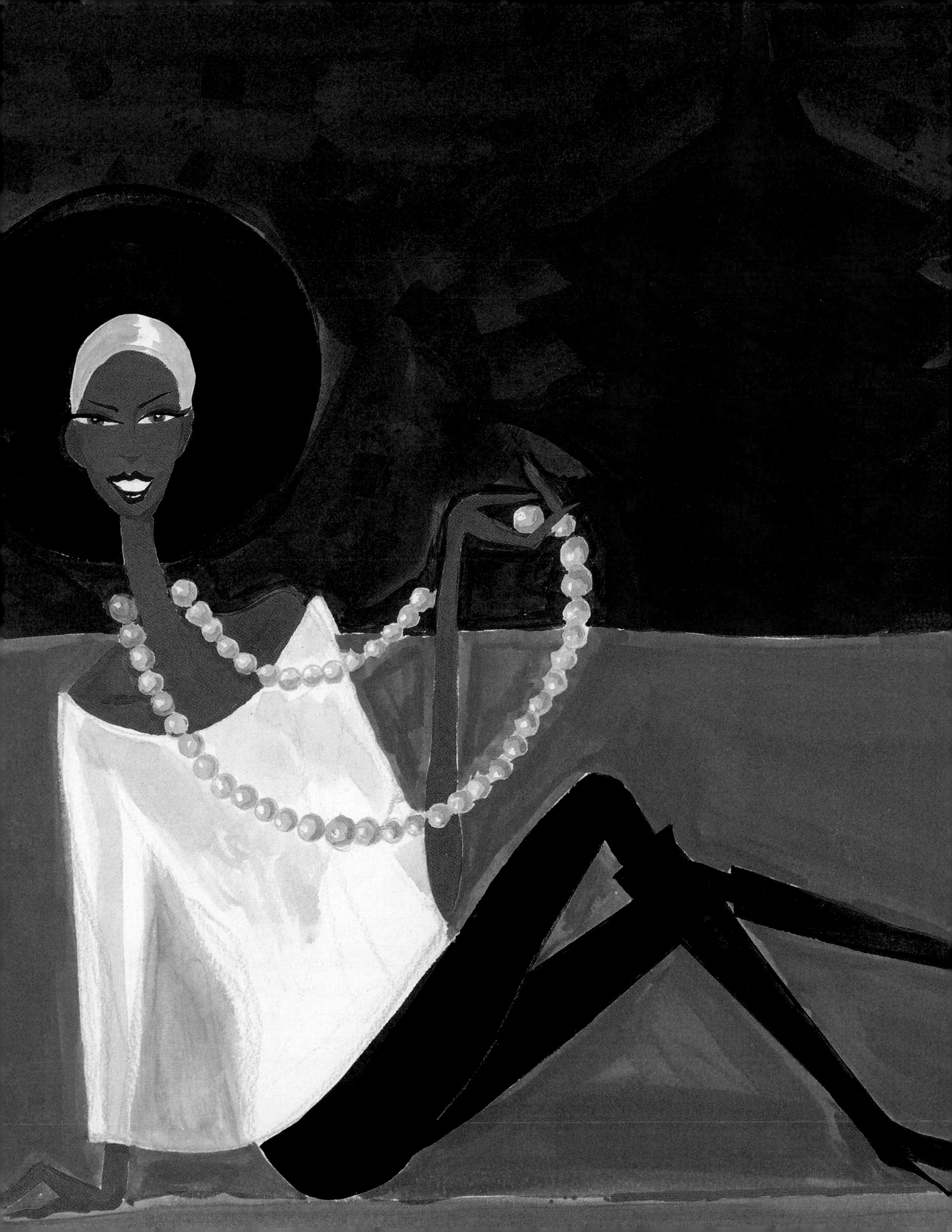

FEBRUARY 9 | LOOK LIKE A WORLD TRAVELER OR AT LEAST A CITIZEN OF THE WORLD.

Shop off the beaten path for ethnic clothing and accessories to add spice to your style. Local Chinatowns, African import stores, and Indian marketplaces offer unique, affordable accessories.

Tell me if you recognize this woman. She has a curious style that always takes you by surprise. You may know her from the local art gallery that she owns, or museum she curates, or possibly from the boutique you pop into every now and again. And although you might not think you could pull off what she's wearing, you appreciate her flair. She often features spicy colors, a touch of menswear, a necklace that looks more like art than jewelry; her glasses have a sliver of attitude, her hair seems a bit less than perfect, and she always seems to have an alluring scent that you have never experienced before. This woman is a total original. Has she traveled the globe? Or has she simply gotten hip to what the savviest women shoppers do? They shop the world market in their backyards.

Nowadays, most cities have ethnic populations that are pronounced and proud, sharing commerce and culture right alongside your local Starbucks. You might find a pocket of trade nestled together, including ethnic grocery stores, spice shops, and interesting clothing shops that offer indigenous fabrics, handmade jewelry, and unique apparel. If not, you can shop the world markets online. Simply type "imported clothing" into any search engine to begin your trip.

Look for extraordinary carved bracelets in wood or marble, beads and stones steeped in history like jade and amber, earrings that dangle and glimmer like royalty, scarves from Indian saris woven with gold thread, and scents that come without fancy packaging but leave your admirers breathless—in a good way! The payoff is often a designer look at a fraction of the price.

Start slow and add just one of your finds to a more understated outfit, like a crisp white blouse and a black skirt. Or with a basic dress that is crying for that special little something. Now you have it from a land far away. And only you know exactly how far you had to go to find it.

FEBRUARY 10 | CELEBRATE YOUR ORIGINALITY.

We have a tendency to compare ourselves to others, believing that their grass is greener and that their great legs, eye color, or height gives them an advantage. Focus on what you've got and celebrate it today. No matter what you have on today's calendar, don't think about what others will think. And don't worry about what others in the room may be wearing. Keep your eyes and mind on creating the best look for you.

Wear the one thing that always makes you feel like a million bucks. It could be a top that hits you perfectly in all the right places, or something as simple as a lip color that makes you feel a bit sexier. Start there to set the tone of self-confidence and carry on with your day feeling that you look and are the best.

FEBRUARY 11 | SHOP SMARTER BY READING SALE SIGNS CAREFULLY TO REALLY KNOW WHAT YOU ARE PAYING FOR.

Sometimes an additional amount off isn't saving you quite as much as you think. Sales are popping up left and right this time of year. Malls, department stores, and boutiques alike are all slashing prices to make room for new merchandise.

Shop the sale racks, but first read the sale signs carefully. For example, it's common to see signs that say:

TAKE AN ADDITIONAL 20% OFF

(THE ALREADY REDUCED PRICE)

Let's say that the previous discount off of a $100 item was 50 percent. What you need to be mindful of is that the total discount won't add up to 70 percent. The item, which costs $50 after the 50 percent discount ($100 – $50), will now cost $40 after the "additional 20 percent off" ($50 – $10), which is actually a total discount of just 60 percent ($100 – $60). The moral of the story is pay attention and ask questions before you head to the register.

FEBRUARY 12 | INVEST IN A PAIR OF BALLERINA FLATS.

There's one thing that can save an outfit and your attitude better than any other: comfortable shoes. Women usually know how long they can wear a particular shoe—from the eight-hour low heels that get you through the day, to the three-hour high heels that help you make a great entrance. But some days you can be caught off guard! You leave for the day, not anticipating a spontaneous evening outing, which leaves you and your aching feet wearing a three-hour shoe for eight hours or more.

Take $100 and spend it on a pair of quality leather or satin ballerina flats (a half size larger maybe to accomodate swollen feet). Choose a basic, neutral, or dark color that will marry well to most anything you are wearing. The best choices: black satin or flesh-tone leather, or vice versa.

Many discount stores will carry ballerina flats starting in the $20 range, in which case I recommend grabbing a few pairs in different colors for different seasons. Sometimes a bright pink pair can look fun and whimsical, taking the onus off you for not wearing heels. They add a quirky vibe that removes the feeling of what people expect you to be in—namely heels!

Stash a pair in your office or in your car. They're compact enough to store in a tote bag. Sneakers run the risk of ruining a dressier outfit, but a pair of ballet flats can work with anything from a business suit to a full skirt and sweater to a ball gown skirt (in a pinch)—and you will garner glares of envy from women suffering through hours being stabbed in their heels. Oh well.

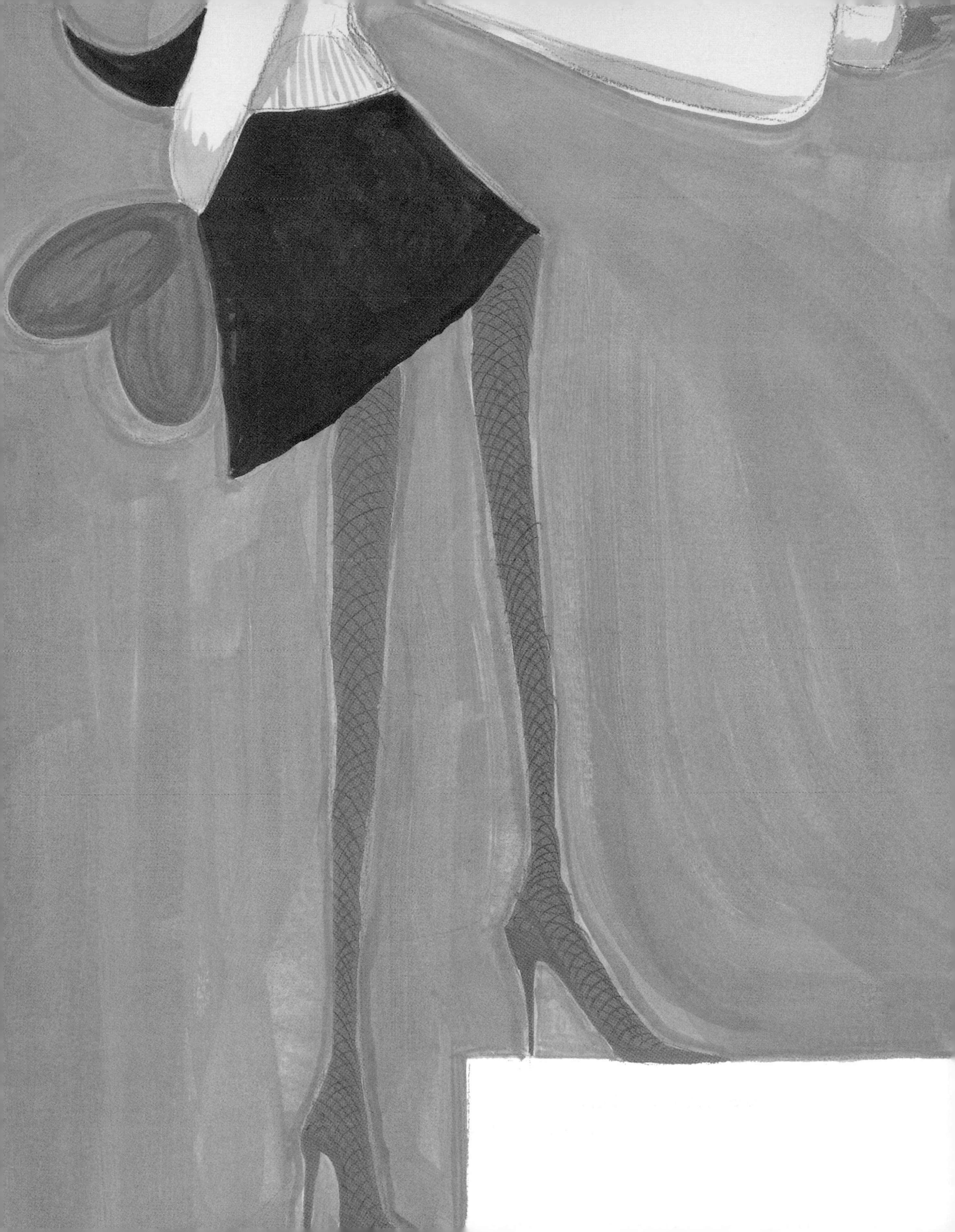

FEBRUARY 13 | LEARN A NEW FASHION TERM.

Piqué *(pee-kay) • Group of durable fabrics characterized by corded effects either warp-wise or filling-wise, most notably created with a waffle texture similar to that of a honeycomb weave. Bird's-eye piqué has a diamond-shaped woven-in dobby pattern. Piqué is used for dresses, blouses, pants, sportswear, handbags, and neckwear.*

Just as the best cooks speak the language of the culinary world—that is, the difference between soufflé and pudding—a fashion-savvy woman knows the vocabulary of the fashion world.

The flirty tennis skirt, the timeless men's short-sleeve polo shirt, and even a classic but common dish towel have something in common: They are usually made of a cotton piqué fabric. Some garments feature a piqué that feels a bit like a microcorduroy, usually garments from England.

For me, piqué signals the start of the warmer seasons, although you can pretty much find it in shirtings year-round. You can feel the texture of a miniature waffle pattern in your hands when you smooth fingers across it, and it has a soft yet firm posture that quietly asks, "Tennis anyone?"

There is something about a woman in a crisp, white piqué blouse that you will never forget. It speaks of authority without looking like you borrowed a shirt from your man's closet. When worn beneath a blazer or suit, a piqué dress shirt's recognizable texture whispers taste and quality in an ever-so-subtle way without screaming it. Either way you spin it, if you want to make a visual statement that speaks of sophistication with a smidge of dressy, it beats plain, combed cotton any day.

FEBRUARY 14 | HAPPY VALENTINE'S DAY!

Celebrate the power of love with an outfit to make Cupid blush. Forget wearing red today or a heart-shaped pin on your lapel. None of these ideas are modern. Try something fresh and unpredictable.

Winter White Pantsuit + Lavender Shell + Camel Boots + Tan Clutch Bag
= Stop, the Love You Save . . .

or

Tan Suede Skirt + Ivory Cowl-neck + Nude Sling-backs + Nude Fishnets
= I Voted for Vixen

or

Floral Full Skirt + Silk Blouse in any Petal Color + Fitted Blazer + Festive Mules
= I Can Be Quite Fresh

FEBRUARY 15 | BE YOUR OWN FASHION EDITOR. STUDY THE RED CARPET LOOKS, DON'T MIMIC THEM.

In our red-carpet-crazed society, we want to see what certain actresses and actors are wearing to movie premieres, award shows, or just going to Starbucks. And whether we want to be or not we're influenced by stars who promote fashion or cosmetics. You've seen the features; this great new bra is Cameron Diaz's favorite undergarment, Halle Berry adores this new lip gloss, and Madonna wears these jeans. Look at what the Hollywood beauties are embracing but to thine own self be true. Take a mental note or two about what speaks to you; jot it down because it speaks to *you*, because you share a characteristic with the star—coloring, age, features—and not because a star endorses it.

FEBRUARY 16 | STEP OUT OF BED OR THE SHOWER LOOKING GREAT.

Try a cashmere robe. The joy of a bathrobe isn't all about absorbing moisture, it is more about the time I like to call the *mise en place* of getting dressed. French for "things in place," this is a term used by master chefs to describe prepping for an elaborate meal. No, you are not anyone's meal, but you can be a feast to the eyes. And these critical postshower and preadornment moments are when the magic takes shape. A time to relax, plan your outfit and make your undergarment selection, apply your makeup (or decide not to), create your hairstyle, or simply sit back and do absolutely nothing in a cushy womb of sorts that allows you to feel ultrafeminine.

As a sale-shopping addict, I know that this is when you chase down high luxury at an affordable price, as most heavier bathrobes are sold for fall and winter seasons. Truth is, they feel just as wonderful during warmer months when you're inside climate-controlled homes. Scour the sale racks first and aim for cashmere if you want a little personal splurge, chunky French terry for sporty luxury that won't ever feel precious, or even simple waffle-knit cotton for the feel of your favorite spa. Get it one size larger for maximum escapism, and grab a color that has the power to take you away each and every time you put it on. For me, that's the brightest white imaginable. For you, think like a queen who has them in all colors but always reaches for her very favorite. That is your color. Now kick back as if her royal servants are just a double-finger-snap away. This is the feeling the robe should deliver. Lastly, snap out of it and start getting ready, you are probably already late. But now, after getting everything "in place" while luxuriating in the right robe, at least you won't look harried.

FEBRUARY 17

TAKE AN EXPERT STYLE CUE FROM JOE ZEE, A TOP NEW YORK STYLE-MAKER, EDITOR IN CHIEF OF *VITALS MAN* AND *VITALS WOMAN*.

What is your best-kept personal style secret for women?
Whether celebrity or model, the rule that I adhere to is to retain their personality. They have to wear the clothes, not the clothes wear them. They should wear something that is them. The women who are able to do this can say that's "not me" and retain their great personal style.

What female celebrity (dead or alive) has kept global style moving forward? What is it about her that makes it happen?
Madonna is someone who influenced fashion. Like her or not, she provokes people to discuss it with her strong and outspoken personality. She has enhanced herself using fashion and style and created a persona. Carolyn Bessette Kennedy was totally understated and chic. She *created* that style. They are both true to who they are.

Why is it so easy for real women to look just as good as the stars on the red carpet today?
There is so much in the media about what is happening, it has been demystified. We've [the media] really broken it down. So-and-so looks good because so-and-so did the hair or [she] is wearing a certain earring. We really break it down so women can take the elements and transfer it to their own lives. They think, I can take that idea and give it a retro spin.

What one style tip would you love other busy people to know that always gets them looking fabulous?
Keep your style simple, classic, and sophisticated, then it's one thing less to do. Pull your hair back in a ponytail. Keep it simple and glamorous without forethought.

FEBRUARY 18 | ADD A GEOMETRIC PRINT TO YOUR LOOK.

Did you pass geometry in high school? Don't be ashamed if you failed or barely got through. Even the women who knew all of its rules and laws fail miserably today when wearing geometric prints.

The rules are much more flexible today when wearing prints that feature uniquely graphic shapes like entwined triangles; lucid, stacked squares in sheer watercolors; and out-of-order circles—not polka dots. These shapes, and other geometrical forms, have been scattered about blouses and skirts for decades, dating back to the geometric designs of the 1920s Art Deco look, when they were commonly outlined in bold black. The French called it "decorative art"—or *art décoratif*, for those who want it proper. It also made a comeback in the Mod 1960s on everything from sweaters to wallpaper for your home.

Now the trick is not *looking* like vintage wallpaper when you opt for a geometric print. And although spring is still weeks away, most women usually feel a yearning for a little liveliness in their ensembles right about now. Geometric prints are a spirited way to transition into a lighter, more whimsical feel without jumping ahead into super-bright colors or lightweight spring fabrics.

THREE WAYS TO ALWAYS LOOK STYLISH IN GEOMETRIC PRINTS

• *Don't pile on geometric shapes.* If you are wearing circles up top, leave the triangles for the next time—not as today's bottom. Opt for solid pants that pull out an unobvious color in the circle pattern for the most modern look. The trick is not looking like wallpaper from the 1970s when you do opt for a geometric print. If you are feeling "printy" from head to toe, try just going head to knee with a chic, printed wrap dress, paired with solid accessories.

• *Graphic prints highlight your shape, since they curve and distort when they hit a "bump."* So look carefully at exactly how those perfect squares fall atop your backside. A wobbly square can be more funny than flattering to followers.

• *Have fun! Be brave and choose a shocking print—but be prudent.* A brazen belt with basic weekend pants or a daringly chic blouse with a tame skirt—a dash will do ya!

FEBRUARY 19 | HAPPY BIRTHDAY, PISCES GIRL.

Whether a size 2 or 22, the fish is always proud of her body. The Pisces woman has a connection to her flesh that is not of worship, but of complete comfort. She always seems to snap back from those holiday dessert pounds just in time for her birthday celebration, because she knows the dress she wants to feature will not forgive.

And this is the same comfort level that puts her at total zen when she struts the beach come summertime. She considers a trip to the tropics if she doesn't already live there. Let those other signs wear the sarongs, caftans, and cover-ups—her skin meeting the sun, sand, and water is like a stylish homecoming in and of itself. She packs lighter than most when taking time off. The power of good clothing speaks to her versatility and fishlike ability to be malleable and spry, darting from work suit to swimsuit with amazing agility.

Sports Illustrated swimwear supermodel Kathy Ireland and the proudly curvy beauty Queen Latifah are stellar examples of the Piscean spirit: open, free, and ever-changing. Take a look at yourself and soak up what you know to be true. You'd have it no other way; even if it all changed tomorrow it would still be perfect.

FEBRUARY 20 | GET TEN-MINUTE STYLE FOR YOUR FUN DATE THAT LOOKS LIKE YOU SPENT HOURS PULLING IT TOGETHER.

Here is a great ten-minute style solution for a fun date night:

Minutes 1:00–2:00:
Identify your best feature, the one you are most proud of, and highlight it—a backless dress, a top that offers shoulders, a suit that reveals a bit of cleavage.

Minutes 3:00–4:00:
Pick one or two accessories that are *really* eye-catching—a clutch or bag that has bold details, a brooch with history, or artful earrings.

Minutes 5:00–6:00:
Choose a shoe that makes you feel sexy—be ready for the dance floor.

(CONTINUED)

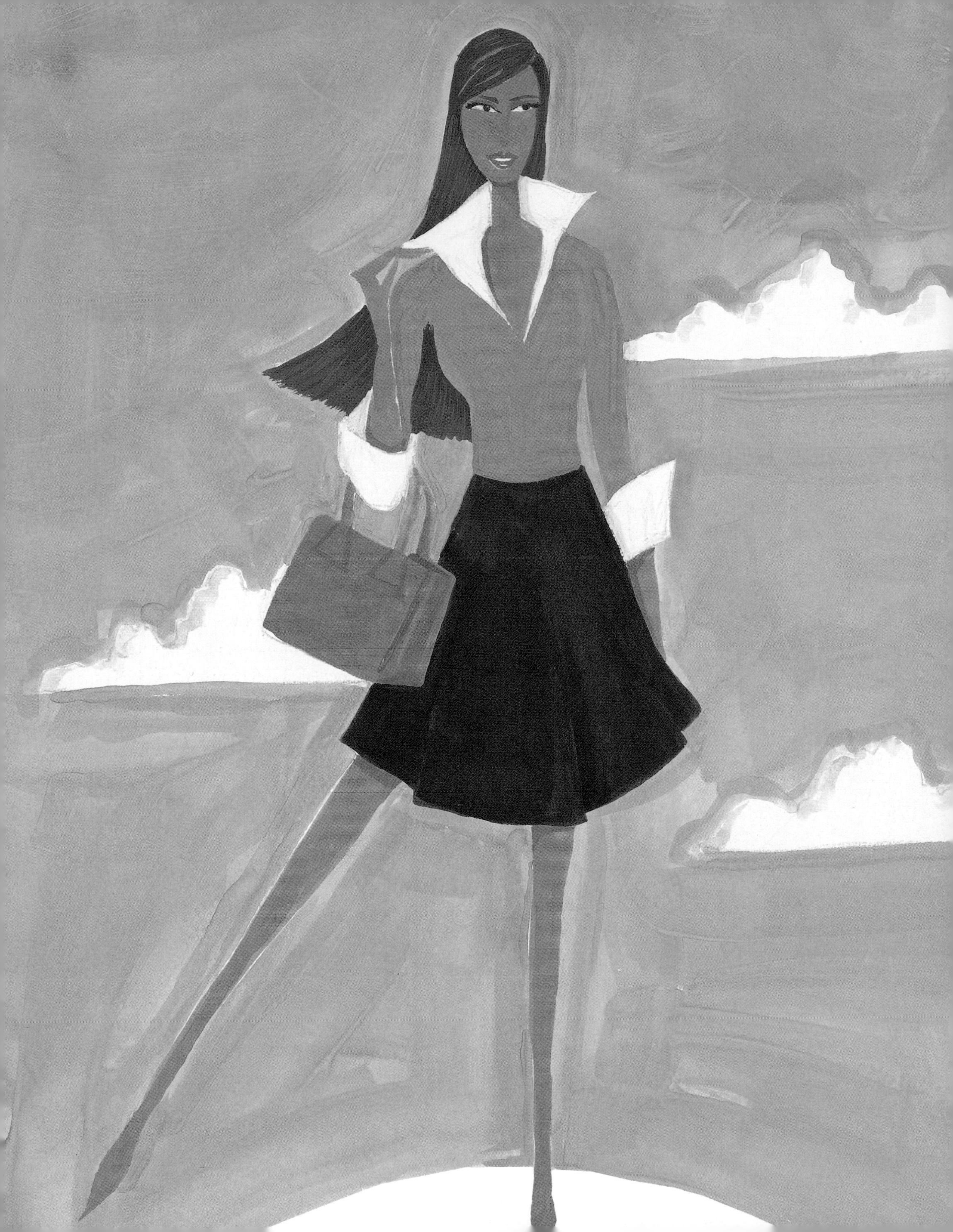

Minutes 7:00–8:00:

Tousled hair can be alluring and low-maintenance. A loose, high French twist works for longer lengths. For short hair, think quick, slick chic. A bold side part, an extra dab of gel to hold, and slick it down tightly defined.

Minutes 9:00–10:00:

Your makeup should shimmer by candlelight, but need not be heavy. Focus on undereye darkness using concealer, all-in-one foundation/powder, go slightly smoky on the eyes, add tinted lip gloss—and off you go!

FEBRUARY 21

TRY CHOCOLATE BROWN AND CLASSIC PINK FOR A LOOK THAT SPEAKS OF SWEETNESS AND RETRO GLAMOUR.

Some days you simply need a fresh take on color combinations to find a great new look. I liken this color combination to the timeless appeal of a scoop of Neopolitan ice cream, with its rich stripes of chocolate, strawberry, and vanilla flavors. This is why it works: The rich brown color grounds the combination (where you may normally choose black or navy), leaving room for a soft accent of pink. If you'd like, you can add a touch of white or ivory to cool and add a breather to the duo. This color combination was very popular in the late 1960s and early 1970s, especially in dress prints and home furnishing patterns. Here are some winning combinations that will make you popular in this decade:

Solid Brown Skirt + Solid Pink V-Neck Sweater + Crisp White Button-Down Shirt

= Neopolitan Gone Cosmopolitan

Pink Tank or Shell + Brown/Cream Pinstriped Pantsuit + Pink High-Heel Sandals

= U. P. Yes!

Brown Sheath Dress + Pink-and-Brown Patterned Neck Scarf + Pink Mules

= Mary Tyler "More"

FEBRUARY 22 | KEEP A FASHION FIRST-AID KIT NEARBY. FROM DRINK SPILLS TO SPILLING CLEAVAGE, YOU CAN CLEAN UP AND LIFT UP IN NO TIME.

Just when you think it is safe to leave the house unprepared is exactly when style accidents happen! The clumsy waiter (or friend), the snug dress that the dry cleaner shrank (or that cheesecake from last week), and the skirt that keeps sticking to your legs like a spoiled child.

Tote a few lightweight style-saving sundries as the ounce of prevention that could be the cure.

Individual stain-removing wipes: Finally! Detergent companies wised up and offered their stain-removing solutions in handy towelettes. So quick, so easy, and no more dipping your napkin in club soda.
Miniature safety pins: Whether pulling together an unexpected tear or lifting the neckline of a wrap dress, the miniature safety pin can make the difference between a great night and an evening of constant tugging and pulling. Look for black pins offered in sewing stores. So chic!
Mini-sewing kit: The one thing to take away from your hotel stays. Enough said.
Topstick or double-sided tape: Originally created to help folliclely challenged men keep their hairpieces in place, this double-sided adhesive can also temporarily lift a hem or keep a dress from revealing your *entire* chest. Just ask Jennifer Lopez.
Dryer sheets: Yes, they freshen up your load of wash when tumbling dry, but gently rubbed against a skirt prevents static cling to your legs and hose. Keep a few handy.

FEBRUARY 23 | PUT DOWN ONE STYLE OR BEAUTY REGIMEN, AND ALLOW IT TO LAST.

"I like to really be dressed up or really undressed. I don't bother with anything in between."
—*Marilyn Monroe*

Norma Jean would just die if she heard this! Or might she be the one who enjoys the "really undressed" part? Who knows?

There is something to be said for an extremist approach to style. "All or nothing" glamour can fuel amazing outfits that look perfectly camera ready and stunning. Reason being, the woman, such as Marilyn Monroe, who gives herself ample days off to pull away from all things artificial and put-upon—

high-heeled shoes, foundation garments, makeup, hosiery, leg shaving, hair styling, jewelry, perfume, and the ubiquitously unnatural fingernail polish, knows a secret.

And although glamour has its perks and advantages, it requires a level of maintenance that, over time, becomes unseen and habitual, fooling many women into thinking that the time and care it takes to achieve their desired result doesn't actually exist. What suffers is the quality of the end result, for out of habit, women are seen in broken-down high-heeled shoes, ill-fitting foundation garments, dated makeup, aging hosiery, hairy legs, flat hair, excessive jewelry, and raggedy fingernails they attempt to keep hidden all day.

Take an honest look at your style and beauty regimens today and see what has really suffered over time from extreme repetition. For instance, are your shoes giving you the same goose bumps that you got when you saw them in the store window? Or is it time to drop them off at the cobbler—or worse yet, the Goodwill drop box?

It may just be one or two of the above. See if you can simply go without some of those things for a spell, just to allow your approach to them to "reset." Hopefully, you'll resume with a rested eye and more precise approach, making you look even better after the style sabbatical.

FEBRUARY 24 | POP STYLE QUIZ.

1. Which fashion designer created the famous wrap dress in 1972?

A. Liz Claiborne
B. Diane von Furstenberg
C. Carolina Herrera
D. Perry Ellis

2. What avenue in New York is known for its numerous fashion designer offices and showrooms?

A. Madison Avenue
B. Fifth Avenue
C. Avenue of the Americas
D. Seventh Avenue

3. Helmut Newton is famous for what critical element of the fashion world?

A. Fashion photography
B. Fashion designer

(CONTINUED)

C. Fashionable accessories
D. Fashionably protective headgear

4. Which of these accessories should never be worn with mules?

A. Toe rings
B. Hosiery
C. Anklets
D. None of the above

(Answers: 1-B, 2-D, 3-A, 4-B)

FEBRUARY 25 | HOW MANY OF THESE TEN ESSENTIAL FLATS DO YOU OWN? MAKE SURE THEY STILL FIT AND FLATTER.

My colleague, early morning shoe-lover Katie Couric, once hipped me to the fact that "when your feet hurt, everything hurts!" And in this day and age of flat shoes that are just as stylish and interesting, there really is no reason to endure the pain that high heels can cause.

Ironically, sometimes the woman in flats is the attention-grabber, because every other woman in the room is wearing heels. When shopping, keep your eye peeled for flats that excite you, so that when you feel the need to stay grounded, they are waiting for you, offering comfort and flair. Keep your closet stocked with a:

Classic loafer
Sexy slide
Driving moccasin
Dressy thong sandal
Girly mule
Cute lounging sneaker
Sparkly slipper
Colorful espadrille
Casual flip-flop
Dressy ballet slipper

FEBRUARY 26 | DRESS FROM SMALL TO BIG.

Grab pants. Snatch a top. Whip out a belt and some shoes, then dive into that jewelry box and search for earrings and a bracelet that works with them all. If that's your habit, reverse the process and flip the script.

Start with the littlest detail that you'll wear and build up to the big pieces for a totally unexpected look. An earring can inspire a total ensemble. Select a small piece that has a story, some character, a history, and unique details to pull from. An oversized bracelet from Morocco, a cameo from your grandmother, or a pair of bright orange socks. Pull it out, whatever it is, and let it be your little guide to everything else.

You may draw on another side of your personality. Is she modest? Is she sexy? Might she be a little daring? Let the little piece tell you the skirt *she* would wear. Let this goddess in the details of your little accessory take you where you might not have ventured if you started your outfit with the dress or the suit.

FEBRUARY 27 | IF YOU DON'T HAVE A DROP-DEAD DRESS FOR YOUR BIG EVENT, INVEST NOW IN THIS SINGULAR SENSATION THAT WILL ALWAYS TURN HEADS.

Is there a dress in your closet that causes jaws to drop when you enter the room? Nicole Kidman's red carpet dress choices command attention at just about every major public event. Elizabeth Taylor's little black dress showed all the men how to trace a curve in *Butterfield 8*. And who will ever forget Michelle Pfeiffer reclined atop the piano in *The Fabulous Baker Boys* in her skintight, flame-red dress, *panting* out "Makin' Whoopee"?

The fit and cut of a dress is what makes it a killer. The fabric, design, color, and detailing can be lightning on a hanger, but unless the fit is pitch perfect, you might as well leave it on the rack.

If your arms are a bit thick, adorn yourself in dresses with lovely sleeves that are a bit translucent. Select empire-waist dresses to lift a modest bustline or to make a petite princess stand taller. Or my favorite, be more of a hip chick and less of a chick with hips by running straight to A-line dresses and skirts.

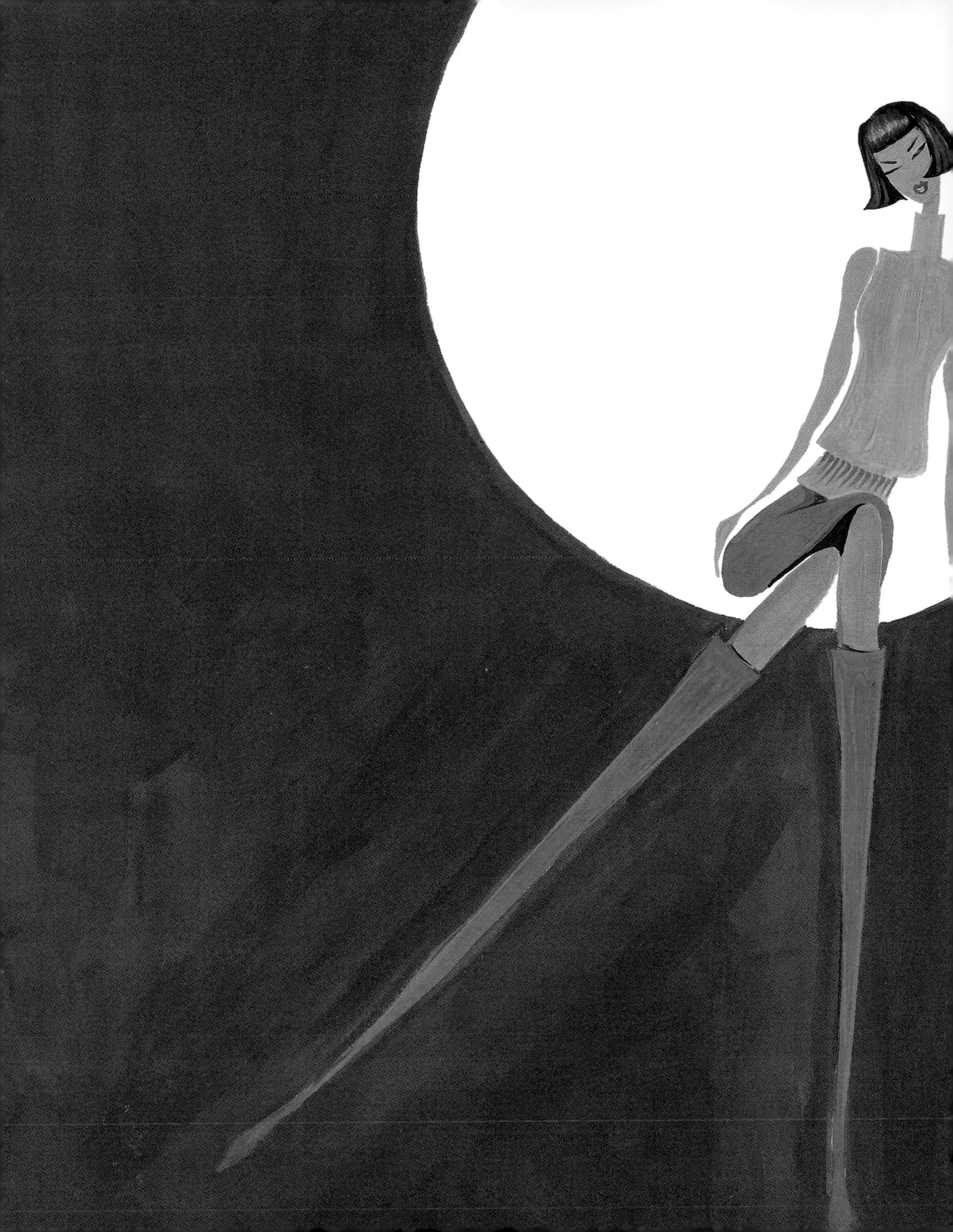

FEBRUARY 28 | CREATE A TIME-SAVING, SUREFIRE, STYLISH OUTFIT COMBINATION.

Top: Bright, spring-color sleeveless sweater (V-neck, turtle, or mock turtle)

Bottom: Dark knee-length skirt

Shoes: Dark sexy knee boot

Accessories: Opaque tights (matching boots and skirt); bright, spring-color handbag

Flex piece: Classic-fitted dark denim jacket

MARCH

"Peek ahead and celebrate spring, if only with colorful outfits."

MARCH 1 | DO SOME SPRING FASHION CLEANING BEFORE THE WEATHER BREAKS AND YOU START THE STYLE SCRAMBLE.

I call it the style scramble. The moment when you are getting dressed for a special occasion. You have about seven minutes left, and you can't find that one special piece of clothing. You should move on and go with another item, but you're determined to find that piece. You just saw it the other day. Sheesh!

The way to avoid moments like this is to be organized and willing to weed out your garden of garments. Take ten minutes to do so today.

MARCH 2 | TAKE AN EXPERT STYLE CUE FROM LEGENDARY BILL BLASS DESIGNER MICHAEL VOLLBRACHT.

What are three fashion essentials every well-dressed woman should own?
Black is a friend. A well-fitted blazer can go anywhere. Never wear cheap shoes. They make your whole outfit look cheap.

What are the biggest mistakes women make when getting dressed?
They don't look at the whole picture. Look at the back view first.

Who is the most stylish woman in existence, in your opinion?
Coco Chanel. She changed fashion, period.

If you could whisper a fail-safe style tip in the ears of women everywhere without them feeling bad by hearing it, what would it be?
Dress for men. Women who do, go further.

MARCH 3 | TRUST A PROFESSIONAL HAIRSTYLIST TO CREATE, NOT JUST TAKE ORDERS.

Their love for the craft may set you free from a style left over from years past.

Why not be the one to shake things up a bit on your next visit, and honor the hardworking hair professional with more than just a folded cash tip! Chances are if you've had your stylist do the same thing to you for years, your stylist has been secretly dying to try something new on you.

Trust them and give them the reins to actually create—within reason. They in turn should explain what they'd like to do and why. What's the worst that could happen? With the advanced hair technology available today, there are so many fixes that you could probably be back to the old, "safe" you, and not be late for your appointment with your manicurist.

MARCH 4 | ON MARCH 4, 1917, JEANETTE RANKIN, PEACE ACTIVIST AND SUFFRAGIST, BECAME THE FIRST WOMAN ELECTED TO THE U.S. HOUSE OF REPRESENTATIVES.

Stylewise, Rankin was a Gibson girl. The look became fashionable in the late 1800s and kept women in "order" well through the early 1900s. The details were unmistakable: tall, slim, perfectly postured, hair coiffed high into a balloonlike chignon or stuffed into a hat with a large feather. The look was a crisply starched blouse paired with a floor-length billowy skirt that fell over a bustle. The foundation was a corset so tight, a woman could probably count her ribs in her reflection without ever touching her body. Yikes!

This objectified and ultrarestrictive look of femininity was in full swing when noted peace activist and suffragist Jeanette Rankin became the first woman to be elected to Congress, paving the way for the 202 women elected to the House of Representatives to date.

In her honor, and in honor of the many women who suffered through objectifying clothes and undergarments for decades, free yourself today! This doesn't mean ditching the bra and running out on the loose. This fashion suggestion is all about knowing and claiming what you genuinely view as beautiful versus that which may have been put in your closet by the opposite sex. Try questioning every piece of clothing

(CONTINUED)

as you dress. Challenge every accessory and each swipe of makeup to ensure that you're featuring it because *you* honestly find it strong, or sexy, or sweet, and not because of any male-centered conditioning. Save this author.

If you can give each item you wear a stamp of approval, then you are representing your self and women everywhere in truth and with total power.

MARCH 5 | DON'T SHOP.

Challenge yourself to really use the clothes you have before you invest in more. You'd be surprised at how many style possibilities are just waiting in your closet. "I dislike anything excessive. It confuses me. I was happier when I had two dresses, both black," said Lucille Ball. She had a point!

Imagine that the outfit you are wearing is one of only three complete outfits that you have to your name. No ifs, ands, or extra belts. Would you toss the jacket or sweater over a chair so lazily, or would you fold it and keep it clear of wrinkles and stains? Might you actually allow your shoes to cool down, dry off, and regain their original shape on cedar shoe trees between wearings? You'd be amazed at how your actions would shift, and your resourcefulness and creativity would blossom.

Sometimes too much of a good thing can get in the way of a great thing: your best style. If you get the itch to shop, recall what you have already. Ask yourself if you've gotten the maximum wear out of what you already have.

MARCH 6 | STAY WITH YOUR SIGNATURE LOOK. THAT IS THE KEY.

"You should wear what you want, be comfortable in what you wear, believe in what you wear, and eventually you are gonna be fabulous and chic!"
—Isaac Mizrahi

Knowing yourself is the first step to having style. Are you most comfortable in sweats and a T-shirt when no one is around? Are you the type who runs to the same solid navy tailored trousers each Monday because it's safe and easy? And what is your presentation standard? Are you perfectly pressed or wrinkle-free enough to get by in the right light? Take some time to figure what your personal style really is.

Pay attention to quality. Even your basic T-shirt can come in pima cotton (a finer quality with an ultrasoft hand) with a shapelier fit and cap sleeves. Navy tailored trousers can be upgraded with leg-lengthening pinstripes, as chunky vintage sailor pants, or even in matte satin for evening if navy is so much your thing. And why be perfectly pressed when you can purposefully choose Irish linen separates that lend themselves beautifully to inherent wrinkling, only to look more island-chic as you pass the hours.

The real you is always the most interesting and certainly the most authentic. This goes for your personality and budding style persona. Trust that it already exists, and is just in need of a brushup. Work *with* your personality and style instincts, not against.

MARCH 7 | GO AHEAD, WEAR STRIPES WITH PLAIDS.

What a boring world it would be if this, of all fashion myths, were in fact a style truth. Just picture it, streets full of pedestrians wearing nothing but safe patterns, cautiously paired with coordinating solids and expected textures. Snore.

We could wave good-bye to such wonderful designers as Christian Lacroix and his quirky, bold plaids worn in a stylish cacophony with traditional ticking stripes. And no longer would we need the services of Brooks Brothers, who are heralded globally for their signature summer patchwork plaids and striped shirt/plaid tie combinations. Farewell to runway and real-way versions.

There is one simple rule to keep in mind for women and the men they dress: When choosing bigger, brazen plaids, balance out the pairing of a stripe by choosing smaller, finer lines. And the rule works back-to-front—the more pronounced the stripe (think awning stripes), the more precious the plaid should be.

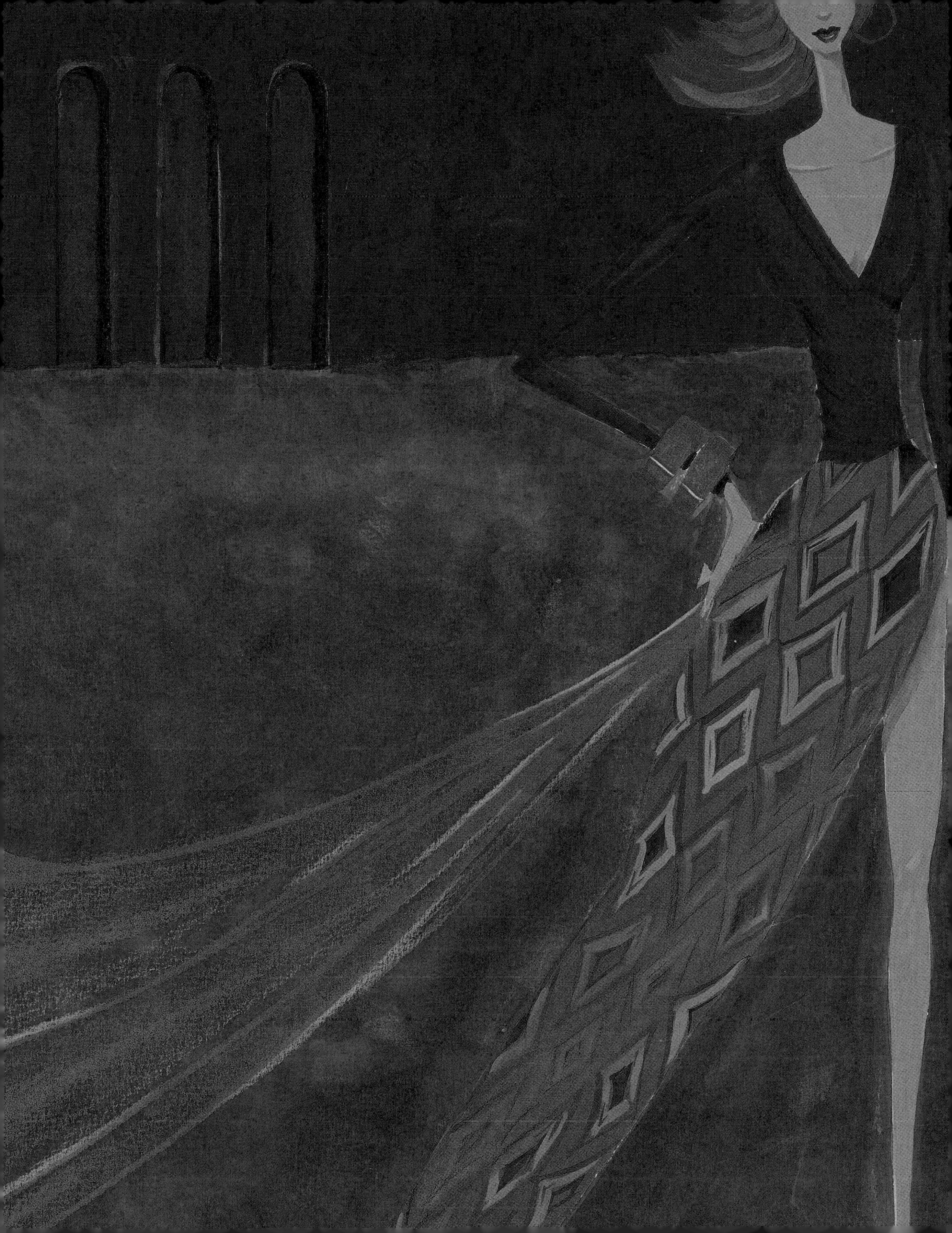

MARCH 8 | ADD AN AFRICAN PRINT TO YOUR LOOK.

The cradle of civilization, Africa, offers a unique and distinct influence on high fashion. The power is in its textiles, which have little to no trend boundaries.

There was a time when African prints were only worn by Africans or people of African descent for traditional ceremonies and rituals. You've seen the majesty of the flowing cloths from the various African countries, wrapped with dignity on the heads of women, or draped sculpturally over the shoulders of proud men. From Ghana's colorfully festive Kente cloth that took the late 1980s by storm to Zaire's brown-and-harvest-toned Kuba cloth that has a story in each imperfect stitch, you can almost tour the entire continent's moods by just studying the cloths indigenous to each region.

Rich, organic, African fabrics and prints can also add interest to your look and fashion mood when worn juxtaposed with more modern silhouettes. Not trying to look too regal is the trick. Glean a nuance from the beloved country and let it shine brighter alongside Western basics.

THREE WAYS TO ALWAYS LOOK STYLISH IN AFRICAN PRINTS

• Be careful of African prints that were "Made in China." The beauty of most African prints and woven fabrics exist in their authenticity. Check for labels; if there are none, it may even be more authentic.

• Be selective about wearing African prints from head to toe—unless you are heading to a gala at the UN or in the Motherland. Choose one wardrobe essential with a print, and let the others be more understated.

• Images of men hunting animals, huts, and safari lodges on canvas are not authentic African prints. Look for rustic, geometric woven prints and patterns that speak of an artisan's hand—those are the versions to wear.

MARCH 9 | TAKE AN EXPERT STYLE CUE FROM TOP AMERICAN DESIGNER CAROLINA HERRERA.

What are the three fashion essentials every well-dressed woman should own?

1. A small handkerchief tied around the handle of the bag, but placed inside.
2. Every woman must have a scent.
3. A ball gown.

What are the biggest mistakes women make when getting dressed?
Excessiveness. Too many ladies try too hard and they appear overdone and uncomfortable.

Who is the most stylish woman in existence, in your opinion?
Marquise de Montespan.

If you could whisper a fail-safe style tip into the ears of women everywhere without them feeling bad by hearing it, what would it be?
If you have great legs you should show them more.

MARCH 10 | INVEST IN A MEDIUM GRAY, YEAR-ROUND PANT OR SKIRT SUIT.

Whether you choose to purchase a true suit (an ensemble with jacket and pants and /or skirt), or separates that are an exact match, the medium gray suit is a style staple.

Black suits are a must for evenings and funerals, navy suits are great for business, and white suits are incredible for warm months and looking red carpet ready without really trying. But there is something about a medium gray suit that rolls all of these into one.

The neutral color welcomes pairing with just about anything from beaded tanks for evening change-outs, to lightly starched button-downs or fine-gauge sweaters for business. Wear the suit pieces from time to time as a separate by adding a leather blazer atop the bottom, or simply use the pants or skirt as a grounding piece to a colorful, sexy evening top that reveals the shoulders. Gray is a style-rich silent partner that is like a chameleon, blending into any mood you are in. Go for quality and be willing to pay maybe $500 and upward.

The investment strategy begins when you lay down those five C-notes, for the value will inevitably come back to you with the amount of use you will get out of the suit together or as separates. It will literally pay for itself over time. In return, you will be consistently covered for work or play, eliminating the need to figure out another way to make those mango pants work again. Your gray suit will know just when to stand out and, more important, when to step back. Finally, you can get to work, be productive, and let a good suit have your back all day, so you can focus on your continued rise to the top.

Choose a year-round super 110's wool, lightweight wool twill, wool crepe, wool gabardine, or even stretch wool, depending on the climate where you live, work, and play. Single- or two-button jackets look the most timeless. And see a tailor before your first wear to get the most impact from a perfect fit.

Five hundred dollars may seem like a bit of a stretch, but I promise you that the number of ways you work this fashion investment may equal—and possibly exceed—it.

MARCH 11 | A "DESIGNER" LABEL DOES NOT EQUAL QUALITY.

Look past labels for quality. There are thousands of brands that offer lesser quality clothing with "designer names" on the label. Some of these are fictitious, created to give a consumer the feeling of purchasing a top-quality item bearing a fancy name. The label is a marketing tool that provides a certain cachet that most shoppers identify with quality, because of the hard work, time, and money put in by authentic top designers.

Be careful when shopping that you are not paying top dollar for a label you only *think* is designer—you could in fact be paying for a garment that simply incorporates a chic label, a *feature* of a designer look. Sometimes the less expensive, no-name route is as far as you should go when seeking out new trends that might not be trendy in a few months.

Investment pieces like dress coats, tailored trousers, and semiformal dresses and gowns are worth spending top dollar on for the best fabric, perfect fit, and expert details and tailoring, of which it takes a proven design leader to truly provide.

MARCH 12 | TAKE AN EXPERT STYLE CUE FROM MAX AZRIA, A TOP FRENCH DESIGNER AND CREATOR OF THE BCBG COLLECTION.

What is your best-kept personal style secret?

Something unexpected that makes you own your look. It could be as simple as an interesting accessory!

What are the three fashion essentials every well-dressed woman should own?

1. A white T-shirt—it works with everything.
2. A pair of denim jeans, because they make any woman look sexy.
3. Something versatile, like a scarf, that can have many uses. For example, you can use it as a belt or wrap it in any number of ways.

What are the biggest mistakes women make when getting dressed?

They usually overdo it and take it too seriously. They don't have enough fun.

Who is the most stylish woman in existence, in your opinion?

The model Helena Christensen. She is effortless!

If you could whisper a fail-safe style tip into the ears of women everywhere without them feeling bad by hearing it, what would it be?

Love yourself because it's at the essence of everything.

MARCH 13 | LEARN A NEW FASHION TERM.

***Jacquard** (jack-card) • Elaborate woven or knitted pattern made on a Jacquard loom, invented by Joseph Marie Jacquard in France in 1801. Fabrics may have a background of plain, rib, satin, or sateen weave with the design usually in satin weave. Some fabrics have specific names such as brocade, damask, and tapestry. Also may be knitted, and then it's called Jacquard knit.*

A fabric process most commonly used for men's neckties, Jacquards can be found just as readily in your own closet—if you look closely. Take a look at that satin skirt you love, with the subtle floral print or polka dots that shimmer and become visible when the light hits just right. Or even the lining of a blazer that has a little more whimsy and character than just plain solid black satin. These pieces are most likely created on a Jacquard loom.

MARCH 14 | GET TEN-MINUTE STYLE FOR A COCKTAIL PARTY.

Here is a great ten-minute style solution for a cocktail fete:

Minutes 1:00–2:00:
Reach for your best, tailored dark suit bottoms, be they pants or a skirt. Find a shoe that you would normally wear for evening—think thin, high, and sparkly.

Minutes 3:00–4:00:
If there is a man in the house, "borrow" his white dress shirt. If not, use a simple solid white blouse. Make sure the collar can stand up tall.

Minutes 5:00–6:00:
Go for a camisole that has femininity (lace details around the bust) to wear beneath. Instead of buttoning the shirt, wrap and tuck it in unbuttoned, or tie it in front.

Minutes 7:00–8:00:
Leave shirt cuffs unbuttoned to feature multiple bold bracelets on one single arm. Add a high stack of pearls or fun bauble necklaces in color, or a huge brooch.

Minutes 9:00–10:00:
Your makeup should be graphic. Focus on undereye darkness using concealer; then add all-in-one foundation/powder, very little color on the eyes, a bold red lip, mascara just on the outer lashes, and exit stage left!

MARCH 15 | PUT THE COATDRESS BACK IN THE CLOSET. TRY WEARING A LONG WRAP SWEATER.

BEFORE WEARING THIS

Some coatdresses were double-breasted, others were single-breasted, sometimes with nautical gold buttons. They became a fashion symbol of the 1980s. But those days and that look are over.

There is a modern alternative.

CONSIDER WEARING

• A long wrap sweater—one that almost hits the knee—that belts at the waist. Choose a lightweight knit in cashmere, merino wool, or gauzy cotton.

• A thin crew or V-neck shell works perfectly beneath it!

• The beauty of the long wrap sweater is its versatility. And unlike the coatdress, you can pop it on over pants or skirt to get the look of a coatdress, but remain in the new millennium. **Turncoat Chic!**

MARCH 16 | COUNT YOUR LUCKY SKIRTS. MAKE SURE THEY STILL FIT AND FLATTER.

You may have tons that you never wear, or you might be hoarding a few for when you drop those pesky ten pounds. If they don't work now, let them go.

Neutral or dark solid A-line skirt
Neutral or dark solid pencil skirt
Neutral or dark solid knee-length straight skirt
Ball gown skirt
Cotton weekend skirt
Vacation wrap skirt
Beaded or embellished skirt
Floral skirt
Winter skirt in tweed or houndstooth
Soft-skin skirt (leather or suede)

MARCH 17 | POP STYLE QUIZ.

1. What is the ideal way to store a knit sweater?

A. On a skirt hanger
B. Folded
C. On a coat hanger
D. In a plastic bag, sealed

2. Which original 1990s supermodel stayed active on the runway longer than the rest?

A. Kate Moss
B. Naomi Campbell
C. Judy Tenuta
D. Roshumba Williams

3. The casual basic store Old Navy is owned by what other major clothing brand?

A. Tommy Hilfiger
B. GAP
C. Michael Kors
D. Army/Navy stores

4. Which former magazine fashion editor had a comeback appearing in Old Navy's quirky 1990s' TV advertisements?

A. Carrie Donovan
B. Diana Vreeland
C. Morgan Fairchild
D. None of the above

(Answers: 1-B, 2-B, 3-B, 4-A)

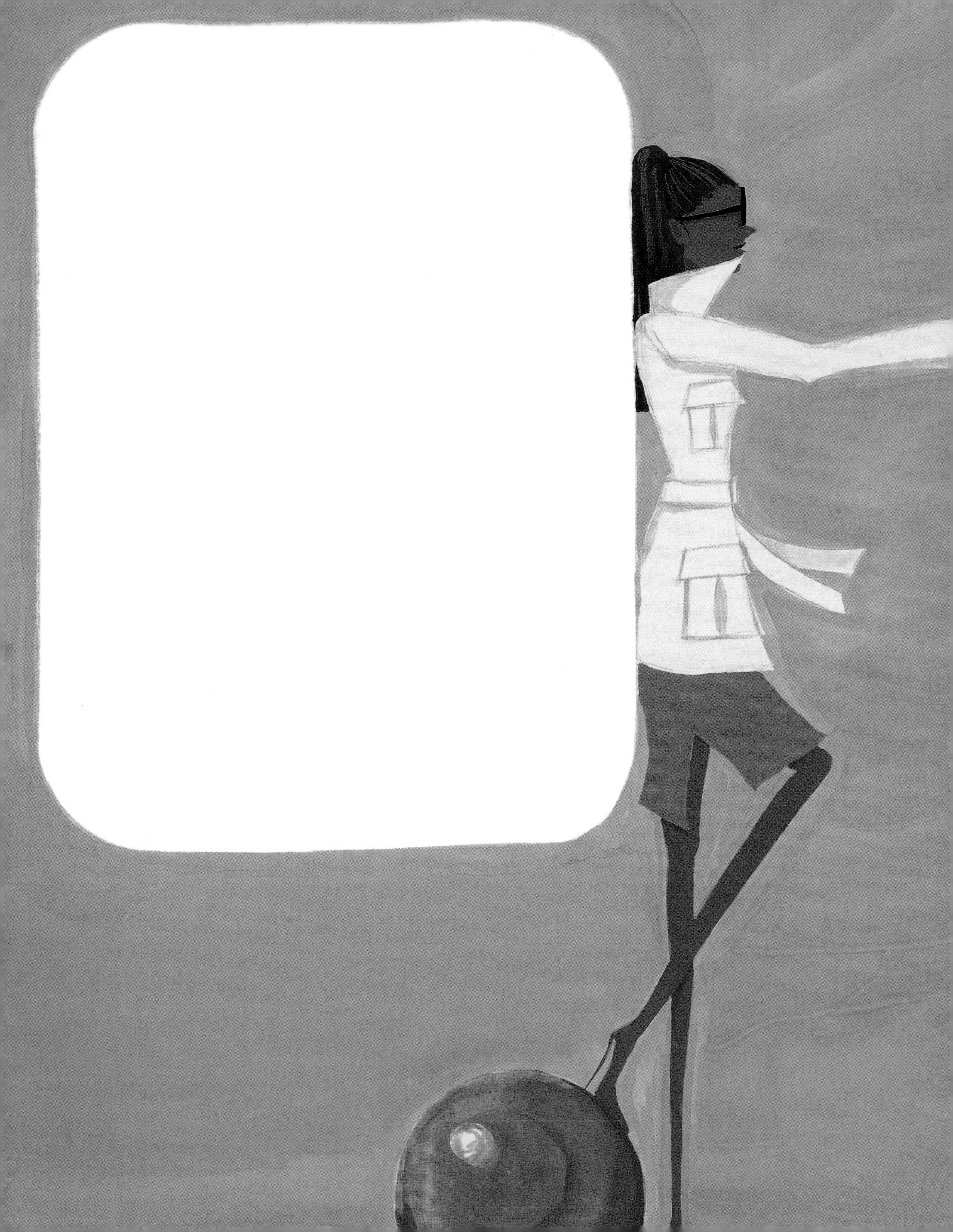

MARCH 18 | IMAGINE A SPRING SAFARI JACKET WITH SKIRTS, PANTS, OR EVEN SHORTS.

Just when you thought you have run out of options for newness in transition weather clothing, the call of the fashion wild beckons you. In the mid-1960s, Dior introduced the safari jacket to women everywhere, and it's been an iffy-weather winner ever since!

Rustic in its rough-hewn flair, usually designed in near-weightless cotton twill or a cotton/linen blend, dyed in a tan, mossy green, or pale neutral tone, the safari jacket was an instant hit with the stylishly sporty female set. And although the fashion versions were less stiff and functional than the genuine article—derived from those worn originally by big-game hunters—the idea was the same. If it gives a nod to the source, today's safari jacket should have patch pockets on the chest (busty women beware) and near the waist, be wrap-belted so it can cinch you within a stylish inch of your life, and have a collar that stands at attention for warmth and attitude.

During transitional spring weather that leaves you chilly today and sweating tomorrow, this jacket beats all. Pair it with a silk shell and softer silk skirt for a look that is office appropriate, or mix it up with cropped pants in a bold color and fun flats to create a look that says "I'll be at the lodge sipping cocktails while the other hunters get dinner." The host of roomy bellows pockets can house everything—thin wallets, single keys, a lipstick, chic mints—without adding bulk to your hips or chest.

MARCH 19 | BANISH THE MORNING NEWS OR STIFLING SILENCE. GET DRESSED TO MUSIC.

Use good music to boost your spirits, especially when getting dressed to face the world.

In this day and age where burning a CD is almost as simple as sending off an e-mail, why not create your own custom CD? Make one for date-night dressing, another for power business days, and a third for getting ready for the weekend.

Here are some classics, some favorites, and some soon-to-be legendary to inspire the start of your music cue for each CD you create. Start dressing from your heart—moved by rhythm and melody.

FOR DATE-NIGHT DRESSING

"Let's Get It On"/Marvin Gaye

"Fever"/Peggy Lee

"At Last"/Etta James

FOR POWER BUSINESS DAYS

"I Will Survive"/Gloria Gaynor

"Strong Enough"/Cher

"Sisters Are Doin' It for Themselves"/Aretha Franklin and Eurythmics

FOR GETTING READY FOR THE WEEKEND

"I Don't Want to Wait"/Paula Cole

"I'm Coming Out"/Diana Ross

"I'm Every Woman"/Rufus featuring Chaka Khan

I'll bet you that "looking out on the morning rain" will never be as difficult again!

MARCH 20 | PEEL BACK THE LAYERS AND THAW YOUR STYLE.

Choose a look that incorporates the colors of nature, and accessories that look like a day of play, not work. That darn groundhog is such a killjoy! He pops his head up and there go your open-toe sandals for another six whole weeks. This is the day you wish you could pop your polished toes and girly shoes into his hole and let him know you made it through, no thanks to him!

Bright Solid Shirt Dress + Nude Heels + Printed Scarf as Belt + Straw Bag

= Daylight Savings

Thin White Button-Down + Grass Green Cardigan + Classic Chinos + Pink Flats

= Last of the Layers

White Jeans + Lemon Yellow Sleeveless Top + Straw Mules + Canvas Tote

= Spring Forward

MARCH 21 | ARIES BIRTHDAY GIRL—YOURS IS A TAKE-CHARGE, SELF-STYLIST PHILOSOPHY.

You are partial to colors very rich in tone and hue—that is, when you're not simply dipped in sexy, mysterious black from tip to toe. Regal tones of red and purple top the list, but you are never afraid to hop into juicy shades of orange and yellow, especially in the warmer months. And since spring is just around the corner, why not use a shot of citrus color today, welcoming your birthday with joy that melts the winter away.

Caution: Even the most inventive Aries can slip up when pairing too many converse style ideas, so be mindful of the fashion statement you are making, limit your pieces, and let the stars do the rest.

Some famously stylish celebrity Aries include Reese Witherspoon and Kate Hudson. Not too shabby style siblings.

MARCH 22

GLAM IT UP FOR THE THEATER IN PERFECT STYLE BY AVOIDING BULKY GARMENTS, CHOOSING FABRICS THAT SHIMMER, AND WEARING YOUR HAIR DOWN AS A GESTURE OF POLITENESS.

Knock! Knock! Knock! Ten minutes to curtain. And all you have on are your undergarments. Dressing appropriately for the theater can give a woman hives if she thinks too hard about it, making her feel as anxious as an actress being called to the stage as she is still zipping up her costume. Not the way to feel as you are about to face the audience or other theatergoers. Theater dressing is about stepping out of your plain self and into someone even more dazzling!

In a time when most women take the dress rules (or lack thereof) from casual Friday, working from home, and an overall casual culture into what they wear for evening events, dressing *up* for the theater is a breath of fresh air! And if done right, it can be fun and feel like a private little fantasy whether you are going to an opening night on Broadway or at a regional playhouse. Honoring the tradition of theater is a worthy reason to glam it up for the night. These are the nights fancy clothes were made for, so go for it!

I believe in four simple style commandments for dressing for the theater. Try as many as you feel inspired to do. Anything is better than seeing yet another woman in jeans and a sweatshirt! You know who you are.

THEATER DRESSING STYLE COMMANDMENTS

- Thou shalt always choose a lighter evening coat or trench when it is chilly outside. Many theaters do not have coat checks, so your lap may become yours. Keep the bulk to a minimum. You may be scooting by a row of people to get to your seat.

- Thou shalt wear your hair down (or in a low chignon) as a gesture of politeness to other theatergoers. Nothing's worse than seeing half a show you paid full price for.

- Thou shalt not wear too many matte clothes. Choose shine that glimmers under marquee lights, during intermission mingling, and whisking off to dinner. Think satin and silk!

- Thou shalt wear heels that slip off easily. The theater is dark, the play sometimes long—why not give your feet a discreet break while getting through multiple acts?

MARCH 23

BE A "MAN MAGNET," EVEN IF YOU ARE MARRIED. PLAY UP YOUR ASSETS LIKE A VIXEN JUST FOR FUN. A LITTLE FLASH, DAZZLE, AND SEX APPEAL CAN MAKE YOU FEEL STRONGER FROM THE INSIDE, WHETHER YOU CATCH A MAN OR NOT.

The 1960s hit television series *Gilligan's Island* had two single female characters who were distinctly different. There was Mary Ann Summers, the sweet country girl who wore gingham and denim, baked homemade pies, and never revealed more than what censors would allow. And there was Ginger Grant, the sexy siren and fallen Hollywood starlet who could jump into a sequin gown faster than she could light a survival fire—and only going without full makeup, a bold beauty mark, and false eyelashes *if* the role called for it.

Who are you more like? If your answer is Ms. Summers, this day's passage is just for you. If your response is Ms. Grant, then you'll most likely agree with what follows, too.

Being a man magnet, if only for a day of fun, is not about disrespectfully revealing and objectifying yourself for the attention of the opposite sex (hey, for that matter, you might not even be attracted to the opposite sex—let's be real, we *are* in the new millennium). This style notion is all about revving up your personal sex appeal to certify what you feel is gorgeous on you (and every woman has at least one gorgeous attribute that never fails), and playing it up in over-the-top Hollywood style! You will feel a little stronger today, walk a bit taller, and take less nonsense from others. And what self-respecting woman wouldn't want that! So it is really all about you, the name just gives you a point of departure.

Choose one of these sexy style essentials from each column, adding them to your outfit for total sizzle. Be careful not to add too many at one time, or it becomes a whole other "hook." And that is something even Mrs. Howell would frown upon:

MAN-TRAP SIZZLERS

Super-high heels with ankle straps
A few faux lashes just on the outside corners
A bustier-inspired top
A fragrance with a chocolate topnote
Shoulders with a shiny finish

MAN-TRAP DROOLERS

Leather pants
Nude lips with a hint of gloss
A backless dress
A pencil skirt (satin if you can)
A peek of lingerie

MARCH 24 | TAKE AN EXPERT STYLE CUE FROM CLASSIC AMERICAN DESIGNER TOMMY HILFIGER.

Tommy Hilfiger's casual approach to fashion has helped place his label in a league of its own—what he describes as "classic, with a twist." Whatever it is, his ads, which are inspired by Americana and music, as well as his clean-cut, simple, and recognizable designs, have led to an empire that is considered one of the highest-ranked publicly traded clothing companies.

What is your best-kept personal style secret?
When building your wardrobe, stick to the classics and accessorize with a few seasonal trends.

What are the three fashion essentials every well-dressed woman should own?
Always start with quality basics and build your wardrobe from there.

A well-dressed woman should own a classic white button shirt, a great pair of well-worn jeans in a flattering fit (for dressing down on a casual day or dressing up with a sexy pair of heels and flirty top for a night out), and a beautiful fitted blazer or classic trench coat for layering. The key is versatility and pieces that transition with your individual lifestyle needs.

What are the biggest mistakes women make when getting dressed?
Trying too hard to follow every trend. You want to look fashionable and put-together, not like you hit every sale rack this season.

Who is the most stylish woman in existence, in your opinion? And what do you appreciate about her look?
Naomi Campbell, Jackie Onassis, and Kate Moss. They all have their own individual styles and know what looks great on them. Naomi and Kate understand how to mix designer with vintage in unique ways. Jackie was the epitome of classic American elegance and taste.

If you could whisper a fail-safe style tip into the ears of women everywhere without them feeling bad by hearing it, what would it be?
Wear what looks *and* feels good on you. If you're not comfortable in what you're wearing, it will show in the way you carry yourself. Comfort and confidence are the key to great style.

MARCH 25 | REACH FOR THE ONE ITEM THAT ALWAYS MAKES YOU FEEL TOTALLY CONFIDENT BEFORE REACHING FOR ANYTHING ELSE.

Creating a winning outfit has a lot to do with fit, color, fabric, and style, all of which can actually be forfeited for how a look makes you feel.

In a pressure-filled world, days that call for fashion armor, a strong yet discreet layer of protection from the world, are fast outweighing the days when what you wear is simply that—what you just happen to be wearing—and that is all. As Stevie Wonder says in his popular song "I Wish," "I wish those days *would* come back once more!"

What is the use of complaining? Life steamrolls onward, and facing it requires immediate style solutions that, for some women, are often created in the wee hours of the morning, when your better half may still be asleep, the light of day is yet to appear, and you're not even exactly sure *what* the weather will bring.

A big presentation ahead, an interview for a new position, a pivotal lunch date with a client, or maybe a weekend event with family you haven't seen in years. These are the instances when before reaching for any of your favorite designers, prints, or patterns, you should be reaching for the one single garment that makes you feel unequivocally confident from the moment you slip a limb into it.

Every woman has at least one of these garments, and even more women own things that don't fit this description. In choosing the latter, you run the noticeable risk of your body reflecting the discomfort and unease you feel all day while facing challenging tasks. And yes, for some, family can be just as much of a challenge as signing on a client.

Take control of the day before it takes control of you by instinctually relying on the one, surefire garment that will surely add a more confident fire to your step and spirit, from the hanger to your hamper.

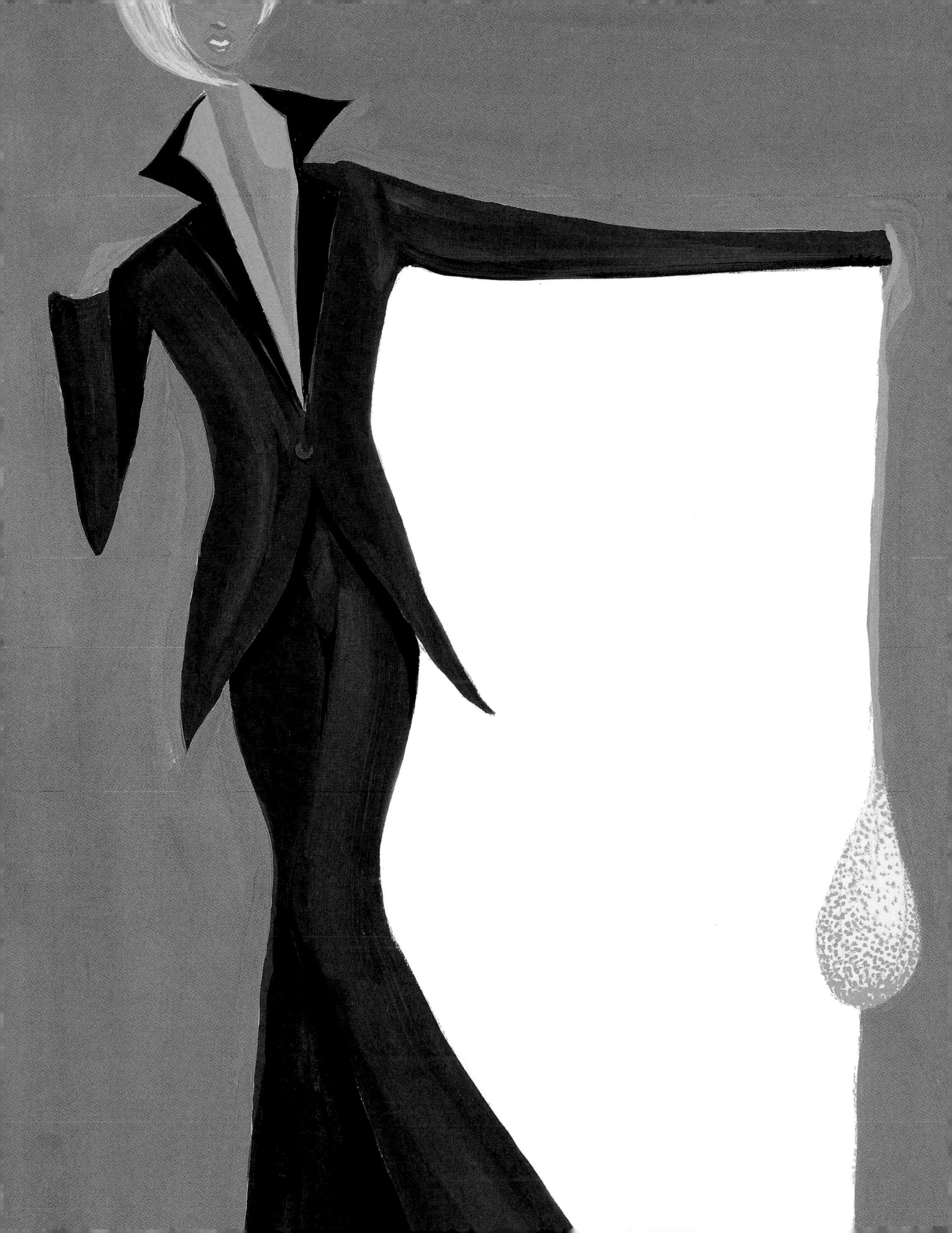

MARCH 26 | WAKE UP YOUR OUTFIT BY ADDING JUST A POP OF BRIGHT, BOLD, UNEXPECTED COLOR AS AN UNDERPINNING OR AN ACCESSORY.

Hold on! Today, before you reach for your black pantsuit and neutral blouse yet again, go for the unexpected. Make a style decision that will get you noticed without overpowering the room. I like to think of this approach as a mini-makeover that any woman can pull off at home, using items you may already have in your closet.

In the fashion industry we call it adding a "pop" of color, and it's a great way to put a stylish twist on an everyday outfit. Think of it as a dose. A splash. A hint. An accent. Not a head-to-toe jolt of hot pink.

Take your black suit for instance. Imagine waking it up with a solid blouse or slim V-neck sweater in cool lavender instead of the usual tan or taupe you automatically reach for. Remember to keep your shoes and handbag solid black. The look is stately and sharp, with a shot of excitement at its heart. Or, with the same black suit, opt for a solid black ribbed turtleneck or a sporty black crewneck T-shirt beneath your jacket, and spike the look with a sexy pair of high heels in lipstick red or watermelon. This is truly a newsflash of color where no one would ever expect to see it.

This clever style trick can draw the eye right to where you want it or, more important, quickly away from where you don't. Used strategically, color equals impact. It relays a level of stylish confidence that makes you memorable. It says you're not afraid to take risks because you know how to pull it off, chicly.

MARCH 27 | UNMATCH YOUR HANDBAG AND SHOES AND JOIN THE MOST STYLISH WOMEN IN THE NEW MILLENNIUM!

Egad! Say it isn't so! Wearing a handbag and shoes that do not match one another? Yes, you read right. Take a breath and read on.

Safety first applies to most active human pursuits. From rock climbing to swimming, we learn it young and the two-word mantra can easily bleed into anything physical we choose to attempt—and make helpful sense.

Dressing to win is not one of those pursuits. Safe dressing sometimes amounts to boring dressing, especially if you want to appear as though you have a point of view, a distinct taste level, and a fashion pulse when facing your day.

By all means, you can sling your mocha brown hobo bag over your shoulder just after you finish reading this, and slip on your identical mocha brown heels, lock your door upon exit, and look put together.

Just know that on this day, and every subsequent day (for now that you know this, you can't act as if you don't), you have the option to find bags, shoes, and, dare I say it, even belts that are different colors. The rule of thumb is to make sure they all complement your clothing. It is as simple as that for modern women who'd rather not look like a page from a mail-order uniform catalog.

Women should look empowered and unique, choosing to express themselves as they see fit. Certain fashion tips apply, others get tossed out with last year's trendy skirt. The idea is having the knowledge at the ready, and selecting what best expresses your mood for the day, week, or year.

Attempt it just once, if only to gauge reactions—yours and the people around you. I promise that the water out there is fine, and you'll get more compliments with an underscored nudge of bravery than you will whispers.

MARCH 28

STOP AND TAKE NOTICE OF WHAT YOU PUT ON FIRST, AND INSTEAD OF THAT ITEM, CREATE YOUR OUTFIT STARTING FROM A TOTALLY DIFFERENT AREA FOR A FRESH LOOK THAT MAY EVEN SURPRISE YOU.

Classically trained actors are taught to study their natural habits and physical tendencies to get in touch with their bodies, ordinary movements, and impulsive expressions, keeping them in a memory reserve for any characters they are challenged to portray. How you brush your hair, how you pour a drink into a glass, or gulp one down, even something as simple as dialing a telephone can inform how you control a character's ability to do the same believably in performance.

The way you reach for your clothing is no different. There is a repetitive sequence that we are either taught in our formative years, or we create on our own, rebelling from what we learned in our upbringing. And just like actors, a woman is creating a character every time she walks out her door to face the world. For some, she is playing a different role daily, and for others, she is a long-standing character who never falters.

Women are infamous shoe worshippers. Ironically, many choose their footwear last each day. And although in cooler months a woman's coat is the first thing people will see, it is usually the last thing she will toss on, hoping it will somewhat complement what she has created beneath it. What defines a woman's style is usually the first item of clothing she reaches for.

And what is that for you? Take a look at what you grab first today, and for the next few days, and watch how it shapes the remainder of your total look.

Sometimes a fresh and unique look isn't about *adding* clothing to your closet, but simply adjusting the *process* by which you put it on. If you faithfully start with a skirt and blouse followed by the perfect shoes and earrings, try selecting your coat first just to see what it inspires you to fit with it. It may be a totally different outfit that surprises even you! You might religiously begin with your jeans on the weekend or for casual nights out, and build the look from the waist up. See what happens when you save the jeans for last, by deciding on your hair and makeup mood first. A smoky eye shadow and pale lip combination may inspire you to put your hair up, and feature that more revealing halter when you would have instinctively reached for that favorite long-sleeve, ribbed turtleneck and your tube of ChapStick. Go ahead, roll the style dice.

Let your limits go by flipping the script and reading the ending first. You just might find out which character you have been dying to play.

MARCH 29 | MAKE GETTING DRESSED MORE FUN AND SIMPLE BY TAKING A MOMENT TO ORGANIZE ALL OF YOUR CLOTHING BY TYPE AND COLOR FAMILY.

The romance between a shopper and her favorite store is a visual one that can ignite all the senses. Clothes shopping in a department store, specialty store chain, or boutique is an experience that is planned out months ahead of your strolling through the doors. Something about the color of the clothing presentation is of an artful palette, blending seamlessly from one wall to another. The music connects to the mood of the season. There may even be strewn around the room enlarged images of women who look the way you have always wanted to look.

It might be the stylishly conceived windows, which draw you in, or the big red sale sign that boasts up to 50 percent off. You may just love the store and always find yourself popping in to see what is new since the last time you dropped your credit card on the counter.

Imagine bottling this feeling and getting the same rush each and every time you step into your very own closet. A place where everything you like is in your size. Everywhere you turn offers another fashion possibility, and the clothes are all "free"—relatively speaking. This is living!

In the same time it takes to fold that week's laundry, you can actually "remerchandise" your closet and dresser to look boutiquelike by simply pairing off your like colors (pinks and reds, neutrals and tans, charcoals and blacks) in neatly folded stacks or hanging areas, and housing similar clothing silhouettes together in their own sections (jackets with blazers, button-down tops near blouses, jeans folded atop corduroys).

The results of this simple shifting will astound you the first time you look to your closet for help, which for most women is every day! It will almost wrap its arms around you to welcome you in, like your favorite store has always done. You will get dressed with more clarity and speed (a wonder for travel), for you now know exactly where everything is at all times. And unlike your choice store, you'll never be looking for assistance or trying to avoid too much assistance, and most important, your size will never be "in the back."

MARCH 30 | CREATE A SEXY "DATE NIGHT" OUTFIT THAT SPARKLES FOR THE EVENING—EVEN IF YOU'VE BEEN MARRIED TO YOUR DATE FOR YEARS.

Remember the excitement you once felt while preparing for an exciting date? How you rushed around to find the perfect, well, everything? You took care to make sure each element looked just right—from your hairstyle to your pedicure. Even the scent you wore was carefully selected. Then, before you stepped out for the evening, you glanced back at your reflection in the mirror and *loved* who you saw smiling back.

Why do women ever stop this magical practice of taking extra time to romance themselves in hopes of romancing that special someone? The answer lies in one word: life—the rigors of which can slowly erode your interest in getting fabulous. Heck, some days it's a challenge to simply function. That's why the date-night look is the perfect remedy, even when it's not actually your first date.

FEATURE YOUR BEST FEATURE

Tastefully show off your best physical feature while leaving room for the imagination. Your sensual shoulders, your beautiful back, those gorgeous gams, even just your pretty smile—choose what feature works best for you, and show it off in styles or with products that highlight it. And remember, when it comes to inspiring romance, a little mystery goes a long way. You don't have to go skimpy to be sexy.

BE SCENT-SATIONAL

Mark the occasion with a glorious new fragrance that will linger in your date's mind. Henceforth, every time they catch a whiff of it, there will be a reminder of you.

GODDESS IN THE DETAILS

Regardless of what you wear, get a fresh manicure, pedicure, and professional haircut and styling. Plain and simple, good grooming goes a long way. People notice the details!

FINE AND FANCY-FREE

Depending on what you have planned, a nice-fitting pair of jeans and a fresh white T-shirt is a stylish, comfortable option. It's an alluring, fun look that doesn't shout high maintenance.

HAVE FUN

Dress for the date's theme. If you are going dancing, wear a skirt with flare and movement (think gentle ruffles or pleats). If you meet over a candlelight dinner, wear something that has a slight reflective

(CONTINUED)

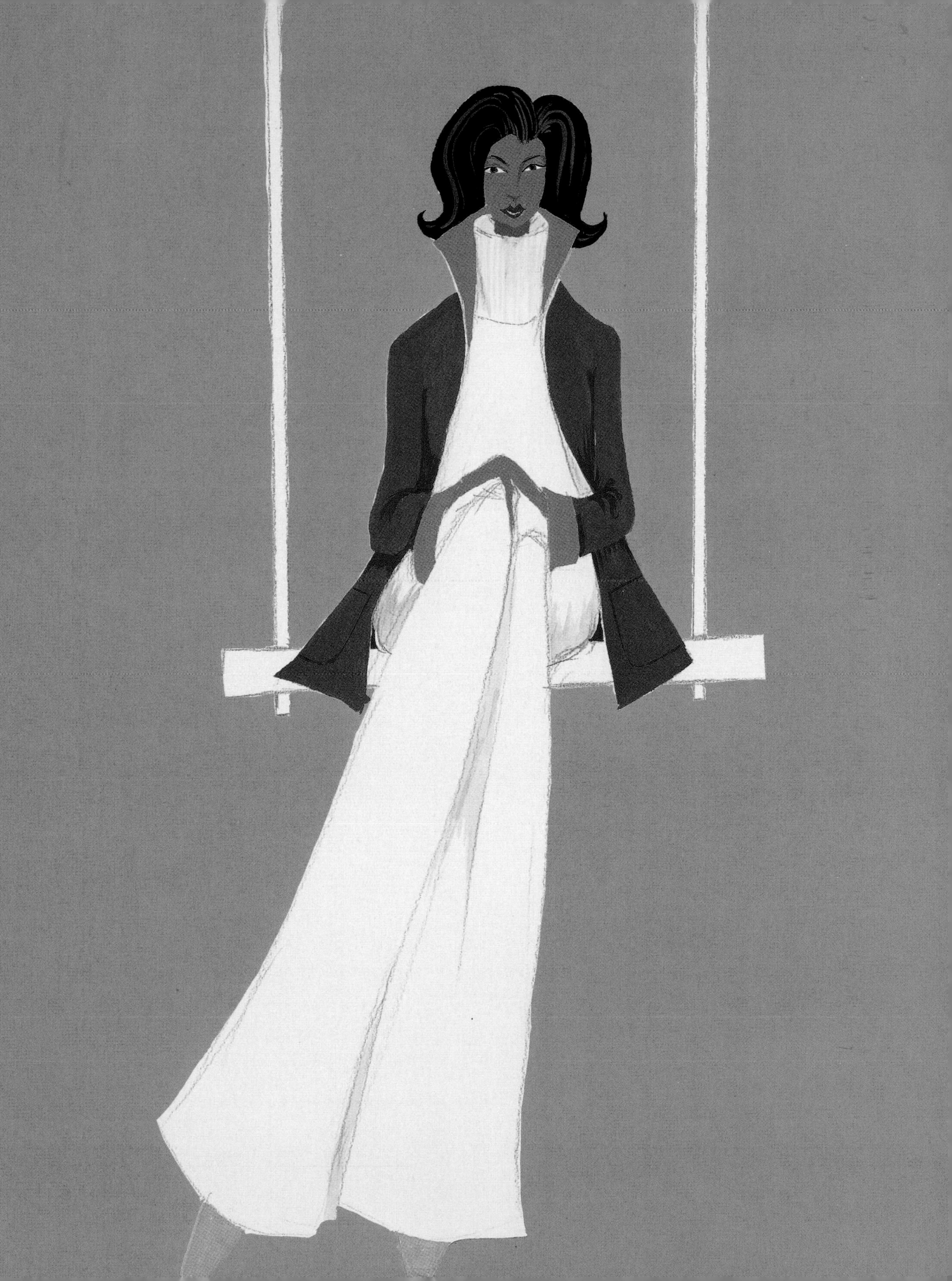

quality above the waist, so you shimmer all night long. Think ahead and play into the night's mood with clothes and accessories that are comfy and appropriate for the occasion.

UNDERNEATH IT ALL

New, alluring underwear will make *you* feel special and fresh—even if your date never gets a peek!

MARCH 31

IF YOU ARE SHORT ON TIME, AND IF ALL ELSE FAILS, CREATE YOUR OWN VERSION OF THIS SUREFIRE, STYLISH OUTFIT COMBINATION AND RUN WITH IT!

It is the last day of the month! If this is one of those days when it seems the clock is jumping ahead ten minutes at a time, and you can't seem to dream up one final, original outfit, here is a fast style solution "cheat sheet" that can get you back on real time—and out the door.

You never really know if an ensemble says exactly what you wanted it to say until you are miles away from your closet and facing your day. Sometimes it fails you and it's too late. Other times you nail it and float through your day unaware of your clothing because when a look works, it leaves you free to focus on more important tasks.

Now is the time to get your last few wears (hopefully) out of your heavier winter clothes and accessories before it's time to exchange them for the lighter, fresher wardrobe that has been packed away all winter long. You may even be transitioning piece by piece, wearing outfits that overlap with items from each season, which is just fine if you do it right.

Get a block of time back right now. Look in your closet and try to match this style equation as best you can with what you *have*. Don't worry if the items you own aren't an exact match. Within this template, choose your own colors and details. Getting the look not so letter perfect gives it a hint of your personal style, which is always better than a carbon copy.

Top: Winter white or white turtleneck
Bottom: Winter white pants or white jeans
Shoes: Flat loafers or moccasins in a bold color
Accessories: Chunky leather belt with bold buckle; sporty tote bag
Flex piece: A quilted three-quarter-length jacket, collar up!

APRIL

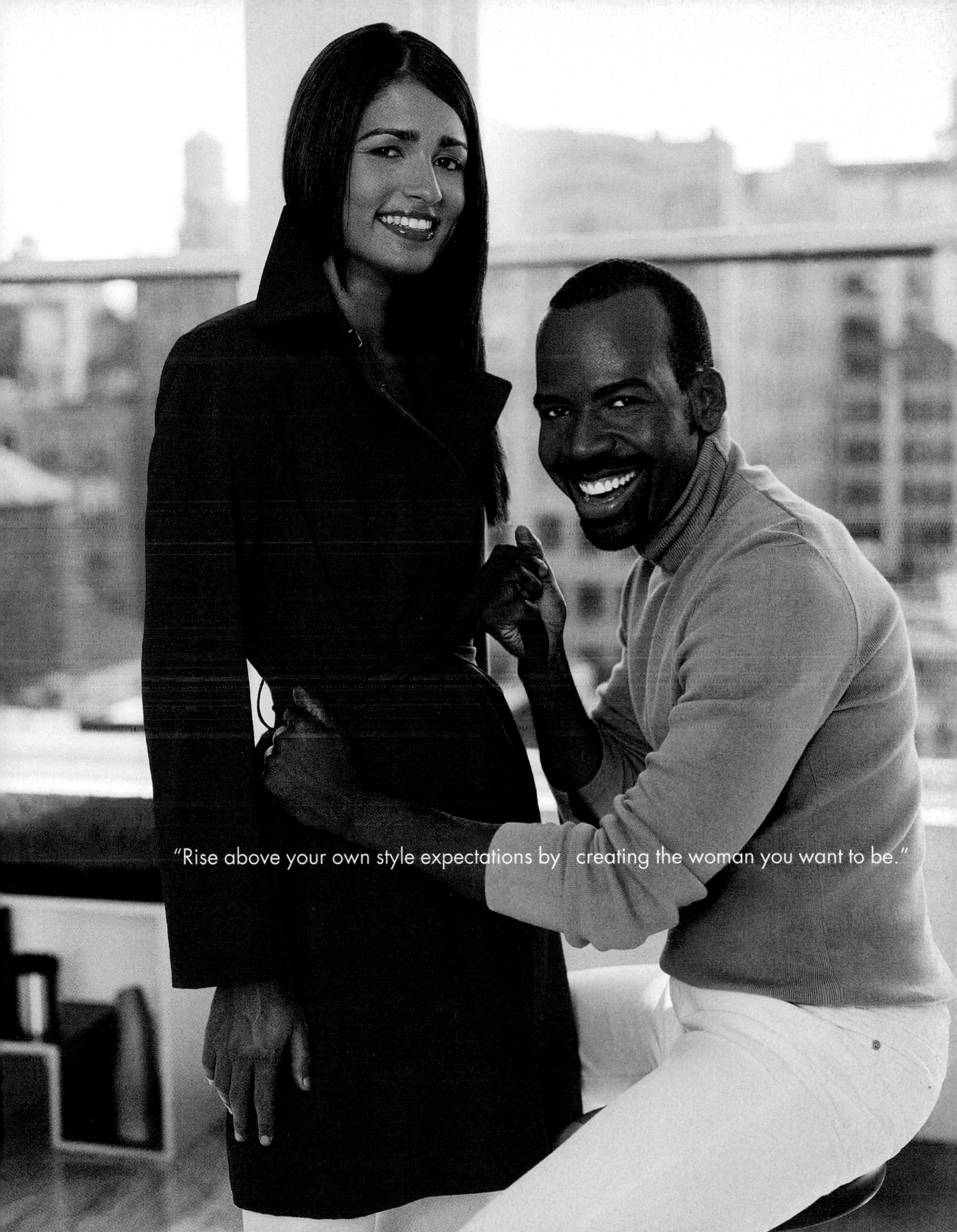
"Rise above your own style expectations by creating the woman you want to be."

APRIL 1

VIEW THE FIRST DAY OF APRIL AS A "RESET" BUTTON FOR THE WARMER MONTHS AHEAD. DAYLIGHT WILL SOON BE EXTENDED, SO USE THE WEEKS AHEAD TO GET READY FOR YOUR TIME IN THE SPOTLIGHT.

Don't be left in the dark this spring—whether in your clothes or in your life! The month ahead welcomes one of my favorite times of year, the beginning of Daylight Saving Time. It usually kicks off on the first Sunday of April, giving you two more weeks of extended daylight to stress over your taxes, which Uncle Sam will expect beneath his pointed finger on the fifteenth. Oh, joy!

Not to fret, though, this is a perfect day to get out of the dark and tackle all things undone, for the darkness and dreariness of winter can assist you in hiding so much. For some women it is a few late-night comfort-food pounds shrouded under layers of dark clothes. For others, it might simply be putting pretty clothes and feminine beauty rituals on a shelf until the world brightens up and defrosts. Well, guess what, today is the day to start shedding the weight and unearthing the allure of your "inner girl."

It is not about starting a binge diet or pulling out your sweet lip glosses and floral-print dresses; it is about being a bit more conscious of what you eat—and maybe choosing a top in color—over instinctively reaching for your safe, secure black clothes. If you can do this and take April days in baby steps, all thirty of them, you will see a cumulative result that will be more than obvious come what may, in May.

If all else fails, one of my favorite looks on all women in the springtime, regardless of age or size, is a long itchy burlap wrap skirt, worn with a sheer white tank top, a few sizes too small, and men's dirty work boots and matching gold belt with purple fringe. April fool! Got ya!

Affirmation:
I will put the dark winter behind me by embracing clothes and a lifestyle that I feel good about in the light.

APRIL 2 | TAKE AN EXPERT STYLE CUE FROM LESLEY JANE SEYMOUR, A TOP NEW YORK STYLE-MAKER AND EDITOR IN CHIEF OF *MARIE CLAIRE.*

What is your best-kept personal style secret?
I'm only five-two but think five-ten when I dress so I never look short. People are surprised!

What female celebrity has kept global style moving forward? What is it about her that makes it happen?
Audrey Hepburn. There isn't a collection that gets made where someone doesn't do an ode to her little shift dresses.

Why is it so easy for real women to look just as good as the stars on the red carpet today?
Knockoffs, plain and simple. I've often said to my fashion team we should call our pages the "Don't Blame Me If You Don't Look Good" story because there is so much that is available at a great price.

As a busy person, what one style tip would you love other busy people to know that always gets you by looking fabulous?
When in doubt—or too busy or tired—grab all black. It's never wrong.

APRIL 3 | THE SABRINA HEEL.

The kitten or "Sabrina" heel is as feminine as it comes in heels. They are usually one and a half to two inches in height, with a distinct girlie curve to it—like a miniature stiletto. They are the perfect happy medium between figure-flattening flats and painful high heels.

The name "Sabrina" stuck to these heels after the effervescent Audrey Hepburn wore them in the 1954 film *Sabrina*. The title character was sweet, pretty, understatedly chic, and, most of all, comfortable.

Pair them with pants, like the signature of the character Sabrina, or with a skirt of just about any shape. Like a kitten, you will remain light on your feet, curiously charming, and stylishly spry.

APRIL 4 | HAPPY BIRTHDAY, MAYA!

A true renaissance woman. At any given time, some of her dreams are nascent, others are in full swing. She paints, she cooks, she gardens, she writes a bit of poetry, she laughs until her sides hurt, she's spirited, she likes to dance all night, and she might even hang glide if she so chooses! Exhausting, yes, but this is her pace, one of self-inspired fun, romance, and joy.

As style is definitely about what you wear, it is also very much about what you feel. Maya Angelou has always felt stylish and beautiful, even when the world may not have deemed her so. Her curves are typical to her African heritage and she celebrates them without apology with her posture and her poems. She's usually noticeably taller than other women in the room, yet her proud carriage and presence turns it into a positive. She never seems to get caught up in what society says she's not. From casually sporting African head wraps atop natural hair, to wearing soft pressed curls, to penning bestselling novels and spirited cookbooks, she ages with grace and continues to reinvent herself through all facets of her style, both the personal and the prose.

Carefree abandon, yes. Reckless abandon, no. Maya Angelou, who was born on this date, is a woman who can experience life's real joys yet also be centered and secure. Who knows if Angelou set out to have a list of titles following her name. What is clear is her ability to live out loud and reinvent without apology.

Use the example of her life to punch up yours, if only for today. Shake up the titles that currently follow your name. Yes, you are a great mother, but you're also an amateur wine connoisseur and kick-butt karaoke champ. Your stylish hobbies and fun pastimes are trademarks of the real you, and may lead to unexpected success and, more important, phenomenal personal fulfillment.

APRIL 5 | DITCH YOUR BLOUSE FOR A DAY.

You've come a long way, baby. By now you probably understand that looking uniquely stylish usually means looking less than conventional. Jumping into the obvious safe clothing pairings is a great route for conservative work environments, sacred events, and the like. But sometimes you have a little leeway to express yourself and want just a hint of wardrobe irreverence with your more serious clothing.

Take the tailored jacket and blouse combination, for example. Women usually think jacket and automatically think blouse. And why wouldn't you? This has been the right, safe solution for decades. A tailored jacket calls for a tailored blouse.

Not this day. The antiblouse is the crisp crewneck or V-neck white T-shirt. You can find them for around $100 at designer stores and boutiques, or you can grab a three-pack of men's (or boy's) undershirts at your local discount store for around $10. The look is basically the look.

Instantly your serious tailored jacket takes a breather. And make sure that when going this route, you pair your T-shirts beneath jackets that have the most structure and are made of the best fabrics (worsted wool, silk, cashmere, leather, suede). This creates a balance.

Now you have a sporty edge that makes you look confident in your clothing, enough so that you don't have to slip into what others expect you to be in, yet you still have the same authority and never appear underdressed. The power is in the decision to pull away from the obvious choice.

APRIL 6 | TAKE AN EXPERT STYLE CUE FROM AVRIL GRAHAM, A TOP NEW YORK STYLE-MAKER, EXECUTIVE FASHION AND BEAUTY EDITOR OF *HARPER'S BAZAAR* MAGAZINE.

What is your best-kept personal style secret?
Always invest in good accessories—a great bag and good shoes will take you anywhere and are instantly noticed.

What are the three fashion essentials every well-dressed woman should own and why?
1. A classic good bag—with no bells and whistles. The "it" bag of the season will be short-lived before it is deemed totally out. The classic will always have longevity.
2. A basic black sheath dress.
3. A well-cut black pant. They are the basics to build upon, can be dressed up or down, layered or worked with the trends of the season.

What are the biggest mistakes women make when getting dressed?
Be honest with yourself. Look at your body—don't be a fashion victim regardless of the trend. Just because a look works on Jennifer Lopez or Sarah Jessica Parker doesn't mean it will look good on you. Have the confidence to sometimes say to yourself this does not work for me.

Who is the most stylish woman in existence, in your opinion? And what do you appreciate about her look?
Jacqueline Onassis. She possessed effortless style—it's innate. All the stylists in the world can't give you this. Whether at a black-tie function, campaigning, playing with her children, or on vacation she exemplified a

(CONTINUED)

woman who always looked fabulous. There is not one photograph of her I can think of, even in unguarded moments, in which she did not look supremely stylish—dressed up or down.

If you could whisper a fail-safe style tip into the ears of women everywhere, without them feeling bad by hearing it, what would it be?
Buy clothes that fit. The memorable fashion icons (Audrey Hepburn, Princess Diana, Grace Kelly) didn't pull at straps, spill out of tops, wear clothing too tight, sleeves too long. Also, don't be swayed by label size—often, different manufacturers have quite different fits.

APRIL 7 | APRIL SHOWERS BRING OUT THE BEAUTIFUL UMBRELLAS.

Splurge a teeny bit today and invest in the best umbrella you can afford that speaks to your taste level and personal style. Chances are, it will be the last one you invest in, and the first one you reach for with pleasure and ease in the next rainstorm. You'll be saying, "Bring it on!"

APRIL 8 | GRAY IS GORGEOUS.

Whether you have strands of silver running through your hair or just a few strands of your youthful color left, remember some best fashion bets to make you glow.

Pinstripes: Dark clothes with pale pinstripes connect beautifully to the tones in gray hair, making them a harmonious part of your overall style.
Heathers: A blurrily speckled knit color treatment that has highs and lows of one tone (think classic gym sweats). Active tops or dressy jersey dresses in oatmeal or gray heather look sporty and chic—while not looking like a forced match to your hair.
Black: When in doubt, super-rich dark black—worn on top or all over—places your gray mane on a pedestal. It registers as worldly and sophisticated. Add chunky silver jewelry for increased chic!

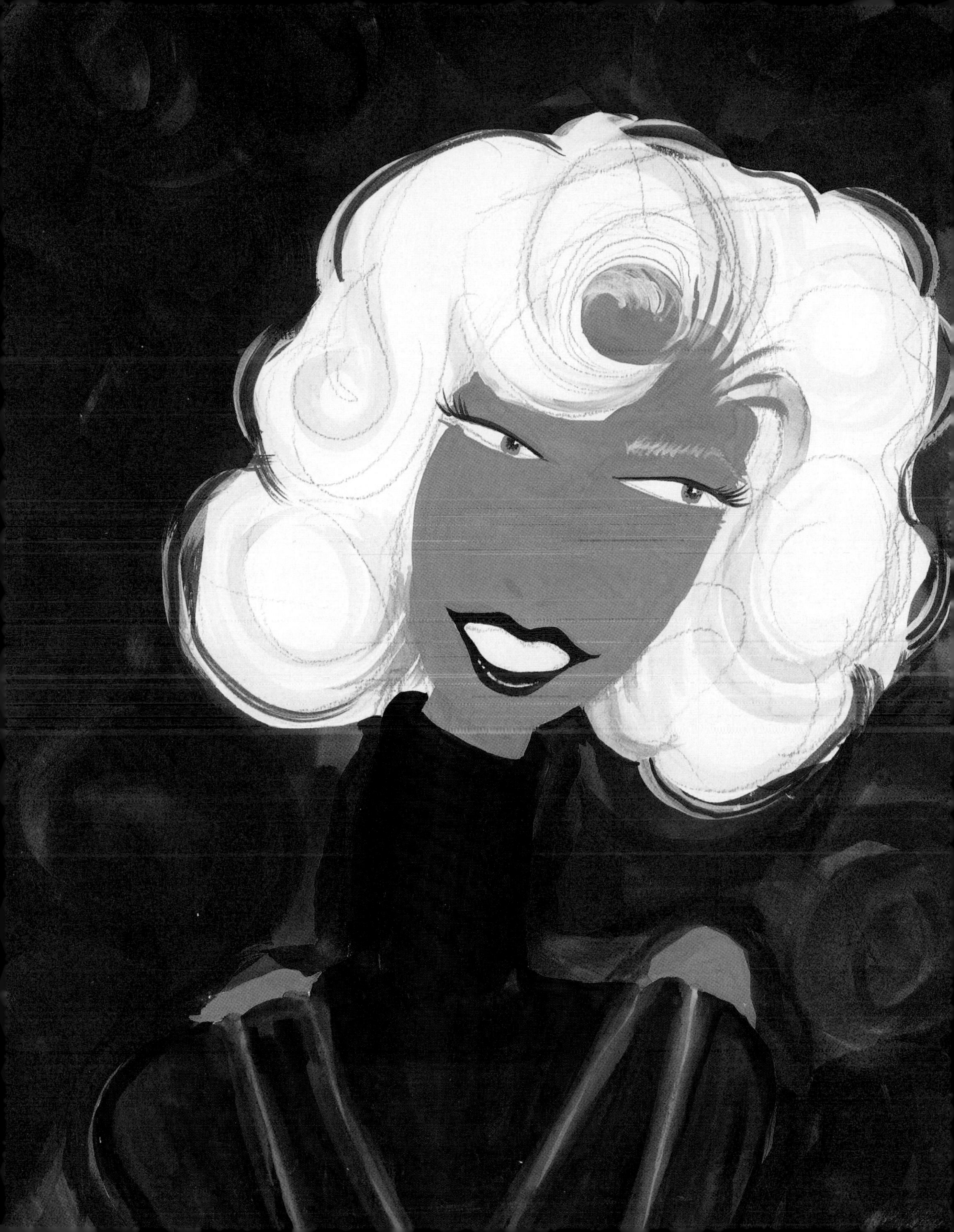

APRIL 9 | BUY A BLACK TRENCH COAT WITH SHEEN.

Being on the go means whizzing in and out of varied climates, different city vibes, and diverse weather conditions. Off a plane straight to a power meeting, from a car right into dinner, or into a taxi going directly to the airport. It is hot one minute outdoors, chilly the next on the flight, misting in that new city, and dressy at a restaurant you thought was all about jeans.

If you are this woman, or hope to be, you must have a black trench coat with a satiny finish. Starting at around $150, you can find a quality name-brand classic trench, and work your way upward of $250 and beyond by looking at even better designer offerings.

This garment works well as a topper, adding a bit of sheen for evening and structure and power for day. It protects from the elements, and stands up to being stuffed into an overhead compartment when you are on the road. If you find a reversible version, so much the better. It can cover a casual outfit in a pinch—dressing it up.

Toss it on, belt it with a strong knot in the front, and raise your collar, and you, too, become a sexy and mysterious citizen of the world.

APRIL 10 | LEARN A NEW FASHION TERM.

Fedora *(fe-do-rah)* • *A felt hat with a medium-sized brim and a high crown with a lengthwise crease from front to back. Originally worn by men but now also styled for women with turned-up back brim. Popularized for men after Victorien Sardou's play* Fedora *was produced in 1882. Became popular again in the 1920s. A staple of most men's haberdasheries, this stately style connoted an upstanding, well-dressed gadabout who knew how to tilt the brim and crease the crown just so. Then Hollywood made it the costume mark of the gangster in the 1930s and 1940s, as well as the private eye in the classic noir films.*

A quality fedora, defined by sharp, clean lines, was a common men's accessory. It would take classic screen idols like Marlene Dietrich, in the 1930s, to liberate women from their expected bell-shaped cloche hats, and modern starlets like Jennifer Lopez to keep this gender-bending accessory trend alive on the red carpet. Their common thread is pairing it with anything but a masculine suit.

For you to get the most impact, juxtapose a fedora with an ultrafeminine ensemble that creates a sexy tension most other women can't quite put their finger on. This is usually because they are expecting a more masculine face beneath the brim. Oh, well, just give them a wink, and tilt your brim like a true gentleman would.

APRIL 11 | TAKE AN EXPERT STYLE CUE FROM ROBERT BURKE, A TOP NEW YORK STYLE-MAKER, VICE PRESIDENT AND SENIOR FASHION DIRECTOR OF BERGDORF GOODMAN.

What are the three fashion essentials every well-dressed woman should own?

1. A sexy pair of shoes
2. A great coat
3. A good fashionable handbag

What are the biggest mistakes women make when getting dressed?
Wearing too many trends at the same time.

Who is the most stylish woman in existence, in your opinion? And what do you appreciate about her look?
C. Z. Guest, a dear friend of mine. She was the epitome of American style. Whether she wore an Oscar de la Renta ball gown or a pair of slacks and a sweater, she always looked appropriate and stylish for the occasion.

If you could whisper a fail-safe style tip into the ears of women everywhere, without them feeling bad by hearing it, what would it be?
Always remember to dress your age.

APRIL 12 | ADD A POLKA-DOT PRINT TO YOUR LOOK.

This timeless print takes its name from a popular dance craze in the 1880s! Even now it remains flirty and springtimelike.

Go for a polka-dot skirt or a semisheer "coin dot" silk chiffon blouse. If not that, then try sweet "Swiss" or "pin" dot pants that fall just above the ankle to bring spirit and a fanciful tone to basic separates.

THREE WAYS TO ALWAYS LOOK STYLISH IN POLKA-DOT PRINTS

•Smaller dots look the most elegant. Larger, more whimsical dots lean toward casual clothes and events. But even then, looking like a game of Twister attacked you is never fashionable.

•Black and white dot prints are a safe way to start dabbling in this classic look. Choose black garments with small white dots or the reverse. Get bolder from there.

•"Ditsy" or imperfectly scattered dots look very modern and sexy. Choose the right dots for your many moods—there are versions for every side of you.

APRIL 13 | LET GO OF OLD HABITS.

"Ten years before its time, a fashion is indecent; ten years after, it is hideous; but a century after, it is romantic."
—James Laver

Style can be fickle. Fashion can be comical. Women often balk at newness in style but hold on to a trend that has long gone south.

Take piercings, for instance. In recent decades, pierced ears were considered a pretty safe style statement, especially if you had one hole in each ear. But there was a time when women with pierced ears were considered "loose" or "fast," leading teens to rebel against their parents' wishes and have their ears pierced at home right in the kitchen or bathroom using a sterilized needle and an ice cube. It was no big deal, the process or the look. Mothers even began to pierce the ears of their newborn babies, so they wouldn't have to consciously endure the pain as a preteen.

In the 1960s, Black American women influenced by African culture embraced piercings as de rigueur. Enter the punk scene of the late 1970s where London-based fashion outcasts sent shock waves around the globe with multiple piercings in each ear. After a while, the practice moved into the mainstream. Cue up to the 1990s when body piercings showed up on the fringe of fashion society. Navel rings, eyebrow piercings—you name the body part and someone has skewered or bejeweled it. Younger people took to it, their elders were outraged!

But generations mature and what was novel becomes typical. There are soccer moms who still have flat stomachs, and let you know it by adding a sweet little navel ring. You'll see a woman who by all appearances works in some sort of financial industry, but every now and then you'll detect a slight lisp triggered by a discreet tongue stud. Oh, behave!

Open your mind to a new trend that shocks you before it becomes *so* last decade.

APRIL 14 | POP STYLE QUIZ.

See how much you really know about looking great. Let the information empower your look and mental style file today, even if you don't get a perfect score!

1. To get the best look when wearing pants tucked into your knee boots, your pant leg of choice should be . . .

A. Stovepipe
B. Capri
C. Slim
D. Cuffed

2. Pants with a wider waistband can disguise what common figure challenge?

A. Long torso
B. Short waist
C. Top-heaviness
D. Thick ankles

3. When helping a man get dressed in a suit, his bottom jacket button should . . .

A. Always be buttoned
B. Never be buttoned
C. Be removed
D. Be mother-of-pearl

4. For the best care of your wardrobe, freshly dry-cleaned clothes in plastic bags should be . . .

A. Removed as soon as you get home to avoid yellowing
B. Kept in bags, and tied at the bottom to keep clean
C. Folded within tied bags, and placed in a cool dry place
D. None of the above

(Answers: 1-C, 2-A, 3-B, 4-A)

APRIL 15 | MAKE SURE YOU AREN'T STUCK IN A PAST DECADE.

Mix timeless classics and new items to keep you stylishly in the present. Take a peek in your closet and see which decade you are known for. If the number of those items outweigh what was purchased in the last ten years, you may need to start purging the trendy items of long ago and purchasing a few of today's new classics to create a balance. Run old items past someone ten years younger. If they balk, maybe it should walk. If they love it, think of it as a classic, or something that has come back around again. You don't want to be like your aunt who got stuck in time. You know the one.

APRIL 16 | SLIP INTO A SLING-BACK HEEL FOR THE MOST IN LADYLIKE VERSATILITY, TAKING YOU FROM POLISHED FOR THE OFFICE TO PRETTY FOR NIGHTS OUT.

If you can invest in only one pair of heels to go with almost anything in your closet from work, to play, to casual evening, you need look no further than a perfect sling-back pump.

Whether pointed toe, open toe, classic pump, or sandal, the sling-back silhouette is one of those that looks just as pretty on the foot as it does on a pedestal.

They cry out to be paired with business pantsuits or to add the perfect punctuation to your pencil or A-line skirt, and are a hopelessly romantic pairing with the sexy jeans that you reserve for girls' night out! Look at them as your "best girlfriend" of shoes, who never lets you down. She can hang out anywhere with you, from stylish charity events to serious, chow down seafood joints.

Use this opportunity to try strapping them on with just about any look for an extra dose of ladylike attitude.

APRIL 17 | GET TEN-MINUTE STYLE FOR AN OUTDOOR WEDDING OR GARDEN EVENT.

Here is a great ten-minute style solution for a wedding or semiformal event:

Minutes 1:00–2:00:
Unearth a colorful, printed skirt that has romance and fun and whimsy (floral, paisley, geometric prints). Go knee length or longer, the fuller the better.

Minutes 3:00–4:00:
Pull out a blazer or suit jacket. Pure white is best, but a soft pastel or pale tan to complement the skirt will work in a pinch. Choose a tank or T-shirt in the exact same color. Select colorful earrings as your only accessory (far from the skirt).

Minutes 5:00–6:00:
Flats work best on grass, but kitten heels can give you a lift and not sink you. Wear a pair that is bright, bold, and fun in a color from your skirt, or go flesh tone.

Minutes 7:00–8:00:
Straw handbags look great all around, or just keep a lipstick, one credit card, keys, ID, and mints in your jacket—for what will you really need a bag for?

Minutes 9:00–10:00:
Your makeup should be au natural. Do spot work with an all-in-one foundation/powder, very little color on the eyes, soft petal lips, clear mascara on lashes and brows—and hit the lawn, fresh and fragranced!

APRIL 18 | WEAR AN A-LINE SKIRT AND ADD A LADYLIKE TWIST TO JUST ABOUT ANY TOP, DIMINISH YOUR HIPS, AND FLIRT WITHOUT EFFORT.

It should really be called the A+ skirt! If I had to give one of the many skirt silhouettes a grade for being super-versatile, classic, and figure-flattering—all in one—it would be the A-line skirt.

The early 1960s gave birth to the A-line skirt and smart women never let it go. The A-line skims the hips slightly, and flares out just in time to make them appear a bit smaller to the eye. Women lacking hips love its power to give shape where there is little to none.

Invest in a timeless A-line in a solid color and year-round fabric. Working women should start with a dark color, where as those choosing versions just for play can opt for a light first-investment piece. Match it with fitted sweaters, untucked tailored blouses, and pretty tanks that are tastefully snug to bring out its best. With a skirt this together, the outfit combinations are almost limitless, from business with pumps, to weekends in playtime flats.

APRIL 19 | BETTER TO BE A BIT OVERDRESSED THAN UNDERDRESSED AND WITHOUT OPTIONS.

We have become casual in our dress and, arguably, in our behavior. There was a time when a woman wouldn't think of leaving her home without her hat *and* gloves. Formal dress and accoutrements were gestures of respect for the room a woman planned to enter, and the people with whom she expected interaction. Times have changed.

Entering a room today is more about a woman's comfort level, not only with her clothes and shoes, but with the people around her. Modern women are less concerned about appearances than ever before, and this is a good thing when it comes to your personality. It means a secure sense of ownership over who you are and not kowtowing to others.

It is easier to peel down an outfit and make it more casual than it is to scramble to find pieces to build up a casual outfit. Once you are out in front of others, the clothes you need are usually not around, whereas removing a tailored jacket, rolling up shirtsleeves, tying a sweater over your shoulders or around your waist all work instant wonders in bringing a look down to earth a bit.

APRIL 20 | MAKE YOUR LEGS APPEAR A BIT LONGER BY WEARING A NUDE SHOE.

Every well-dressed woman needs a pair of nude, high-heeled dress shoes. Nude means that the color of the shoe should be a strikingly close match to your particular skin tone. I proudly prescribe this look for women who want to add the illusion of length to their legs by wearing a shoe that doesn't match an outfit to perfection or compete with an understated outfit. Think about it: Sometimes a grass green dress and matching grass green shoes can leave you looking stumpy. And what are your options? Black shoes are too heavy. Metallics, yes, if they are in this season. Need I continue?

The look of a soft, natural nude shoe is, all at once, rich, organic, and elegant. Choose a traditional pump, a sexy sling-back, a strappy high-heeled sandal, or a Sabrina heel—the choice is yours. This nude or neutral approach is a surefire shoe that is great for travel because of its versatility. It allows you to wear and repeat, without the chance of looking like you are wearing *those* shoes again. You can pack a lighter bag with one great pair of shoes that will go with just about anything, because they go with *you*. They almost disappear from your feet.

APRIL 21 | HAPPY BIRTHDAY, TAURUS GIRL—ORIGINAL, UNDERSTATED, LOVING QUALITY OVER QUANTITY.

Many Taurus women like to think of themselves as classic dressers, embracing style from a place of quality over quantity. You know a good fabric, sometimes without even touching it. You'd prefer an amazing, simply cut dress created by a local tailor, where you are actually a part of the design process, to a designer-label version found in twelve or more sizes at a swanky department store.

Compliments come frequently to you. As a very practical earth sign, you take them with a grain of salt, offering a polite thanks as if you really have no idea how good you really look. This is exactly why your clarity in matters of aesthetics never seems to fail you. Think of it as a cosmetic karma of sorts.

Trust it today and stick to your tried-and-true fashion essentials: earth tone colors, amazing tailoring, and just the right accessory worn for flair—but never too much.

A few of your bullish celebrity sisters of style are Cate Blanchett and Renée Zellweger. They seem to share similar traits when they stand before the flashbulbs. You, too, can work it like it's the Oscars!

APRIL 22 | IF YOU CAN ROCK THE MICROMINI SKIRT AND HEELS, TRY ADDING A "SKORT" AND KITTEN HEELS TO YOUR ARSENAL.

The heels simply let you know why *certain* working girls prefer this look, as you *should* be paid for standing around on stilts this high.

The micromini and high heel combo is for the few who are slim enough to be complimented by wearing it. The rest of us can enjoy looking at those who wear it right and opt for a skort and kitten heels. This outfit can vacillate from sexy to sporty in a flash, and is much more age appropriate. Keep a pair of tennis sneakers in your bag-of-the-moment, just in case you need to dash.

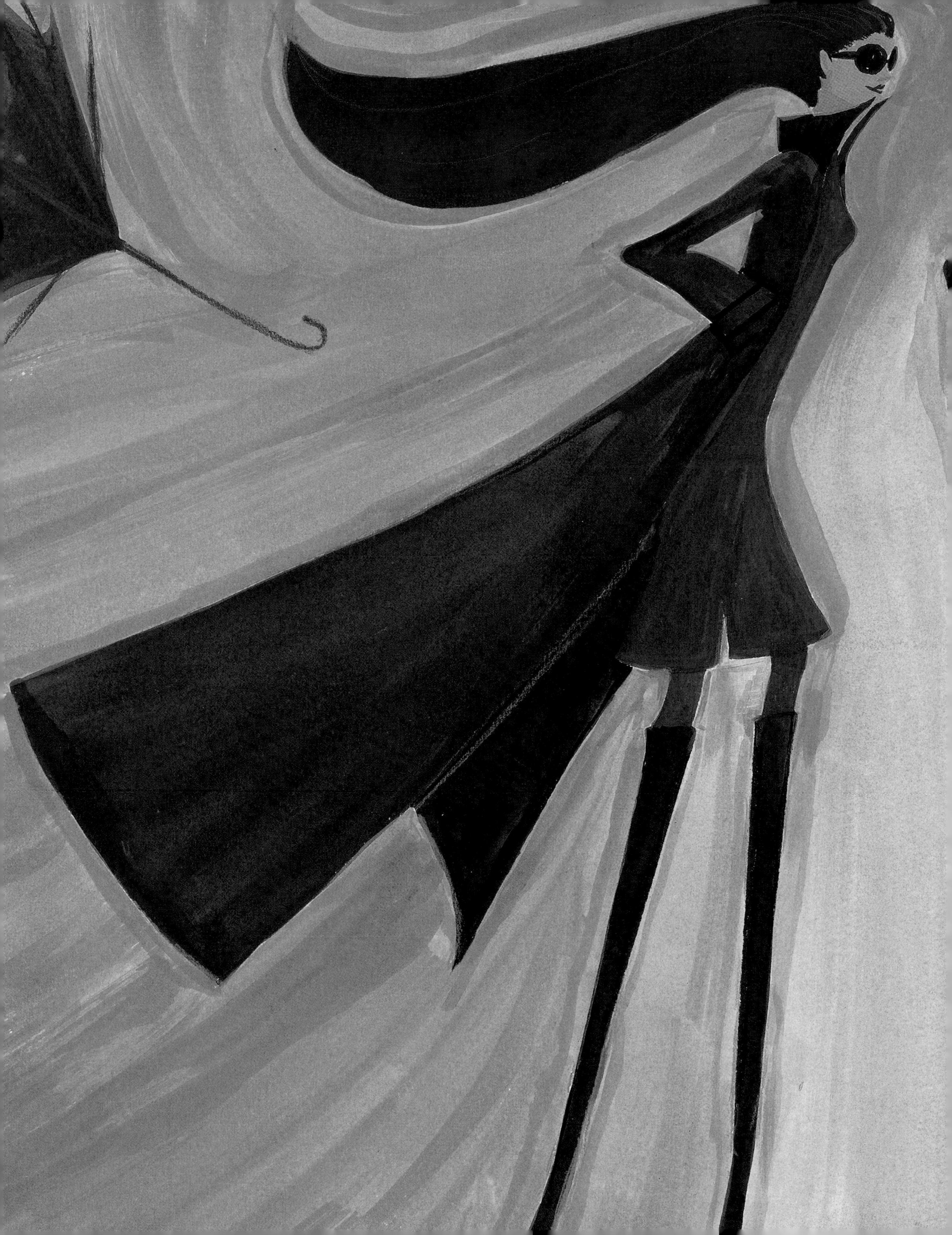

APRIL 23 | JUMP INTO A BLACK AND NAVY ENSEMBLE.

Experiment with this color combination for a look that speaks of European chic and a fashion runway sensibility. Some days you simply need a fresh take on color to achieve a new look. It is not about running out to purchase an entirely new outfit, just mingling items you already own in a way that appears new to others and, most important, feels fresh and new to you. You can do this right now with the combination of black and navy.

For many years this unexpected pairing looked like a major fashion mistake, as if you were getting dressed in the dark, mistaking your black clothes for the navy—and vice versa. Fashion right now is all about flipping on the lights and intentionally coupling these dark cousins with a well-appointed approach. The trick is wearing a balanced amount of each.

Women in Paris and Italy have long known how modern and sophisticated this grouping can appear if done right. Picture yourself at a romantic sidewalk café sipping from a dainty white cup, legs crossed, looking just as good as any woman who walks by, model or not. Ask the French house of Chloé, where the marriage of coal black and midnight navy have graced its runways as a rule. Here are a few ways to do it on a real budget, using what you may already own:

Black Silk Blouse + Navy Pleated Knee-Length Skirt + Navy Hose and Shoes

= Am I Blue

Black Pantsuit + Navy Scarf-Tie Blouse + Thin Strappy Heels in Black or Navy

= Business as Unusual

Black Trench Coat + Navy Sweater + Navy Cropped Pants/Tights + Black Knee Boots

= 'Round Midnight

APRIL 24

SLIP INTO A FLATTERING FLORAL PRINT THAT SAYS "PRETTY" AND "POLISHED," WITHOUT BRINGING ATTENTION TO AREAS ON YOUR BODY YOU WANT TO DOWNPLAY.

When I began my career in the fashion industry, I heard an idiom in the design room where I worked that has always stayed with me: Unflattering prints were called "flowered" prints while the gorgeous counterpart was called a "floral" print.

Look at your floral in a three-way mirror, or create a two-way mirror in any room by holding up a compact to review the back. Notice exactly where your Poppies pose, your Posies rise, and your Roses bloom. If any of these lovely garden varieties hit you where, as my mother says, "the good Lord split you," or on any other modest area, it may be time to remove them from your backyard.

Gorgeous floral prints should welcome in spring with a burst of ladylike femininity and fun! Pair a pastel floral top with pale pants and a shoe in a color from your print's petals, or wear a jewel-toned flirty floral skirt with a white boatneck sweater to let the world know what time it is. Keep it fun, and not funny, as the giggles might be at your expense if the flowers are signaling unwanted attention.

APRIL 25

CLAIM YOUR TWENTIES AND FEATURE A STYLE THAT BEST SUITS YOU, OR PASS ALONG AN AGE-EMPOWERING TIP TO A WOMAN WHO REALLY NEEDS IT—OLDER OR YOUNGER.

Ask any woman over thirty if she took her twenties style for granted, and the answer will be a resounding "yes!" Hey, these are the only twenties you'll get, so let them roar!

Many women look back at their twenty-something bodies and wish they'd had more fashion fun when carbs didn't matter as much! Your bustline keeps up with you. Your hair is as close to "wash and go" as it will ever be. And the skin you are in is the skin women twice your age are trying to buy in a jar. Look at these blessings in the mirror and savor them, starting today!

This is the season of your life to celebrate your natural-born assets, while you have them, through fashion, playing with bold color, touches of shine, and flirty separates that will define your decade of freedom and discovery.

You'll also want to take the time to find style essentials in these years; your perfect jean cut, your ideal cocktail dress, and that killer skirt suit that keeps all eyes on you—or lands you on the fast track within your career. Once you identify these perfect items, you may push yourself to always fit into them, which isn't always a bad thing, if you are honest about what looks best as you age. Many women who invest in good-quality clothing in the twenties take their favorite labels and good habits along with them through life, making sure they stay as close to their original size as they can. Hey, it's worth the old college try!

QUICK STYLE LIST: THE TOP FIVE TWENTY-SOMETHING STYLE ESSENTIALS:

Perfect-fitting jeans
Your ideal little black dress
A killer pant- or skirt suit
One color that looks amazing on you
Your best high heels

APRIL 26 | EVEN IF YOU ARE FLYING COACH, DRESS LIKE YOU ARE BOOKED IN FIRST CLASS.

Flying in style is a vestige of eras gone by. There was a time when a woman wouldn't dare travel in anything less than heels, a well-made leather vanity bag, and her travel gloves. These outfit ideas and accessories aren't very practical today, but there is a more comfortable and less fussy alternative to consider.

My favorite travel ensembles begin with the feet. Whether loafers in leather or suede, driving moccasins or lace-free sneakers, always choose slip-ons over traditional lace-ups. They come off easily when faced with security checkpoints, and when your legroom begins to let up.

As for bottoms, choose pants that are wrinkle-friendly, like tailored, worsted wool pants; merino wool, velour, or cashmere drawstring pants; or dark denim that contains a bit of Lycra for ease of movement

(CONTINUED)

(not basic cotton sweats). Avoid linens at all costs, heavy cotton twill (like chinos), and fussy fine fabrics (such as silks). Remember, wrinkle-friendly fabrics will usually look just as good when you rise as they did when you sat down. Getting off crisp is as important, if not more important, as getting on in style.

On top, layer relatively thin knit tops so you can peel down—or stack up, as cabin temperatures also tend to shift while flying. Travel vessels of any kind can be quite chilly—or quite hot. So dress prepared with options. For matters of style, the sweater set is the answer. You have the coverage when you need it, and quick freedom when you don't. I say splurge on cashmere or really soft lamb's wool for the cutest and most comfy trip.

APRIL 27

PUSH YOUR DENIM JACKET OVER THE TOP BY COUPLING IT WITH ANYTHING OUT OF THE ORDINARY—FROM PENCIL SKIRTS TO POSH SATIN PANTS.

Levi's has been designing and manufacturing jeans for guys since the latter part of the 1800s. They launched their more tapered "Levi's for Gals" collection in 1969. You can thank Bruce Springsteen for reigniting the international denim craze in the 1980s when he donned one of the sexiest pairs of dungarees ever captured on an album cover. And let's not forget Madonna's "Lucky Star" era—where denim was the core element of any of the decade's defining ensembles. Today, you will find some version of the waist-length denim jacket in the closets of women around the globe.

Fronts that are zip closed, washes and rinses that go from near-black indigo to faded blue, tapered numbers that give an ultrafeminine shape, and the glitzy fur-lined renditions with matching fur collars—whether you choose fun faux or the real thing—the options abound.

Gone are the days of simply tossing on your matching jean. In fact, matching jeans are the last thing you might want to wear with your denim jacket.

Pull out the skirts and pants. That is the pile that you will start with. Take your pick from what you may have: satin pencil pants and kitten heels, perfect-pleated skirts and motorcycle boots, stovepipe tweed trousers and open-toe pumps, colorful cargo pants and suede mules, satin-striped tuxedo pants and canvas sneakers. And if these wacky combinations don't spark some ideas, take this as a shopping checklist to get the most out of your anxious, underutilized denim jacket.

APRIL 28 | BALANCE YOUR WARDROBE WITH LASTING, HIGH-QUALITY CLASSIC ITEMS, AND MIX IT WITH FUN, INEXPENSIVE TRENDY ITEMS.

When it comes to clothes, what is a classic? The items you can look at and say you'd wear ten years from now as proudly as you would today.

Ideally, your closet should have a balance of classic and trendy items that can coexist flawlessly. Trends are best worn as a way to add a spark of current style to your more traditional classic pieces. This season it may be a crocheted poncho in warm autumnal tones, or an ornate antique brooch. Next season, you are nothing without a floppy houndstooth newsboy cap, brightly colored opaque tights, or a buckle-heavy handbag.

If one thing remains constant in fashion, it is that trends will definitely come and go, sometimes changing faster than you can find them. They burst onto the scene like a hot new musical group with a big number-one hit—only to be banished into relative obscurity when the next new thing hits the stores. Think of ultratrendy items as being somewhat disposable—depending on how specific they are, they're usually finished after one season. So it's better to spend less on these items. Look for these flash-in-the-pan fashions on sale racks, in discount stores, or even vintage and secondhand stores if it's retro that's enjoying a revival. Just be sure to grab them at the lowest price possible without sacrificing too much in the quality department.

Think of your classics as the meat and potatoes of your wardrobe. Don't be afraid to invest in the best-quality pieces you can afford. By doing so you'll have the cornerstone of a stylish wardrobe from season to season and year to year.

APRIL 29 | FEATURE YOUR DÉCOLLETAGE.

An irresistible area that almost always looks good whether you are currently loving your body or not. Most men will never say it, for they probably don't know the area even has a name.

The oftentimes forgotten region of a woman's body, the area where the shoulders and upper chest can be prominently highlighted by the low top edge of a dress or blouse, is called your décolletage.

(CONTINUED)

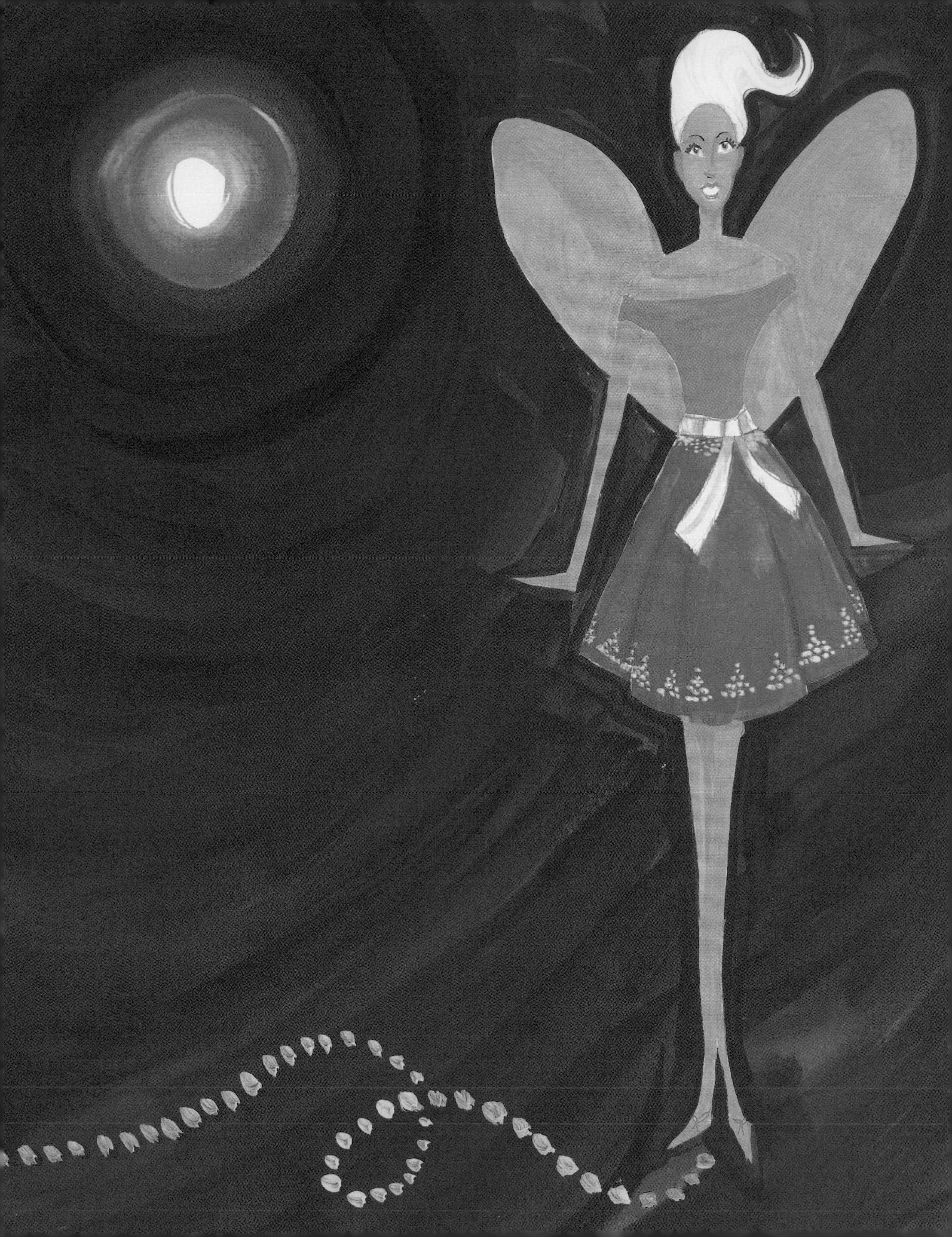

French women have known the power of this understatedly sexy area since forever! And slowly, women everywhere who don't want to compete with breast-enhanced counterparts choose this naturally sculpted and alluring zone to play up.

The indent of a collarbone and shoulder blade; the soft, rounded shoulder; and just a promise of the bustline is what drives men crazy—for you aren't really revealing anything, while actually saying a whole lot!

Strapless dresses, oversized cowl-neck sweaters, 1950s-style portrait-collar suits and ballet-neck dresses all highlight the décolletage perfectly.

If this is the area you're featuring, the best way is to cover most of the rest of your body—within reason. This brings a visual vertical thrust straight up to the area. You can also dust on a bit of one of the many shimmer creams or body powders for a subtle glimmering effect to just *that* area. With or without a necklace, this zone sparkles!

APRIL 30 | CREATE YOUR OWN VERSION OF THIS SURE-FIRE, STYLISH OUTFIT COMBINATION AND RUN WITH IT!

Top: Fitted solid top that offers up shoulders

Bottom: Fuller printed skirt that swells at the hem

Shoes: Sling-backs or sexy mules

Accessories: A preppy grosgrain ribbon left loose or tied into a bow; hosiery with attitude (think flesh-toned fishnets); classic sparkly studs

Flex piece: Shrunken fine-gauge cardigan sweater (to drape open over your shoulders)

MAY

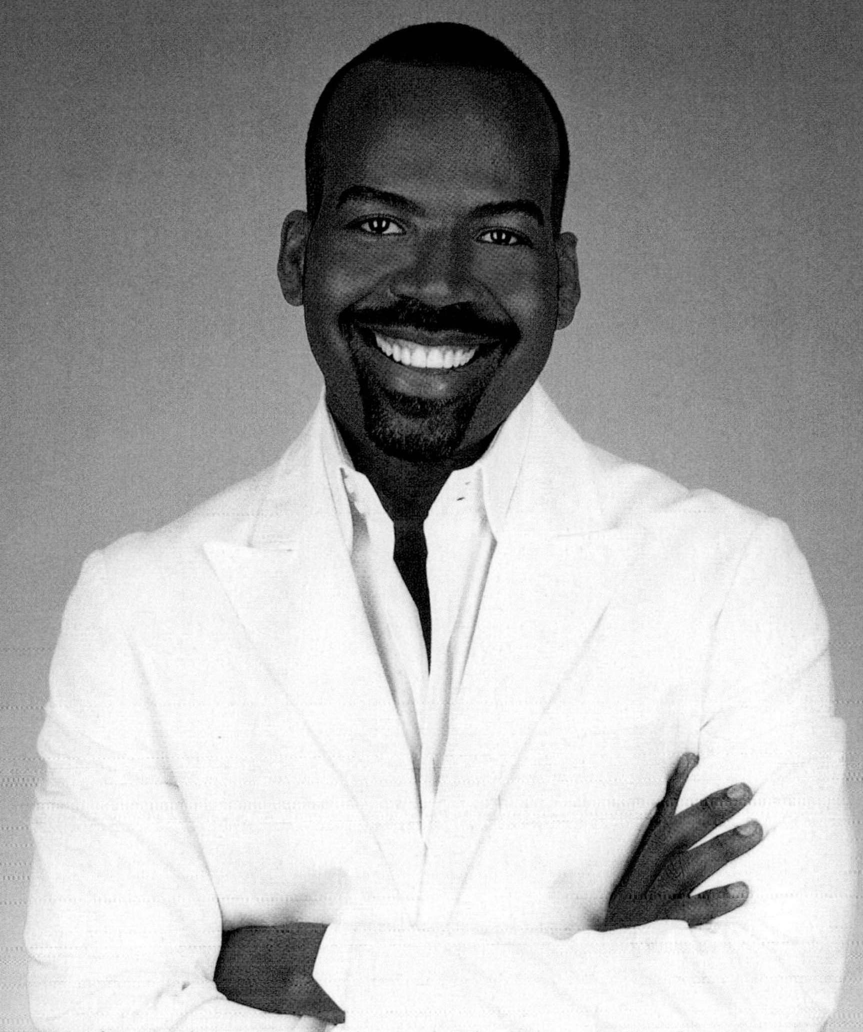

"Try to enjoy getting dressed. It may be the only dedicated time for yourself all day."

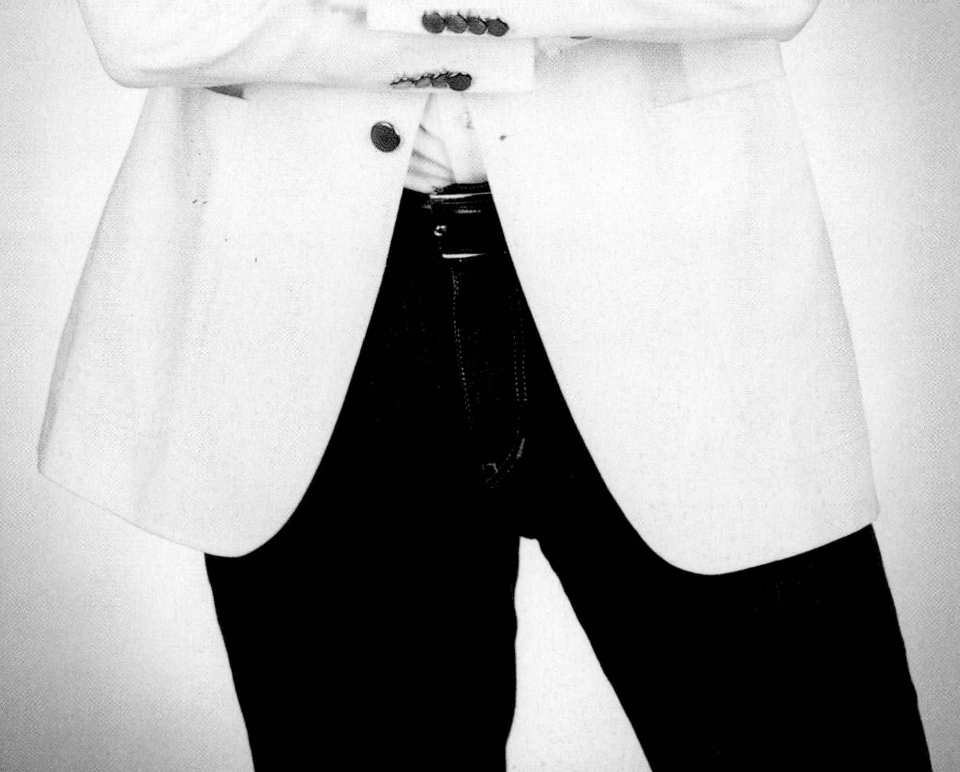

MAY 1 | TAKE TIME OUT TO THANK MOM ALL MONTH LONG FOR HELPING YOU STAND TALL—WITH OR WITHOUT HEELS.

Mom always said, "Bundle up, it's chilly out there," along with scores of other protective style warnings. From "always pack a sweater," to "never leave home without clean undergarments," sometimes you wish she didn't have a tip for every climate and situation.

Besides the proverbial May flowers, this month is known for many important things—from the unofficial kickoff of summer, Memorial Day, where we should remember those who have died in our nation's service, to a day just for moms when the abundant flora of the season actually gets put to good use.

This is a great month, and an even better day to make note of some of the life lessons passed along from those before us, especially moms. Think of three fashion fundamentals that you clearly remember coming from your mom's loving voice. Do you still use them day to day? Have you passed them along to your daughter or son? Do you laugh a bit when you find yourself saying them on instinct? If they still apply, identify them and refresh their importance in your life by honoring her with a simple thanks.

Jot them in a card today, and pop it in the mail just in time for her to get it on Mother's Day, or simply tack them on your fridge in her memory. Sometimes a silly reflection such as this can bring you closer, or make you feel as if she's right here watching over you, making sure you remember to "button one more of those shirt buttons, young lady!"

MAY 2 | TAKE AN EXPERT BEAUTY CUE FROM KEN PAVÉS, A TOP CELEBRITY HAIRSTYLIST.

What is your best-kept beauty secret?

My best beauty secret! The most beautiful thing a woman can be is confident! My job is to celebrate a woman's own special uniqueness and make her feel beautiful in her own skin! I don't try to change women, only enhance them. Taking what she feels are her most beautiful features and framing them with her hair.

What are the three hair-care and hair-styling essentials that every woman should own? Why?

The key to beautiful hair is healthy hair. My three hair essentials are:

1. A sulfate-free shampoo like Pavés Professional No Sulfates Allowed
2. A great everyday nourishing conditioner, with 100 percent pure essential oils, like Pavés Professional Un-Damaged Goods Milk
3. A Mason Pearson mixed-bristle brush

What are the biggest mistakes women make when styling their hair?

1. Applying product to just their crown and not evenly distributing the product through their hair.
2. Getting stuck in a "rut" and styling an updated cut in the same way they styled their old style. This makes any current cut look dated.
3. Creating volume only in the front of their hair since they don't see it from behind.
4. Following any trend too literally. Trends should only influence your style—less is more.
5. Believing that when you turn a certain age you have to get your mother's haircut. Do not eliminate sexy from your vocabulary.

Who is the most stylish woman in existence? And what do you appreciate about her look?

Brigitte Bardot embodied a nonproduced sex appeal and is the major influence in all of my work. She had an iconic sexual confidence that I think being a woman is all about!

If you could whisper a fail-safe hair-care tip into the ears of women everywhere, without them feeling bad by hearing it, what would it be?

Classic, simple looks are always in style. Grace Kelly and Jackie Onassis were always up to date with their style but it was always simple, chic, and as a result timeless. Remember healthy.

MAY 3 | HAVE YOUR SHOES SHINED RIGHT ALONGSIDE THE BOYS—JUST REMEMBER TO WEAR PANTS!

Crossing the great style divide between womenswear and menswear is a trip few women take. The ones who do are unafraid to mix a little gender-bending style into their closets for the days they don't want to look like every other woman who raided the same mall. Works for some, a sacrilege for others.

One area of menswear a woman can take a cue from is the art of the professional shoeshine. Especially this time of year, when the leftover salt from winter streets and spring showers can almost eat through your best leather shoes.

Carve out ten minutes the next time you need a lift, and sit down for the shine of your life. And remember two *tips:* one for you, make it a pant day, and one for your shoeshine man—at least 50 percent of the shine cost, it will still only run you a few dollars. After the shine, you'll feel like you can run to your corner office.

MAY 4 | MAKE SURE YOU LOOK GOOD COMING *AND* GOING. ENTRANCES AND EXITS COUNT EQUALLY—ARE YOU PUTTING EQUAL TIME INTO EACH?

My best friend, pianist Craig Rose, once told me a music philosophy that strangely spoke volumes about style. "The most important part of any song is the beginning—and the end," he said.

Think about it. You've seen it a million times when a diva hits the stage to tell a story in song. The moment she opens her mouth to sing she has your total attention. Usually within three bars, anyone who recognizes the tune will let her know by applauding, sanctioning her choice. They are with her.

Somewhere in the middle the story takes over, and what she's saying becomes slightly more important than how she's singing it—that is, if she's a great singer. Even if she isn't, the audience usually hangs in there.

As the music hits a crescendo, her posture cues the audience to the big finish. Could be one elegant arm rising high into the air, or even a soulful "doubled-over in pain" body fold—but you know it is coming. The last note swirls from her mouth and ends on a crisp consonant, and the crowd goes through the roof! Great beginning, great end.

Does the outfit you have in mind for this day have the same appeal? This doesn't mean you should be zipping yourself into a sequined gown before jumping into the carpool, it simply means to check your backside, just as carefully as you do your front. Look at three areas to self-police. It only takes a minute.

Is it interesting (a fun kick pleat or slit in your skirt), is it finished (no loose threads or tags showing through translucent fabrics), and does it fit properly (often gravity hits you first where you're not looking)?

If these three categories get a resounding "yes," feel free to exit the stage while the crowd is still on their feet, for there they will remain.

MAY 5 | TAKE AN EXPERT STYLE CUE FROM NICOLE FISCHELIS, A TOP NEW YORK STYLE-MAKER, VICE PRESIDENT AND FASHION DIRECTOR OF MACY'S EAST.

What is your best-kept personal style secret?
I have been wearing the same blue mascara and red lipstick for years. My fragrances are natural essences, and I will never reveal any of my sources.

What are the three fashion essentials every well-dressed woman should own?
A perfectly cut pantsuit, a great trench coat, and a fabulous form-fitting skirt to emphasize the legs and show off the shoes.

What are the biggest mistakes women make when getting dressed?
Thinking fashion and not style. Style remains, fashion passes. Buying a brand because it's trendy rather than making sure it's relevant to your personality and lifestyle.

Who is the most stylish woman in existence, in your opinion?
Forties-era movie stars. They were elegant and very seductive. I also like the elegance and sophistication of the Chinese actress Maggie Cheung and the new sensuality of the Bollywood actresses.

If you could whisper a fail-safe style tip into the ears of women everywhere, without them feeling bad by hearing it, what would it be?
Make your flaw your asset! Do not try to be who you are not!

MAY 6

PUT YOUR FACIAL POSTURE IN CHECK BY LIFTING IT UP A SMIDGE. WATCH IT GIVE A LIFT TO YOUR PERSONAL STYLE IN A WAY YOU NEVER COULD IMAGINE.

"Beauty is power; a smile is its sword."
—Charles Reade, novelist

I'd like to offer a very personal piece of style advice that has helped me look better as a television personality facing millions of viewers. For women and men, there is a small nuance of style that oftentimes goes forgotten because, unlike on-camera professionals, most average folk would never even think to focus on it. I call it facial posture. That is, how you hold your face when unaware of any onlookers. Like right at this very moment.

Try relaxing your face as if you never read what is above, and take a look at yourself in a complete, natural, resting position. What do you see?

For me, my natural resting position is a frown of sorts. My eyes sag a bit, the outer corners of my mouth head south, and my cheeks droop right in line. I don't *feel* a bit sad or angry, but if you were to pass me running errands, or going about my day, you would think I am having an *awful* day.

From working in front of the camera, I began to see my face in a resting position while awaiting a question from a co-host, interviewer, or interviewee. I looked like a mildly upset man who would perk up when speaking, only to return to the mad side.

I soon learned how to hold my face and all the muscles in it pleasantly when not speaking, and sometimes even when speaking, to create a more inviting mug for viewers to really want to listen to. In working on perfecting this over the years, I also found that it made what I *wore* look better, and what I said translate a bit easier as those on-screen with me reacted to the sunnier look in my eyes.

Take this idea and process is carefully. I am not sanctioning walking the streets with a huge, lottery grin on your face all day long. Just a subtly more pleasant expression. To start, try thinking happier thoughts during your downtime. This exercise is about not allowing what you can control to subtract from all the hard work you are attempting to put into your personal style each and every day, without you even realizing it.

MAY 7 | TAKE AN EXPERT STYLE CUE FROM REEM ACRA, A TOP AMERICAN BRIDAL DESIGNER.

What is your best-kept personal style secret?
Layering different colors and different lengths and always accessorizing with a jeweled piece of fabric, whether it is a tie or a scarf.

What are the three fashion essentials every well-dressed woman should own?
1. High heels
2. A short black dress
3. A fabulous ring

What are the biggest mistakes women make when getting dressed?
The biggest mistake is when they are dressing to look like someone else. It means they are not in touch with their bodies and what suits them. They need to figure out what is the best length, the best shapes, the best colors for them and then follow the trend within what suits them.

Who is the most stylish woman in existence in your opinion? And what do you appreciate about her look?
Audrey Hepburn. She had her own individual style and carried it with grace.

If you could whisper a fail-safe style tip into the ears of women everywhere, without them feeling bad by hearing it, what would it be?
You need to carry what you are wearing with allure no matter what it is you are carrying.

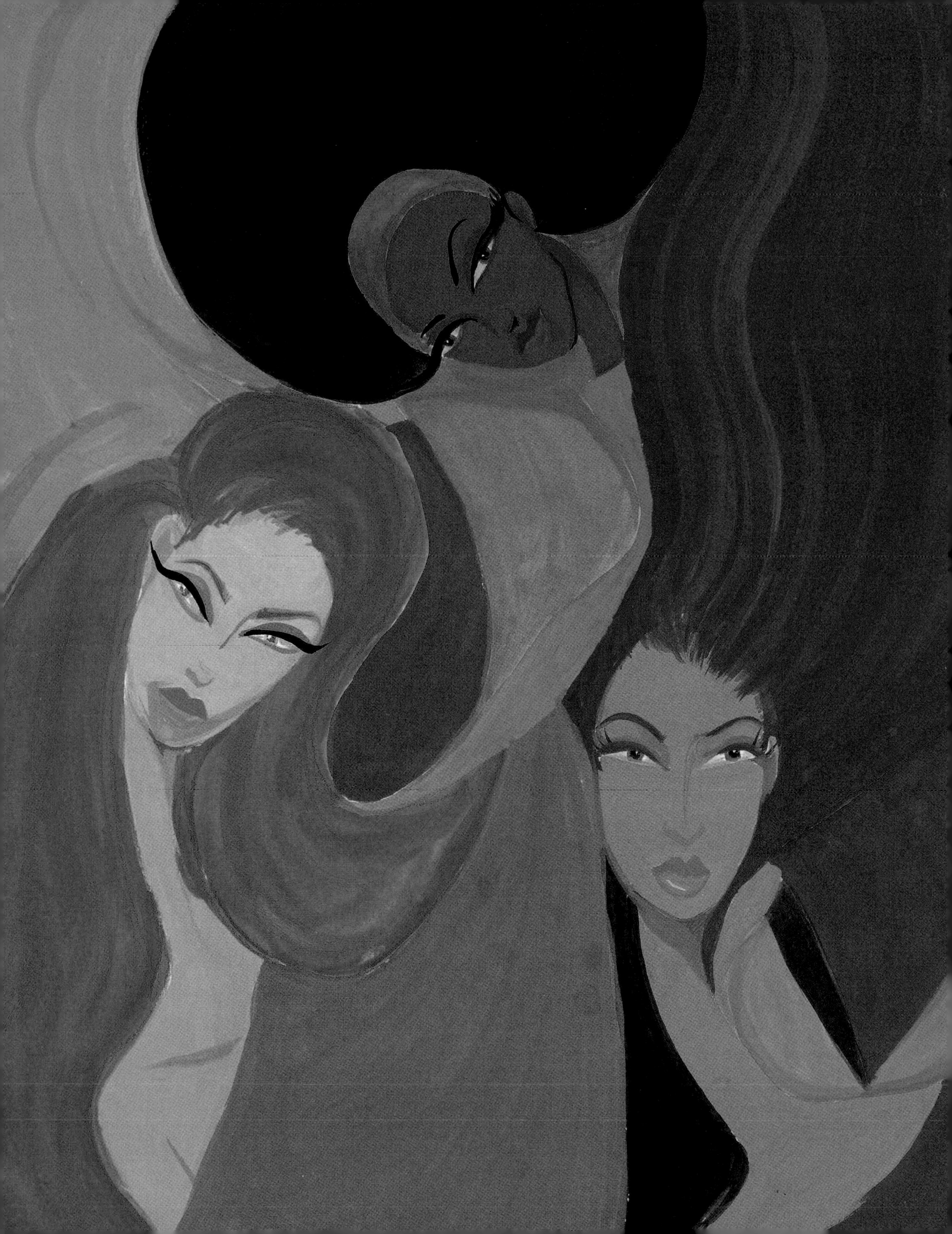

MAY 8 | CREATE PERFECT FASHION COLOR BALANCE BY PAIRING THE RIGHT GARMENTS TO BRING OUT YOUR HAIR COLOR.

How your clothing color relates to your hair color, be it natural or from a bottle, plays an important role in your overall style equation.

A woman can usually stand in a mirror with a new garment and viscerally react to whether it looks good or not. What is more difficult is understanding why. It may not be the shape of the garment, the fabric, or the fit, but simply the color as it corresponds to your hair color.

Knowing which color families work best with your particular hair color can save you a lot of time and frustration and lead you exactly to where you should be shopping. You'll look up and know exactly what your best palette is, and just about everything in your closet will eventually complement you color-wise. That is, if you don't decide to make a drastic hair color change.

Commit at least three colors from your hair color group to memory for future shopping trips, or even for selecting your most flattering top to wear right now. See if you notice the *instant* visual marriage.

BRUNETTE/BLACK

Fuchsia
Lipstick red
Black
Cool pastels
Bleach white
Turquoise
Cool reds
Royal blue
Citrus yellow
'50s hot pink

CLASSIC BLONDE

Tones of gray
Orange
Gentle earth tones
Chocolate browns
Peachy tones
Classic camel
Navy
Grassy green

REDHEAD

Mint green
Ruddy oranges
Earth tones
Brown family
Classic camel
Grass green
Orange
Pale gold

MAY 9 | TAKE AN EXPERT STYLE CUE FROM MONIQUE LHUILLIER, A TOP CELEBRITY DESIGNER.

What is your best-kept personal style secret?
I get everything tailored to fit me right so I own the look and don't look like I'm playing dress-up from my mother's closet.

What are the three fashion essentials every well-dressed woman should own?
1. A great bag will make any outfit.
2. A pair of diamond studs. I can't live without mine.
3. A great pair of shoes, because if they are great they will last for seasons!

What are the biggest mistakes women make when getting dressed?
Overaccessorizing!

Who is the most stylish woman in existence, in your opinion? And what do you appreciate about her look?
Kate Moss. I love how she mixes pieces together. Her style is so unique and always her own.

If you could whisper a fail-safe style tip into the ears of women everywhere, without them feeling bad by hearing it, what would it be?
Don't follow the runway trends so literally. And you shouldn't push a trend that doesn't work for you.

MAY 10 | INVESTING IN A PERFECT BLACK DRESS.

There is no way around it. The perfect black dress is by far the smartest style investment a woman can splurge on. My advice: Spend as close to $1,000 as you can possibly afford to ensure that this dress might be the only one you ever need to invest in. And if this means $400 for you, so be it. Just stretch financially a bit with this purchase, for if selected properly, the perfect black dress will stretch your wardrobe and personal style to the next level of chic.

You've seen it done in knee-length for decades, from Audrey Hepburn's definitive 1961 sleeveless, knee-length legend in *Breakfast at Tiffany's*, and Elizabeth Taylor's more vampy version in *Butterfield* 8 just one year earlier, to real women today taking their cues for longer evening shapes from such style notables as Julia Roberts, Susan Sarandon, and Jennifer Aniston, who choose perfect black dresses for many a red-carpet affair, including the pinnacle, the Oscars.

When deciding on which silhouette to choose, consider maximum versatility. Opt for a dress that can take you from semi-formal all the way down to business-laced evening affairs. For this, choose a tailored style that fits your body with pronounced shape and fit, in a fabric that looks more elegant than casual.

Since you are splurging, throw caution to the wind and check out cashmere first, and work your way down to wool gabardine or crepe, or super-100s wool.

Think about a measured amount of sex appeal that you can either rev up or cool down when deciding on the cut. The sleeveless boatneck is a safe start for first try-ons, then plunging deeper in the front or back if you want to show more skin. The perfect sleeveless sheath for you may even be in lightweight viscose rayon for a chic, alluring, and elegant drape. Either way, go for a timeless straight hem, avoiding the froufrou.

If evening events are more of what you need your noir stunner for, look to slim, body-conscious, flowing bias-cut silk charmeuse with a deep-V neckline and mirroring V-shaped back.

The experience of finding the perfect dress should be just that—a truly memorable experience, thus my (somewhat) limited guidelines. Make a day of it, as if you were searching for the single gal's equivalent of a wedding dress, and try on loads of them.

You will know it when you see it, if it makes your eyes light up in a way they never have when gazing into a three-way mirror.

And if $1,000 is, in fact, your price ceiling, buy the dress that is $900 and save a cool C-note for masterful tailoring so that your off-the-rack stunner will look more like it was custom made.

MAY 11 | LEARN A NEW FASHION TERM.

Tortoiseshell • *1. Mottled yellowish to brown substance from the horny plates of sea turtles native to the Cayman Islands, Celebes, and New Guinea. Used for ornamental combs, jewelry, buckles, eyeglass frames, etc. 2. Pattern similar to genuine tortoiseshell used for printed fabrics and plastic eyeglass frames.*

From belts and stylish combs, to earrings, bracelets, and hair bands, one of America's most classic and recognizable patterns is the wealthy, preppy look of tortoiseshell. Its unique and interesting character and luxurious beauty speaks of to-the-manner-born richness, probably due to its popularity in the mid- to late nineteenth century on jewelry and furniture. Authentic tortoiseshell was softened with high heat, and then inlaid with gold and/or silver in floral or geometric patterns. Many classic Victorian pieces and some Mexican jewelry are set with tortoiseshell that has been inlaid with metal or mother-of-pearl. A decadent mix.

Tortoiseshell is for those who seek classic, elegant accessory accents as foolproof as a simple diamond or sterling silver. Trust the look of plastic, simulated tortoiseshell, as well as the real thing, on everything from designer handbag handles and chic eyewear, to preppy barrettes and cuff bracelets, not to mention home furnishings that speak of a rich traditional design.

Tip: When adding a touch of tortoiseshell to your look, choose carefully, as plastic usually has a regular and repeating pattern, whereas genuine tortoiseshell has a random pattern. I say go vintage and choose the genuine article.

MAY 12 | LOOK AT WOMEN AROUND YOU AND BE MORE APPRECIATIVE OF THEIR UNIQUE TASTES.

"Taste is the mind's tact."
—Chevalier de Boufflers

You may consider yourself a style seeker, or you may not care at all, opting for comfort over style. Well, guess what? You still have taste.

Taste is no different from the buds on your tongue preferring sweet over sour. There is no right or wrong, simply a preference.

What happens as people begin to define their taste is where judgment comes in. One's own predilections in clothes, home furnishings, hairstyles, and even fragrances begin to become so specific, that anything that doesn't fit into the realm of the chosen mood is not valid or tasteful to you.

Identifying and honing in on your own taste is something that can make life easier. Removing judgment of what others choose is what real taste and tact are all about.

At the end of the day, no one really has *good* taste. We are simply people who express ourselves through inanimate objects, from clothes to vases, which speak in ways we cannot. Be open. You may learn something.

MAY 13

EVERYTHING YOU WEAR CANNOT SHINE. CHOOSE ONE SEXY ITEM, ONE SIGNATURE ACCESSORY, OR JUST ONE QUIRKY ELEMENT AND PULL BACK ON THE REST OF YOUR LOOK.

Calling all gypsies! You know exactly who you are. You've got an arsenal of clothes and accessories that are your "favorites." Sentimental brooches, retro-patterned scarves, dangling earrings-of-the-moment, ornate belts that wrap and twist, clever hats, funky hair bands, exotic necklaces, your "eclectic" watch, charm-filled bracelets, silky wraps, handbags large enough to fit a small country, and your never-leave-home-without-them sunglasses are almost like your trusted friends in the morning. You pick from them lovingly to be at your side for special occasions. It is a pleasure to see them. They make you feel secure.

Following the philosophy created by designer Coco Chanel, I challenge you to leave one of those things behind before you walk out the door today—just one. It may be difficult. Most women begin to feel an emotional attachment to what I deem "personality accessories" that they collect over the years, not realizing how many of them they are actually featuring at once, out of sheer habit and emotional attachment. Personality accessories are the fashion trimmings, which, over time, come to define who you are—or who you aspire to be. And each and every woman has her own personal reasons; a special cameo passed down from an aunt, those sweet little "huggy" earrings that fit your ear exactly the way they did on the first date with your husband, or a ten-year-old neckerchief that is just so very soft—they've become a portable security blanket of sorts. As special as these items may be, they have a tendency to all gather together, creating a cacophony of style statements that aren't very easy on the eye—for they are all speaking at once—and not one gets heard clearly.

Use today as a testing ground to allow your favorite pantsuit to shine on its own by adding just a beautiful pair of tasteful heels and a sophisticated watch. Or let that party dress that takes ten pounds off you steal the attention when you walk in, avoiding the chance of your brooch, wrap, pinky ring, and hair-clip elbowing in for first place. Save your boldest personality accessories for occasions when they can spruce up an easy T-shirt-and-jean combo, or add a smidgen of verve to a somber little black dress. This will give them the attention you feel they deserve.

MAY 14 | ADD A CLASSIC PUCCI PRINT TO YOUR LOOK.

Designer Emilio Pucci had an unlikely rise to fashion fame. Beginning his career as a member of the Italian Olympic ski team, he was pictured in *Harper's Bazaar* on the slopes wearing his own designs. Readers and clothing manufacturers took notice. As fashion legend would have it, he was invited to create the same colorful winter clothes for women to be sold in New York City.

He established his own fashion house in the early 1950s, in his Palazzo Pucci in Florence. The designer's famed "Palazzo pajamas" in noncrushable silk jersey were almost instantly adored by notables like Grace Kelly, Lauren Bacall, and Elizabeth Taylor—becoming a sort of jet-set uniform.

Pucci's strengths were as a colorist of kaleidoscopic, swirling patterns in brilliant hues and outlined in black, based on medieval Italian banners, Op Art, and funky psychedelia—matched with an inventive use of fabrics. Many say that the motley Pucci print captured the mood of the 1960s on fabric. Now, whether buying it new or vintage, the look speaks of wealth, sophistication, fun . . . and a retro-Italian elegance that will never go out of style.

THREE WAYS TO ALWAYS LOOK STYLISH IN CLASSIC PUCCI PRINTS

- Start with a scarf or a men's necktie that can be used around the neck or as a flirty belt. The Pucci print is a cinch for springtime flair—ladies who have had style for decades will recognize it—and immediately know that you are in the know.

- Pucci-print tops and skirts make great partners to white separates. Most versions have strong doses of white outlining and repeating in and around the twisted color shapes. Pair with bleach white blazers, Palazzo pants, or simple white T-shirts to add a sporty edge.

- Careful of cheap imitations! Invest in the real deal for maximum fashion impact. Those who know, know.

MAY 15 | GET TEN-MINUTE STYLE FOR AN ART GALLERY OPENING OR ANY CREATIVE EVENT.

Your closet should have you ready for anything, including events that you may only attend once every couple of years. Let's say you received a last-minute invite to an art world gala, a night at a museum, or even a local fashion show.

Do as the creative pros do for these types of occasions and whip together a stylish look worthy of a painting. The trick is not looking too studied or contrived. Your clothes should look as if you have the courage to risk originality.

Minutes 1:00–2:00:
Go straight to your leather, suede, or shine (silk shantung is great) on the bottom (skirts or pants). Go classic, no fringe or fussy details.

Minutes 3:00–4:00:
Select a matte top to cool things down a bit. Dark fitted turtlenecks, sleeveless knit tops, and simple solid white T-shirts worn beneath jackets rock!

Minutes 5:00–6:00:
Take a thin scarf in a bright color and wear it in an unexpected place. Work it around your waist, thrown around your neck aviator style, or flowing from your neck down your back.

Minutes 7:00–8:00:
Grab your most interesting flats (embellished or bright) or go with the highest heels you can stand in. It's only an hour or two. Go for it!

Minutes 9:00–10:00:
Your makeup should be artful and a bit dramatic. Do full coverage with an all-in-one foundation/powder, play up your eyes, lips, or cheeks (not all three) with a strong color, and be on your way!

MAY 16 | POP STYLE QUIZ.

1. Which is the best lengthening cocktail dress shape for petite women?

A. Strapless
B. Long-sleeve wrap
C. Classic sheath
D. None of the above

2. How long should one's sleeves be on a properly fitted overcoat?

A. Long enough to expose the entire wrist
B. Long enough to cuff several inches
C. Long enough to cover the entire wrist
D. Long enough to cover the hand in cold weather

3. Which is the best eyeglass shape for a round face?

A. Round
B. Slightly square
C. Cat
D. Any of the above

4. The midi- or tea-length skirt can dazzle or daunt. If not careful, its midleg length can do which of the following shape killers?

A. Make your legs look thicker
B. Make your hips looks wider
C. Add volume to your ankles
D. Make your shoulders look masculine

(Answers: 1-A, 2-C, 3-A, 4-A)

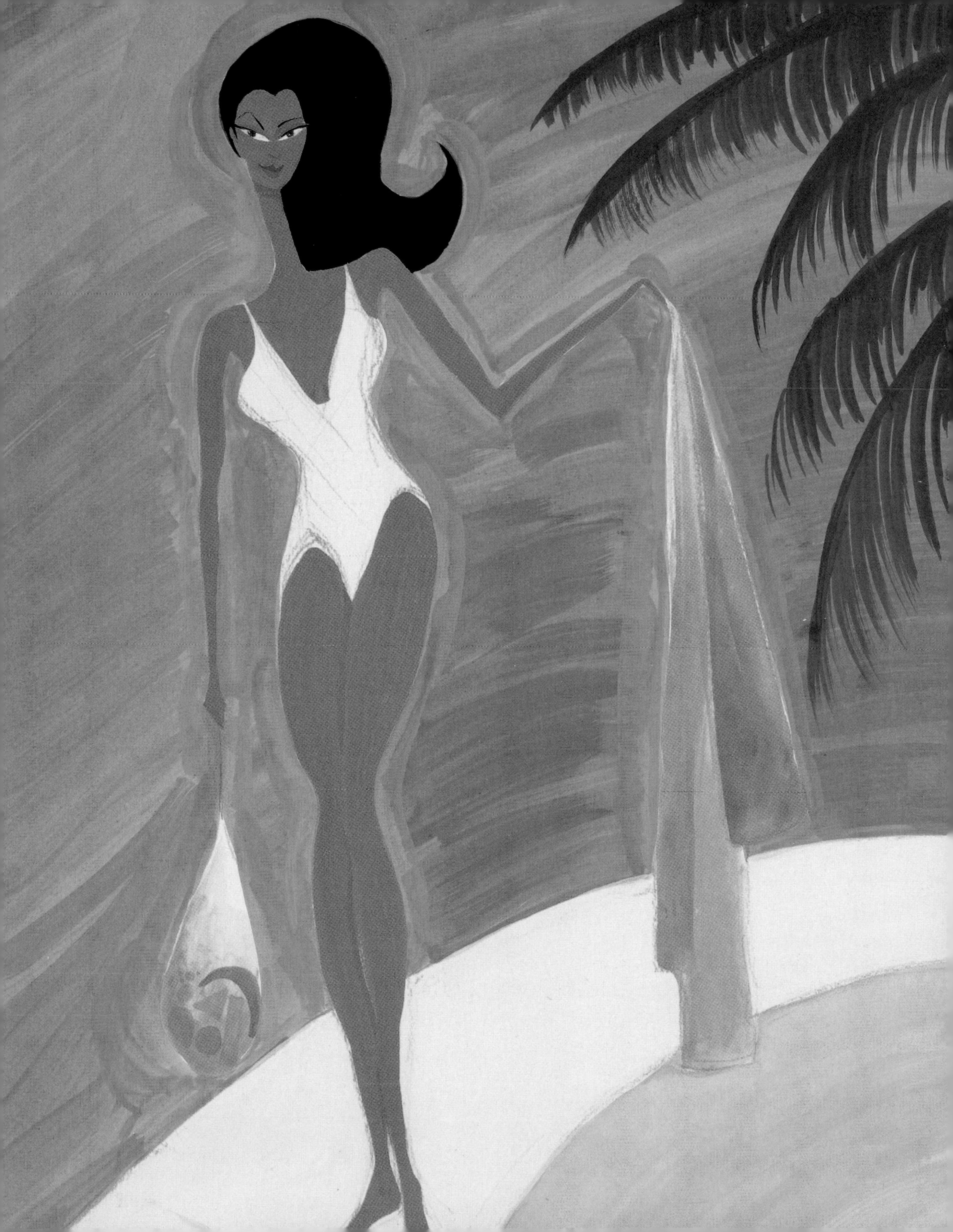

MAY 17 | FOR "HIPPY CHICKS": TRY A SWIMSUIT WITH "HIGH CUT" LEGS.

Swimsuits should now be on standby. Another trick is looking for suits that have a gradient color treatment (fading from one color to another). Select the version that has a darker tone on the bottom. (*Bonus tip:* Sarongs don't hide as much as you may think: If anything, a big wrap can bring more attention to all you're trying to camouflage.) *More sun, less self-consciousness!*

MAY 18 | MAKE YOUR JEANS LOOK AS IF YOU JUST STEPPED OFF A FASHION SHOW RUNWAY BY PAIRING THEM WITH AN UNEXPECTED EVENING TOP OR TAILORED JACKET.

Individual fashion trends live and die pretty quickly, but then resurface as if they are new. Low-slung pants that bare your private zones might be de rigueur today but so passé tomorrow. The cycle of fashion takes no prisoners, unless you are the type to save everything you've ever purchased.

One soon-to-be-classic fashion trend you *should* hold on to is the pairing of your head-turning blue jeans with an unexpected nighttime top or tailored jacket.

Most stylish women know that their jeans are the casual centerpiece of their wardrobes. When you find a pair that fits, it seems as if the heavens are opening right there in the dressing room and the choir is singing the Hallelujah chorus! Lifting your assets exactly where they should be, holding and shaping your legs to what you knew they always could be, and grazing the floor precisely—calling for no alterations. This is the harmony that should inspire you to buy that very jean in every wash and color on the display.

This is also the jean that will welcome not only your sweet T-shirts and weekend sweatshirts but also your tailored tweed blazers in the fall, and your nipped-waist cotton jackets in the spring. The jeans that contrast so beautifully with the tops in your closet—you know the ones. Ladylike printed silk blouses, evening tanks adorned with shimmery little bugle beads, or that sleeveless red cashmere turtleneck that hugs your every curve. These are just the tops to create the sexy juxtaposition to pull this look off.

(CONTINUED)

Complete the look with a sassy flat shoe with personality (think kitten heels or ballet flats in velvet, satin, or supple suede), or a sexy, sky-high pump for nights out on the town.

I like to call this look a "downtown" take on the casual suit. And every town or city has a downtown area—or one nearby. Listen for the music, look for the neon lights that are glowing after midnight, and keep an eye open for the cars meant to be shown off—and you are facing in the right direction to wear your entrance-making jeans and unconventional tops. The night will be yours. This stylish combo will be the reason.

MAY 19 | BREAK DOWN THE WALLS OF YOUR STYLE INSECURITIES AND LEND A HAND TO ANOTHER. IT WILL ONLY MAKE YOU LOOK EVEN BETTER IN THE END.

"Truly elegant taste is generally accompanied with an excellency of heart."
—Henry Fielding

When someone asks you where you purchased a new garment that you are wearing, what do you answer? Be truthful. Do you offer up the name of the store and the designer or manufacturer's name, helping the admirer get her own if interested? Or do you fabricate a story that throws her off the scent? You know some of the more popular options: "Oh, this old thing," or "I can't seem to remember." Hmmmm.

The most stylish women on the planet draw from a wellspring of confidence before ever putting on anything man-made. They know that lipstick is genius for enhancing your mouth, making it supple and polished so it can play right into your fashion mood for the day. And the right pair of shoes can not only lift your body and posture to a more statuesque place, but they can also lift your spirits. But none of this matters if you are not confident enough to realize that it is you, the unique, original being, flaws and all, who makes any aesthetic artifice come to life and do the work it was designed to do.

Knowing this fully and with complete self-assurance is what allows some women to share their style successes with any woman who asks. And you know, sometimes it takes a lot of nerve to ask.

If you aren't one of those women who can share freely, why not try it just once the next time you are asked? There is no need to challenge yourself to do it forever, just try it once and see how it makes *you* feel. My prediction is that you will experience a freedom from what you *thought* was style safety, when you see the gratitude on the other woman's face. Like quickly ripping off a Band-Aid, it won't hurt as much as you thought, and the next time you won't even think about it.

And if you see a woman who took your advice and ran straight to the store to buy an exact match, the onus is off you, for you both know who is the fashion leader, and who is the follower.

MAY 20 | HAPPY BIRTHDAY, ACE PILOT AMELIA EARHART.

Amelia Earhart, the first woman to successfully fly across the Atlantic, took to the skies in 1932. She flew from Harbor Grace, Newfoundland, to Paris. Brutal north winds, intensely icy conditions, and mechanical challenges beset the flight and forced her to land in a pasture near Londonderry, Ireland. Earhart herself felt the flight proved that men and women were equal in "jobs requiring intelligence, coordination, speed, coolness and willpower." Amen.

What monumental challenge have you been avoiding? Maybe your style can help you to conquer it—or at least take the first small steps.

What would you wear if you were living your dreams?

Honor the courage of Amelia Earhart on this day and take your own dreams to the pilot seat with the help of a little style. Sometimes, if you can picture yourself in the role, the image you witness can help you make it happen. Self-actualization, some call it. I'm sure Amelia would agree with this full-throttle.

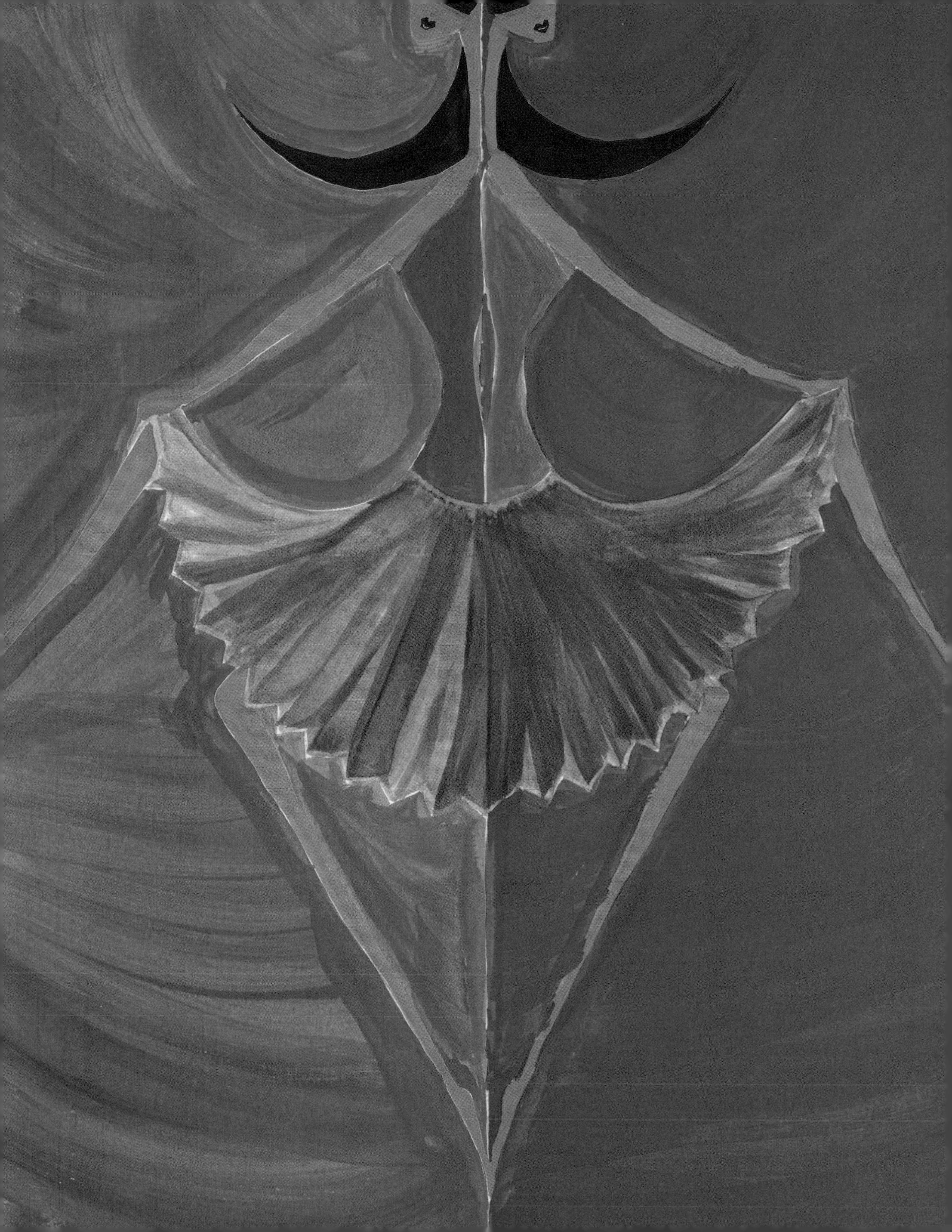

MAY 21 | HAPPY BIRTHDAY, GEMINI GIRL.

The Twins are notoriously good communicators. You say exactly what you mean. You mean precisely what you say. The message is always clear and full of fashionable intent. From sexy to sophisticated, coy to cutting-edge, your closet is stocked with every element to pull off your point.

You may find that many women envy your ability to draw a crowd, even when not trying. Most great communicators can do this, whether on a soapbox or center podium at a huge auditorium. Fashion is no exception.

Color for you leans toward tones of the bluest of oceans and greenest of lush pastures, but you will never be predictable, especially as your date of birth approaches. You love to toss on that perfect little tangerine skirt, just to keep observers guessing. Let this year's greet-the-summer ensemble be the one they really remember. The stars are talkin' heat from day one!

You share your twin-vision for style with Courteney Cox and Elizabeth Hurley, although none of you would ever admit to sharing anything with anyone, especially inspiration for outfits. So be glad there are two of you for every one.

MAY 22 | MAKE A SINGLE STRAND OF PEARLS YOUR FINISHING TOUCH.

But don't wear them too seriously. Let them add a wink of retro elegance to something very right now. Don't be afraid of an accessory legend. A single strand of pearls has been a stalwart signifier of taste and elegance for decades. Women looking to build an accessory collection of classically timeless wardrobe accents have always invested in them before anything else if they weren't lucky enough to have them passed down.

Successfully mixing pearls into your fashion repertoire means knowing when you match them with commensurately classic clothing, and when to contrast them with trends loaded with funk! You just need to have them on standby for anything from a strapless evening gown in solid satin, or your tweed suit jacket/distressed jeans/sexy silk top combo. A single strand of pearls will put the right punctuation on the end of your style statement.

When looking for your single strand, keep these pointers in mind:

•The larger the real pearl, the more you will pay—and the richer you'll look.

•When going *real,* pass up pearls that resemble dull, cloudy white balls.

•Today's cultured pearls come in a myriad of nontraditional colors from warm rosé to sexy black. Rosé or silver/white pearls tend to look best on fair-skinned women, and cream or gold-toned pearls are ultraflattering to darker complexions.

•For a more modern twist on classic pearls, look for pearls from the East. Tahitian cultured are identifiable by their exotic, unique colors ranging from light gray to black, greens, and purples. Those from Japan and Indonesia are cultured pearls grown against the inside shell of an oyster and have modern-looking, flat backs. They really shine on earrings and rings.

•Perfectly round real pearls are the most costly and sought after, although there are other shapes to choose from.

•Remember, pearls can add years when worn atop serious, tailored clothing. And add youth and fun to jeans and separates. Choose wisely!

MAY 23 | STEP OUTSIDE YOUR REGIONAL STYLE HABITS.

The cowboy boot is an icon of Texas. The viva la glam black suit is the uniform of New York City's trendy set. L.A. rocks hair that boasts sunny highlights and sexy length. Most regions of America have some signature style or beauty culture.

Work it, but don't get stuck in it. If you are a stubborn city woman try a touch of country chic, switching the usual black pants for a floor-length peasant dress and flats. Stuck Southern beauties may want to explore a bit of L.A. chic and let a little skin show where they usually never would dare. And Midwestern gals who layer up for warmth and comfort may try looking to Miami (at least when indoors) and stop at a single fitted top for a romantic dinner. Try to identify your regional style signature and mix it up a bit. If only for one fun day or night.

MAY 24 | CLOTHING SHOULD WORK *FOR* YOU.

"I believe that function should dictate the style.
Function is always a beautiful departure for style."
—Diane von Furstenberg

MAY 25 | GO BASIC.

Take a break from color. Going black and white can almost erase the dateline from your appearance, especially since it looks great in just about any season, can be sported in any fabric combination, and is appropriate for day or night. What more could you ask for? Check out these graphically colorful ways to go color*less*, using basics you might already have in your closet:

White Dress Pants + Black Velvet Blazer + Black Camisole + Black Sling-backs
= Chic Checkered Past
Black Turtleneck + White Trench Coat + White A-line Skirt + Black Knee Boots
= O-R-E-Ohhh!
Black Jeans + White Safari Jacket + Black Shell and Flats + White Clutch Bag
= A-to-Zebra Style

MAY 26 | DIG OUT THAT OLD BRIDESMAID'S DRESS AND BRING IT TO A TAILOR TO DISCOVER ITS POSSIBILITIES.

The lavender, puffed-sleeved princess dress in silk chintz, the strapless ball gown with the bride's favorite appliqué up the side of the bustier, or the quintessential, sequined jacketed number—they were meant to be worn again. How? Take in your dress, or graveyard of dresses for some, to what I call the fashion emergency room—a seasoned tailor—and keep these tips in mind.

SALVAGE WHAT YOU CAN

That lavender princess dress with what seems like nothing to salvage might simply become a flirty spring/summer miniskirt. Let your tailor dream and offer options you don't have the experience to know you don't know.

GARISH GOWNS MAKE FOR GLAMOROUS BALL GOWN *SKIRTS*

Your tailor can remove the upper portion of any dress and add a clean French waist to the remainder. Now you have an evening skirt that you can wear forever!

SIMPLIFY THE SURFACE

Beading, ruffles, and even bows and ribbons can be professionally removed by a tailor and make the dress look as if they never existed. All of a sudden that jacket becomes your favorite little unique bolero to wear with your jeans.

MAY 27 | CLAIM YOUR THIRTIES AND FEATURE STYLE THAT BEST SUITS YOU, OR PASS ALONG AN AGE-EMPOWERING TIP TO A WOMAN WHO REALLY NEEDS IT—OLDER OR YOUNGER.

Your wardrobe should reflect the balance that becomes more evident in your life every year after the big three-oh. From new moms who focus on snapping back their figures, to women who are the main squeeze, the first rule of thumb is placing quality before quantity—unlike you may have shopped in your twenties. High-quality style classics should outweigh the thrifty trends that you dispose of after a few wears and washes. For many thirtysomething women, these are your primary earning career years, and your wardrobe should reflect that you want every dollar's worth that you are entitled to. Sending this message sometimes means looking like you really don't need the money. Or to put it simply, fake it, till you make it.

When shopping during these years, invest in power items that reflect your every mood. And your power shouldn't only be reserved for boardroom style. From an updated cashmere sweater set for weekends in the wine country, to a fits-like-a-glove pair of leather pants for those nights when dinner might turn into breakfast.

Always keep an eye on the styles of the twenty-something set as a gauge on what's cool as well as what you should avoid wearing.

STYLE QUICK LIST: THE TOP FIVE THIRTYSOMETHING STYLE ESSENTIALS

The "corner office" business suit

Cashmere

A great handbag

A drop-dead dress for evenings out

Workout clothes for function and fashion

MAY 28

BE AWARE OF PROPORTION—BULKY TOPS CALL FOR SLIMMER BOTTOMS, FITTED TOPS CAN WELCOME FULLER SKIRTS AND PANTS—THE RIGHT CONTRASTS CAN MAKE AN OUTFIT SHINE.

Remember the 1980s, when big, oversized sweaters ruled the fashion runways and stores from coast to coast in just about every mall? They hung from the shoulders, slouched around the thigh, bloused around any waist you may have had, and added at least five to ten visual pounds to even the Twiggy-est of women. What a look to forget. Even though this display was a proportion extreme that should be erased from our collective style memories, it started from the correct theory: If you go full on top, go slimmer on the bottom.

Fast forward to the new millennium and you will see women facing the same conundrum with their heavy winter sweaters and generously cut, warm winter pants and skirts. Many simply succumb to the elements and bulk up in full-cut clothes from head to toe, tossing any fashion dictates to the chilly winds, only to pass a mirror and see a close cousin to anyone in the Michelin family, maybe even the "man" himself.

Fitted pencil skirts and cigarette pants look amazing when matched with loose, open bottom sweaters, blouses, and even tunics that float around the top half. Slender tops and jackets that skim close to the upper body scream to be coupled with classic, high waist, Katharine Hepburn–inspired stovepipe pants, fuller A-line skirts, or floor-length ball gown skirts for evening wear.

MAY 29 | PLAY UP YOUR ASSETS.

Focus on what you have always loved about your body instead of what features get the most attention.

Take as long a look at your compliment-grabbing assets as you would of your shortcomings. Is it your smile? Might it be your flawless shoulders and supple skin that always glow when you let them see the light of day? Maybe it is all about your perfectly elegant forearms, wrists, and hands that rival that of any model in any jewelry advertisement? You know what it is, and you always have. It is the one you feel certain will never let you down.

Use this day not to let *it* down by selecting a chic new lip color that puts your smile center stage. Or go from day to night in a top that reveals your camera-ready shoulders while cloaking the rest of you. Or simply push up the sleeves to your sweater or jacket and don a fun vintage bracelet so your arms get the work done—and get a few compliments along the way.

MAY 30 | VINTAGE CLOTHING.

Have you ever noticed that some women look as if they've stepped right out of a fashion magazine? Their look is perfectly appointed in shape and color, cleverly fitted in areas that most women don't give much attention to anymore, and boasts a certain elegance that speaks to a true ladylike air. It might be an easy cocktail dress that features a bow at the waist in plush velvet. Or it might be a portrait-collar jacket in grassy green reminiscent of Jacqueline Kennedy in the 1960s—except this version is paired with jeans and a beaded clutch.

When you are stopped in your tracks by a garment that is like nothing you have ever seen, it may, in fact, be a classic vintage garment, or a new version that is inspired by an original created decades ago. Fashion designers of every ilk look to the past when they set out to create what they want their customers to wear. From vintage stores and consignment shops, to thrift shops and swap meets, vintage clothes offer both professional tastemakers and real women the option of having a unique stamp and original edge to their creations and personal style.

For you it may simply be a whimsical 1960s Pucci print silk neck scarf that you nabbed from your mother's closet. Today you may wear it as a sash belt with dark tailored pants and a denim jacket. If you don't own anything vintage, today is the day. You may choose a pair of 1940s stovepipe pants with four-inch cuffs, reminiscent of Joan Crawford. The idea is to dress in the times gone by without looking like you're wearing a costume.

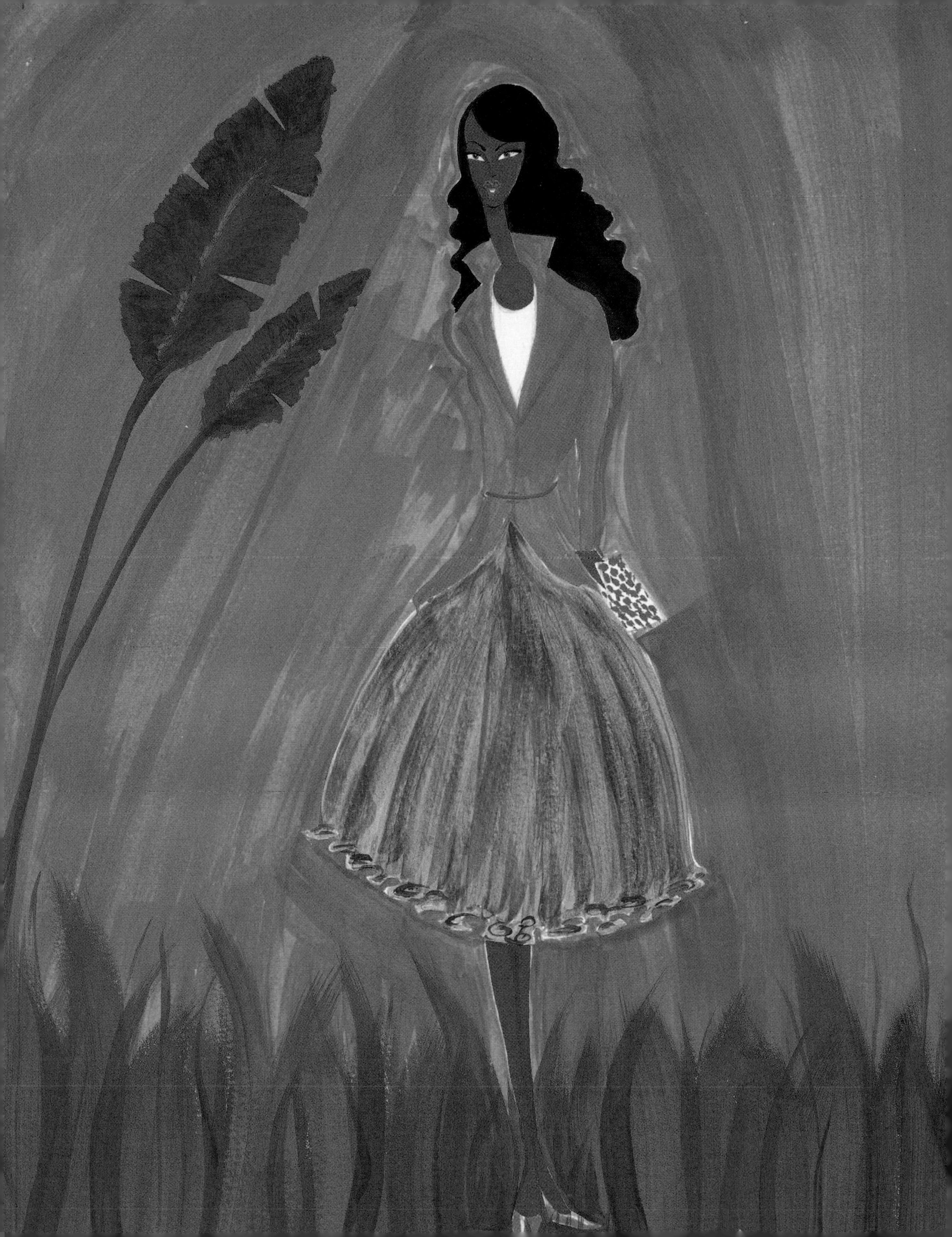

MAY 31 | FAST FASHION (FOOD).

A sneakily busy event month, May has a tendency to be like December because your social calendar can fill up quickly—Mother's Day, graduation ceremonies, weddings, garden events, and early summer celebrations toward the month's end. And no one ever gave the heads-up that it is mini-holiday season!

Look in your closet and try to match this style suggestion as best as you can with what you have. Don't worry if the items you own aren't an exact match. Within this template, choose your own colors and details. Getting the look not so letter perfect gives it a hint of your personal style, which is always better than a carbon copy:

Top: Pale solid blazer or suit jacket; basic white T-shirt or men's tank top
Bottom: Flouncy skirt (pleated, ruffled, or tiered)
Shoes: High-heeled sandals or espadrilles
Accessories: Fun clutch (usually meant for evening); all-over body bronzer (to welcome bare spring legs); drop earrings
Flex piece: Superskinny belt worn with a jacket (to give a 1940s edge to the look)

JUNE

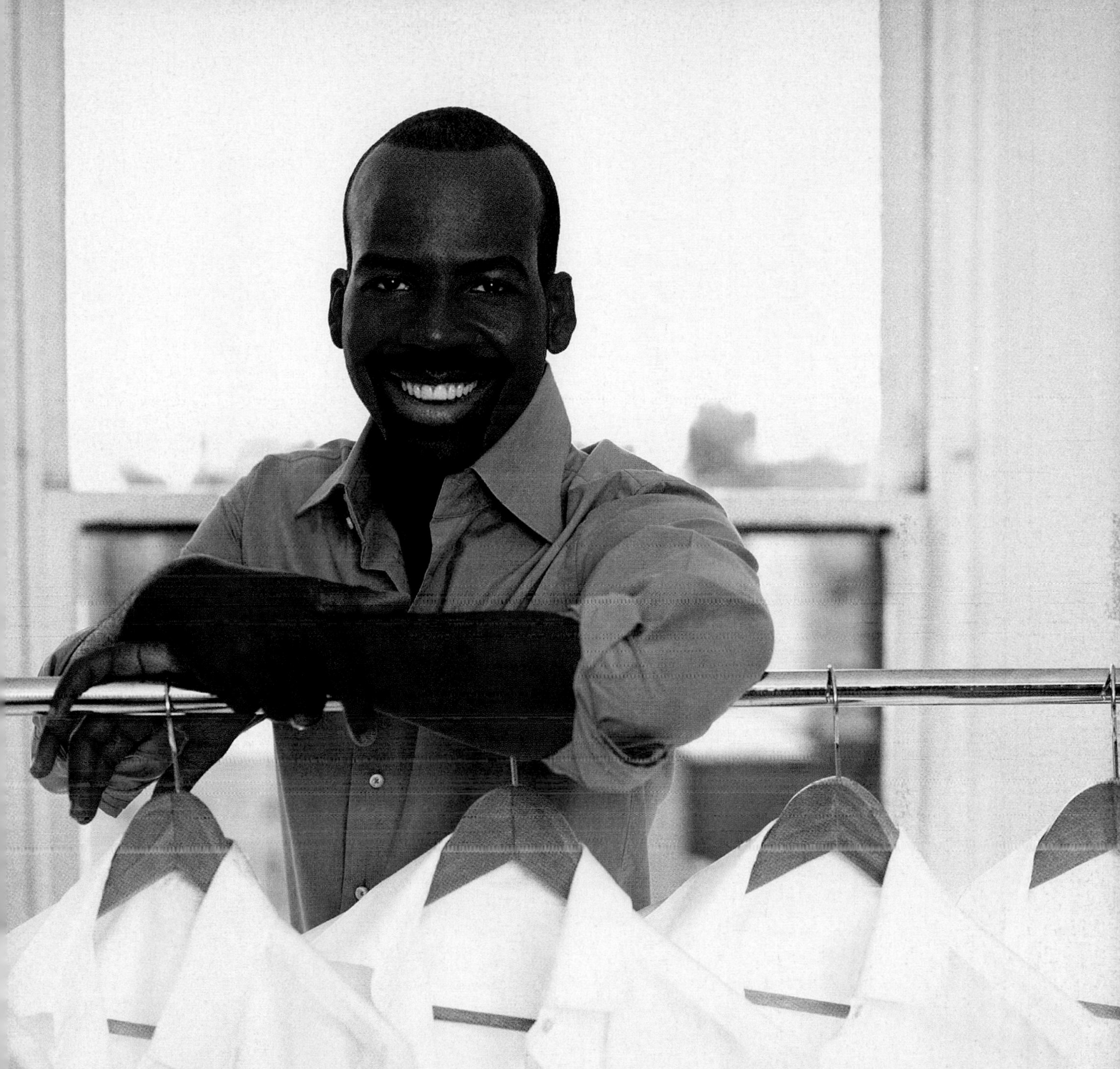

"Let the sun be your best accessory, highlighting your natural glow."

JUNE 1 | STOCK UP ON SUMMER ESSENTIALS NOW.

Summertime, and the livin' is easy, especially if you are fully stocked with warm-weather requisites. You want low maintenance, high style. Swipe on lip gloss versus a regimen of lipstick. You can pull your hair back, glide on a little sunscreen, and hop into any convertible faster than you put down the phone from which the invite came.

Take a look at this list of ten summer basics:

Sunscreen
Waterproof makeup
Flattering swimsuit
Alluring beach cover-up
Page-turner of a book
Oversized tote bag
Colorful rubber flip-flops
Flirty sundress
Great camera
Fun straw hat

Affirmation:
I will leave behind some of my usual fuss, be ready for the sun in minutes, and remember that my usual primping never seems to matter poolside anyway.

JUNE 2 | SHOP "GREEN." GIVE SOMETHING BACK TO THE EARTH.

The first week of June traditionally marks the time when the UN uses World Environment Day to stimulate awareness of the environment and enhance political attention and public action.

More and more style-conscious women are becoming ecoconscious as well, opting for quality green products from head to toe, helping the earth by wearing goods that have an environmental integrity base from product manufacture through shipping. From art to underwear, free-standing stores, catalogs, and online shopping sites offer a plethora of ecofriendly, unassuming style options. Many offer fashion-forward clothes and accessories that *didn't* and *won't* harm the environment.

A great way to navigate is to check out a directory of stores that qualify as sanctioned "green" shopping sites. One of my favorites is greenmatters.com. It offers online shopping sources for everything from activewear to underwear.

There is a legendary adage of the Shenandoah Indians: "We are made from Mother Earth and we go back to Mother Earth." Do your part this day by trying to pay a nod of respect to the land on which you stand in those stylish shoes, and at least try on a pair that is more ecofriendly.

JUNE 3

TAKE AN EXPERT STYLE CUE FROM KELLY KILLOREN BENSIMON, A TOP NEW YORK STYLE-MAKER, EDITOR OF *ELLE ACCESSORIES MAGAZINE*, AND AUTHOR OF *AMERICAN STYLE* AND *IN THE SPIRIT OF THE HAMPTONS.*

What is your best-kept style secret?
Fashion is about trends, and style is a reflection of your life. Wear what makes you feel like you. Confidence always leads the way.

What are the three fashion essentials every well-dressed woman should own?
Tight black pants, gold high heels, and ballerina flats.

Black pants are the ultimate staple. They can go disco dancing or meet the in-laws at the country club. Tight always shows the curves. Curves are good.

Gold high heels are the sexiest shoes ever and they act like a nude shoe, for they go with everything, but they have a little seventies flair I love.

And every woman should have a pair of ballerina shoes. They work nicely with pants, jeans, skirts, and all dresses.

What are the biggest mistakes women make when getting dressed?
Biggest mistake is when women mix trends. Stick with one theme. It is so beautiful to see a woman with a strong sensibility like: boho, modernist, or minimalist.

Who is the most stylish woman around?
My style icon is Miuccia Prada. She doesn't follow rules and she embraces who she is. I love that!

If you could whisper a fail-safe style tip into the ears of women everywhere, without them feeling bad by hearing it, what would it be?
My secret is: Wear a girdle if you feel it will give you a better line. It is all in the underpinnings—just ask Marilyn Monroe.

JUNE 4 | LEATHER OR SUEDE IN THE SUMMERTIME?

With the advent of new textile technologies, leather and suede are now breathable and of paper-thin weight. So you can wear them now, as well as in the winter. Summer-weight leather and suede can be found on designer runways and in department stores alike. Also gently lined skirts—these look more like a sateen-finished fabric than what you'd expect of a skirt in leather. The new millennium ushered in a fabric phenomenon most women would cringe over: washable leathers and suede. These are not to be mistaken for leatherette—a nonbreathable misnomer for fabrics made in imitation leather.

Pulling off any skin in the heat of the summer works best when you feature only a piece of it. Maybe just a skirt with a cotton tank or cami, or even a fun pair of tissue-thin leather capris for a night out dancing, matched with a crocheted top.

The look is hotter for now than you'd imagine and as cool as cool can be.

JUNE 5 | A TATTOO. IS IT REALLY YOU?

More and more stylish, sophisticated celebrities are adding fuel to the tattoo revolution. It makes the skin art form even more alluring when you witness such unassuming and seemingly elegant starlets going under the needle. Oscar-winning actress Angelina Jolie has a tribal dragon tattoo (note: seemingly elegant). TV star Alyssa Milano has a reported seven different markings in places that rarely see daylight. Producer and actress Drew Barrymore has a butterfly tattoo just beneath her navel. Hollywood sex goddess Pamela Anderson sports a tough, barbed-wire armband tattoo. Sweet Sarah Michelle Gellar has a Tao symbol near her ankle. And this list would not be complete without a mention of the ever controversial Britney Spears's lower back fairy tattoo. *Seemingly* elegance at its best!

The choice is yours, but is a tattoo what you really want to do to express yourself? Take a breather and think before getting inked. Although the look may feel sexy at the moment, and look cool for a few years, your life and style will evolve. Consider that the area you choose to paint may not always be as firm as it is today. And you may be working at a firm that has a very different outlook than you do today.

JUNE 6 | BRIGHTEN THOSE PEARLY WHITES!

Gritting teeth for anger, showing all of your teeth for extreme joy, and closing top to bottom for a classic "eek!" when alarmed. Do your teeth speak for you? Are they saying what you want?

A bright, fresh smile can make a simple shirt and casual pants appear a bit fresher. Some dentists also believe that shifting your tooth color closer to white can create an illusion to the eye of onlookers, where your skin actually looks a bit warmer, thus a free little tan without ever packing a bag. And young people usually have teeth that are naturally whiter, for they haven't experienced the ills of adult life, from coffee to cocktails with cranberry juice and every evil in between. So you may look a bit younger by whitening your smile, kiddo!

Do yourself a mini-makeover favor, without ever buying a stitch of clothing, visiting a salon, or stepping foot in a gym. Research a professional tooth whitening service and get an estimate and consultation. Run it past your dentist to make sure it is safe for your teeth, and ask him or her for other, less expensive, over-the-counter options they might recommend. See what fits your budget, and go for it.

Trust that you will instantly feel lighter and refreshed, and getting dressed may not be such a hassle, as a gorgeous, bright smile can really make any little thing you toss on look a bit newer.

Be careful not to overdo it, as many of our Hollywood sisters do, not realizing that teeth *should* have a smidge of color. Remember, only Chiclets gum should be blindingly bleached white and perfectly rectangular. Not a good look on a real woman. A naturally white look is best, as if you have been brushing and flossing after every meal since you first learned how. Hey, who's to say you haven't? Don't ask, don't tell!

JUNE 7 | LEARN A NEW FASHION TERM.

Haute couture *(oht koo-toor) • A French term that applies to custom-made clothes by top designers. Der. French, "highest-quality dressmaking." Is used throughout the fashion industry to represent original styles, the ultimate in fine sewing and tailoring, made of expensive fabrics. The designs are shown in collections twice a year—spring/summer and fall/winter.*

Simply put, haute couture is the legendary art of one-of-a-kind, made-to-order fashion (traditionally for the wealthiest of clientele) of the finest fabrics and masterful craftsmanship available—from numerous designer sketches, hours of fabric and trim research, multiple painstaking client fittings, expert sewing, hand-finishing, and masterful embellishment work (e.g., beading done one bead at a time by hand).

Most wealthy clients of the haute couture set are worldly women who will pay the tens of thousands of dollars for each garment for the security of not seeing any dress similar to theirs coming and going into a gala or society event. The designers they choose are usually selected members of a Parisian association called the *Chambre Syndicale de la Couture Parisienne*, which was founded in 1868 and regulates its members in regard to piracy of styles and various promotional activities.

Other European cities, particularly London, Rome, Florence, Zurich, and Madrid, have since developed their own couture industries, all of which have emulated the Paris haute couture system.

Lesson over. But one more thing: Sorry, ladies, but fun American labels such as Juicy Couture don't hold beads here. Think more along the lines of Christian Dior Couture for the real deal when you are ready to wait about a month, and use what amounts to a house down-payment for that special night and a must-have dress.

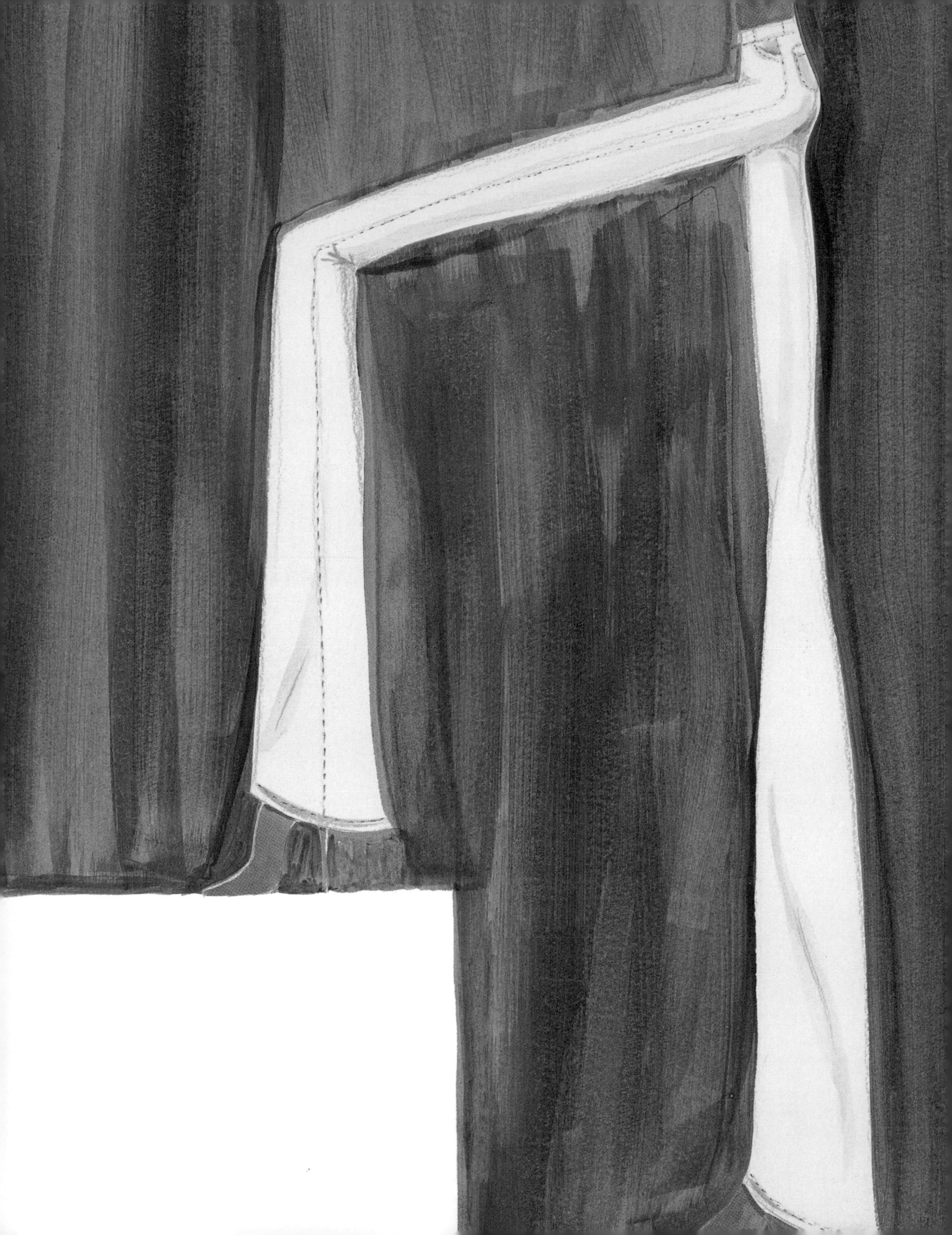

JUNE 8 | WHITE JEANS.

If I had the power of a billionaire, I would ship a pair of white jeans to every woman alive. She could be a svelte size six, or a curvy woman proudly working a sixteen and beyond—everybody gets a jean!

If fitted properly—which means enough room in the seat for bending and walking without any panty lines, and ample leg room so no one mistakes them for stirrups—a classic, five-pocket, bleach white jean is the common style denominator of fresh spring outfits. From super casual to dress casual, they'll serve you as loyally as your favorite tan khakis, blue jeans, or dark trousers. The difference is, they stand alone and go with almost anything, year-round.

White jeans bring a pure, blank, and bright burst to a head-to-toe look, and unlike other casual bottoms, don't equate into the color relation with any separate you pair them with. They're as close to universal as you can get, next to your natural bare legs.

You will see that they are mentioned throughout the book in outfit ideas from January to December, for I truly believe that the white jean is just that fun, powerful, and versatile. Hopefully, by year's end you will feel the same.

JUNE 9 | TAKE AN EXPERT BEAUTY CUE FROM NICK BAROSE, A TOP MAKEUP ARTIST AND BEAUTY GURU.

New York City–based celebrity makeup artist Nick Barose first entered the beauty scene while assisting makeup legend Kevyn Aucoin. Since then, he has been featured in major fashion magazines ranging from *Harper's Bazaar* and *In Style* to *Marie Claire*, *Shop Etc.*, and *Glamour*. Nick has worked with dozens of celebrities including Kim Cattrall, Tara Reid, Zoe Saldana, Scarlett Johansson, Kirsten Dunst, Brooke Shields, and Joss Stone.

Please share your best-kept makeup secret.
Putting on liquid foundation with a foundation brush. It allows for more control and you can layer on in certain spots that may need more coverage. Sponges eat up foundation and are a waste because they get thrown out often.

Name the three makeup essentials every woman should own.
1. A good liquid foundation that blends like second skin and is not oily. Some can double up as concealer if you layer it.
2. Translucent pressed powder to help cut down shine and keep your face from looking greasy.
3. A set of five makeup brushes that include one for concealer, powder, blush, [and] lip color, and one that allows you to apply eye shadow and liner as well as fill in brows.

What are the biggest makeup mistakes most women make?
A lot of times I see women with foundation or powder that doesn't match. At night you can get away with it but in broad daylight you see everything. Try to do your makeup next to a window where daylight is filtering in rather than in a badly lit bathroom.

Who is the most stylish woman around?
Actress Kim Cattrall. What I like about her is that she knows what look is right for her. You'll never see her in clothes, makeup, or hairstyles that are too trendy. She adds small elements, like playing up her lip color or wearing an interesting piece of jewelry to keep her look different without overdoing it.

Is there one fail-safe makeup tip all women should know?
Makeup is fun and there's no need to be intimidated by it. If you try something and it doesn't work for you, start over. It's not *Nip/Tuck*! Have fun.

JUNE 10 | POP STYLE QUIZ.

1. Which swimsuit idea can give a fuller look to women with modest busts?

A. One piece
B. Bandeau top with slight padding
C. The tankini
D. One piece with high-cut legs

2. Which number do you add to your American women's size to quickly convert it to an Italian size?

A. 34
B. 2
C. 7.5
D. The same size number

3. Which is the best color to wear to highlight an amazing tan?

A. Orange
B. White
C. Turquoise
D. Celadon green

4. If not careful, pleated pants can do what to your midsection?

A. Add volume
B. Add width
C. Flatten it
D. None of the above

(Answers: 1-B, 2-A, 3-B, 4-A)

JUNE 11 | IF YOUR TOP IS FINISHED, UNTUCK IT.

Enjoy a day of relaxed elegance, and possibly hide a flaw or two. Most dressy tops can look just as good untucked as they do tucked. If the seams are finished, you will not look slovenly or unkempt, just easy and confident. This release will also help to conceal a waistline or backside you may not love today, and until it looks the way you'd like it to.

JUNE 12 | HAPPY FATHER'S DAY.

As Father's Day approaches, it is time to let Dad know that you are grateful for his support, and equally glad that he had no problem saying no to things that you now know a teen should never be caught dead in. You probably thought of it as style deprivation back in the day, but now hopefully understand that it was his way of fostering *life* preservation.

Your first heels, the day you were finally allowed to try a little makeup, the wedding dress you dreamed of, or maybe just your favorite barrettes kept fully stocked—he probably had a silent financial hand in all of it. So whether you're "Daddy's Little Girl" or not, when confidently getting dressed on *this* day, and as we approach *his* day, be prepared to thank him for something he'd never imagine: your totally together image.

JUNE 13 | JUMP INTO A GRASS GREEN AND BRIGHT WHITE ENSEMBLE.

The sporty combination of grass green and bright white is an idyllic example of welcoming the warm weather. The look speaks of a day of tennis at a swanky country club, a now retro-chic tracksuit worn by an athlete at the 1976 Olympics, or just a perfectly manicured lawn against the clearest of skies. Can't you just smell the fresh air? That is what observers will feel when you breeze in wearing your green-and-white ensemble a bit later today. Here are a few style solutions that will make others green with envy:

White Jeans + Green Cotton Blazer + White Ribbed Tank + White Sneakers
= She's a Bit Green
Green Turtleneck + White Trench Coat + White Knee-Length Skirt + Nude Heels
= Spring Forward
White Cotton Button-Down + Green Slim Belt + White Pants or Skirt + Nude Flat
= "Money" in the Middle

JUNE 14 | TRY A DIFFERENT TAKE ON JEANS AND A T-SHIRT.

There is nothing more American than the crisp, clean look of a great-fitting pair of jeans and a T-shirt! The pairing of the two is a timeless statement that can go from the sidewalk to the catwalk when worn with interesting twists.

With jeans, you should have at least three blue washes in your closet and one solid white. A dark indigo or black, a classic medium blue, and a washed down, lighter blue. Within these three tones you will have the ability to use them for everything from just hanging around (lighter), to casual events (medium), to dinner or nighttime fun (dark).

As for T-shirts, my favorite choice is crisp, classic white. And if you choose to invest in a number of tees, the whites should certainly outweigh the colored tees and printed or design T-shirts.

Here are a few of my favorite style equations that are simple and bring a touch of the unexpected to a basic jean and T-shirt combination:

Dark Jeans + Black T-shirt + Slim Colorful Blazer and Boots
= Dazzling for Dinner
Medium-Colored Jeans + Gray T-shirt + Grosgrain Ribbon Belt and Sneaks
= Prep in Your Step
Light-Colored Jeans + White T-shirt + Cardigan and Driving Moccasins
= Modern Ivy League
Dark Jeans + V-neck T-shirt + Metallic Belt and Heels
= Retro Disco

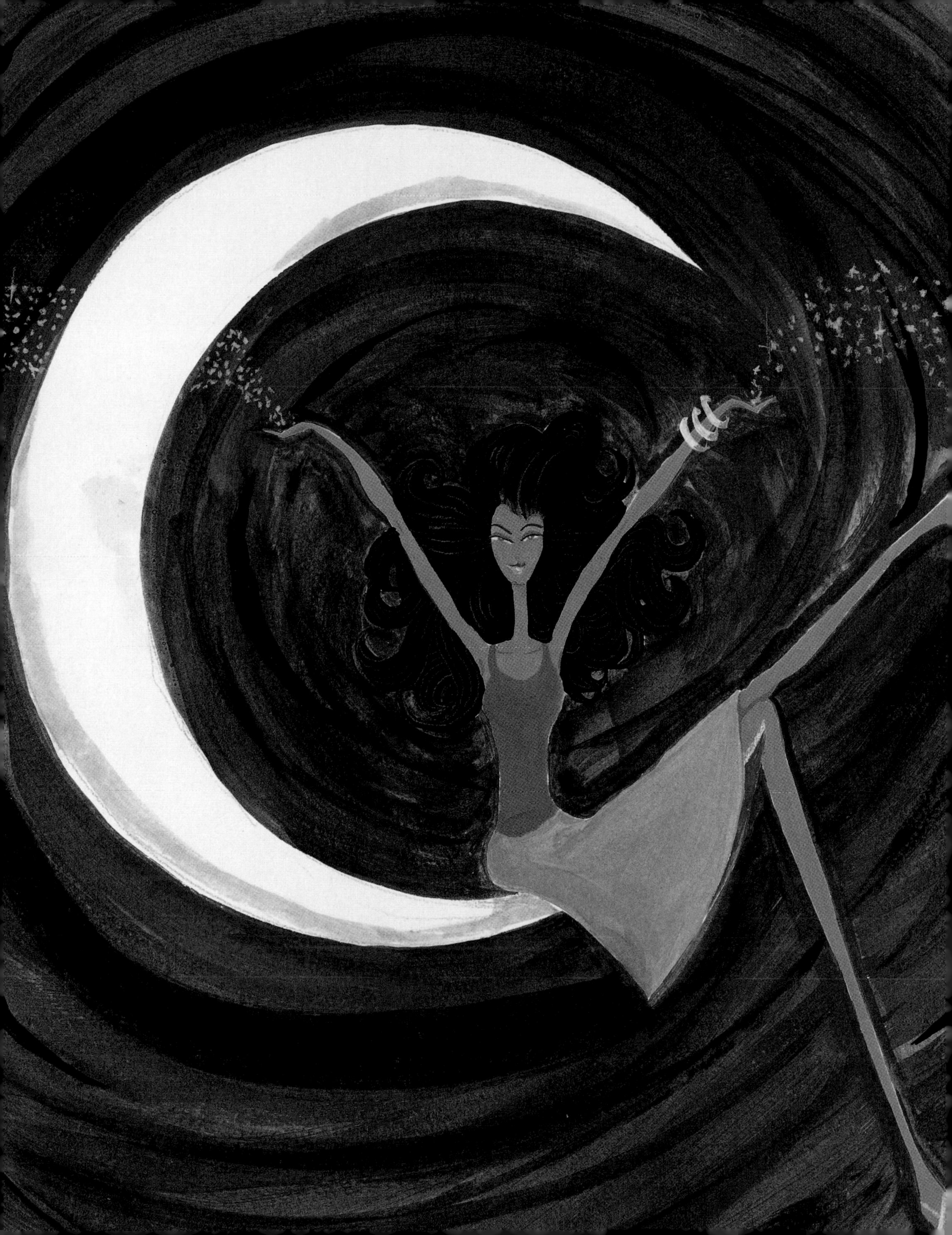

JUNE 15 | JUMP INTO AN ORANGE AND HOT PINK ENSEMBLE.

Juicy, irreverent, and almost shocking! Marrying hot pink and orange takes its cues from the look and feel of the French Riviera and the classic exteriors of buildings on Caribbean islands or Bermuda, where seeing two bold saturated colors such as these right beside each other is actually quite normal.

Think of the bright umbrellas that line the beaches of Nice, or the chapels and storefronts that line cobblestone Caribbean streets, that make you feel as if you are passing an array of juicy Popsicles! Mixing your boldest pinks and most saturated oranges should infuse this feeling into your bones on a day when the sun's just not shining or even on a starry summer night. Add a splash of bright white or tan accessories to cool down this combo if it's too shocking for you. Here are a few of my favorite ways to make it all work together:

White Drawstring Pants + Orange Caftan + Pink Flats + Straw Bag
= Sunny Delight

Pink Knee-Length Skirt + Orange Tank Top + White Bangles and Thong Sandals
= The Juice Is Loose

Orange Capri Pants + Pink Sweater Set + Orange-and-Pink Striped Espadrilles
= Totally Fresh Squeezed

JUNE 16 | GIVE YOUR FEET A BREAK AND YOUR TRADITIONAL OUTFIT A LIFT WITH ESPADRILLES.

Take it from the stylish French women: Pretty ensembles begin and end with expressive shoe choices that keep an observing eye excited, and allow the wearer to feel beautiful. The espadrille, a rope-soled shoe with a canvas upper (usually in bright summer colors) is one of the more casual examples of this idea, as made popular by the French in the 1940s.

Soft. Organic. Ultrafeminine. Natural in their sole material and fabrication, you will never be closer to earth, unless tipping around barefoot, since you are wearing products grown directly from the soil. Yet

(CONTINUED)

the glamour and whimsy of an espadrille is very obvious. Many styles have long, girly laces threaded through the top of the shoe, crossed, to be tied around the ankle. Colors like Matisse red, papaya, and azure blue are considered basic colors when shopping for espadrilles in France, even today—not to mention the colorful awning-inspired stripes and fun prints, which can tell a story of summer romance at beachfront cafés just by looking at them!

Imagine strutting your stuff in a pale linen pantsuit, a bright pastel tank underpinning, straw bag, and espadrilles that complement your tank of choice. Or espadrilles dyed in candy stripes, worn with a white cotton skirt and tie-front silk top in grass green. They're fun and feminine, and that's the way you have to think when wearing them, for they will bring this out in you. And your feet will let out a sigh of relief.

Finding an espadrille to suit your warm-weather mood may be a challenge. Since their humble beginnings, there are now many stylish incarnations, from flats to super-high sexy versions. In the 1980s we were introduced to the pump version or wedge-heeled options that made women teeter but still showed up all over the pages of fashion magazines and remain available even today. They are especially great when you want a shot of color on your feet and haven't had a moment to grab a pedicure.

JUNE 17 | TAKE AN EXPERT STYLE CUE FROM NANETTE LEPORE, A TOP CELEBRITY DESIGNER.

What is your best-kept personal style secret?
My secret is to always mix things up with style. Blend a little soft and feminine with a little sexy and a little tough. A woman is more stylish, more interesting and more mysterious when she combines different moods in her wardrobe choices. My secret to finding that perfect mix of style is picking up clothing and accessories in unexpected places and exotic locales for unique additions to my closet.

What are the three fashion essentials every well-dressed woman should own?
1. A fabulous entrance-making coat is a necessity for party-hopping throughout the night. You'll make a fashionable entrance at every stop and can slip out before even having to take it off.
2. Don't forget what's underneath. A colorful, lacy bra gives an element of surprise to any evening dress.
3. It is all about the shoes! Glittery, strappy, over-the-top heels offer the perfect finishing touch whether wearing your favorite jean or your essential little black dress.

Who is the most stylish woman in existence, in your opinion? And what do you appreciate about her look?
My early fashion memories have always been about the women in my family. I remember my mom's penchant for mod bikinis and quirky sunglasses. My aunt Sandra's bouffant hairdo and cool sixties style along with her mom, who had the best leopard-print chiffon blouse. My grandmother, who wore sheer nylon tops with fancy slips. My sister, who is the original gypsy with her layered bright shawls. And most currently, my daughter Violet, with her madcap mixing and matching.

If you could whisper a fail-safe style tip into the ears of women everywhere, without them feeling bad by hearing it, what would it be?
It's okay to show a little cleavage, just don't be trashy!

JUNE 18 | RIDE, SALLY, RIDE!

June 18, 1983: Sally Ride becomes America's first woman astronaut.

Twenty-seven years old and armed with B.A., B.S., and master's degrees, Sally Ride was a Ph.D. candidate looking for postdoctoral work in astrophysics when she read about NASA's call for astronauts in the Stanford University paper. She took a chance and applied. And although over eight thousand men and women did the same, in hopes of landing a spot in the NASA space program, less than forty were accepted, just half a dozen were women. Sally made the cut!

After joining NASA in 1977, Ride underwent extensive flight training and embraced it as a hobby as well. During the second and third flights of the space shuttle *Columbia* (November 1981 and March 1982), Ride was the communications officer.

In 1983, the now *Dr.* Sally Ride became the first ever American woman in space on board the shuttle *Challenger*, and she amassed more than 343 hours of spaceflight by her retirement from NASA in 1987.

Sally Ride took chances and made history on this very day because of a less than calculated risk. Taking style chances are certainly not comparable to that of exploring outer space, yet the principles are similar, in that you might be the first woman in your circle to actually step out of the box and take a chance. Hey, you might even start a trend instead of just following one. One woman has the power to

(CONTINUED)

do this, for she can inspire another, and another, and the look becomes alive. Or should I say *launched*, in honor of Sally.

Ditch your itchy hosiery today and go barelegged for a more youthful look, put your hair down when everyone knows you by your ponytail, or simply wear your favorite shoes with your handbag of the moment, even if it's not an exact match. Take a style chance and see where it leads you, or simply how it *frees* you. For Sally, her chance led her to a place that was out of this world. Honor her work today by looking at your world a little differently. Ride, Sally, ride!

JUNE 19

TRY A BIT OF QUICK AT-HOME TAILORING TO UPDATE WARDROBE ESSENTIALS. CHANGING BUTTON COLORS, REMOVING EMBELLISHMENTS, OR CREATING A NEW HEM LENGTH CAN MEAN A TOTAL NEW LOOK.

Over the years, I have heard countless women say this one phrase when looking at a garment that they seem to like, but are on the fence about: "Wow, that top would be perfect, if it wasn't for ______." Could be a fabric rosette attached to the lapel of a jacket, the big white buttons affixed to a dark duster, or something as simple as the length of capri pants.

This is no reason not to buy a new garment that you simple adore. Or worse yet, banish a perfectly good quality piece of clothing to the back of your closet, never to be seen again.

Although professional tailors are the best friends of the most stylish women on the planet, most busy women striving for improved style rarely have the time to visit them. Tailors are usually reserved for larger, more complex sewing tasks that require a seasoned craftsperson. This is when quick at-home tailoring comes in handy.

Use this day to see what garments in your closet are out of rotation simply because of the details. Small particulars can be changed with a little needle and thread, a seam ripper, or some stitch witchery (fusion tape) that's applied with an iron.

Removing large or dated buttons from jackets and pants and replacing them with chic updates can be done while watching your favorite thirty-minute TV show, and can be quite cathartic. Old long pants can be instantly made into fresher, younger capri pants by taking up the length, and hot pressing in a new one, in about the same time it takes to iron them for work. And you would be shocked to see what a $4 seam ripper can remove, from 1980s shoulder epaulets to ruffles attached to a summer dress. Enter a cleaner, simpler garment that is now timeless.

Whip out your sewing kit, no matter how small. Attack just one garment for starters, and see what comes out of it. The worst that could happen is that it returns to the gloomy rear of your wardrobe. Just call your self "Miss Tailor" today, but without the baggage of the seven husbands!

JUNE 20 | DRESS LIKE A CELEBRITY BY WEARING A SOLID WHITE PANTSUIT AND OWN JUST ABOUT ANY ROOM YOU STEP INTO!

She'll wear it to a red carpet event, even if it's just a regional theater opening night. She'll keep it on reserve for the nights when she knows that every other woman will run to their trusty little black dress. She also knows that white clothes can be worn year-round in season-appropriate fabric weights, which always sets her apart. She is the woman who ignites the murmurs as she enters (and exits) the room. And her white pantsuit is her best fashion friend when it is time to shine. Today, this woman can be you.

Before you put on another drab evening ensemble that is composed of matchy-matchy color separates, another conservatively patterned pantsuit in a tone of autumn, or, worse yet, another safe black cocktail dress that you might see a semblance of on another woman within feet of you, prioritize a white suit into your wardrobe of ideas.

And there is a white suit option for every woman: from the daring woman with a modest bustline who can slink into a white pantsuit and a nude or white camisole, giving the look of nothing on at all; to the curvy, full-figured woman concerned about tapering her shape, who should choose white zip-front jackets and pants with a touch of stretch in the fabric to offer ease, movement, and support—especially on top. This is a style solution that is worth spending a half-day to find, if you haven't already made the investment.

From Podunk to Pasadena, and Paris to Poughkeepsie, the power of this wardrobe staple is universal and somewhat undervalued. It gives you a clean, stellar look ready for any room ahead, and any velvet rope that is trying to keep you out. For with the right attitude, a crisp white suit, and the look of star power, all you'll hear at the next blockade is "Right this way, miss!"

JUNE 21 | THE FIRST DAY OF SUMMER, DRESS IN EASY PIECES THAT GET YOU OUT INTO THE SUN FAST.

With summer arriving on this very day, pull the emergency brake on grabbing your multiple layers of cold-weather armor and think about limiting the number of pieces you can wear to a maximum of three. By starting now you will be perfectly conditioned when the phone rings with an invitation for that spontaneous beach day. You'll save more summer time and grab-and-go like you've been doing it all year long.

Think three easy pieces at all times and watch how your time in the sun increases, leaving you feeling lighter and low maintenance and looking youthful. Check out these three-for-three summer launch looks:

Faded Blue Jeans + Oversized Sherbet-Colored Men's Button-Down + Straw Flip-Flops

= My Boyfriend's Back

White Shorts + White Caftan + Nude Slides and Red Toes

= All White With Me

Purple Tank Layered with an Orange Tank + Chino Skirt + Multicolor Mules

= Juicy Cute

JUNE 22 | HAPPY BIRTHDAY, CANCER GIRL.

Crabs are of the yang energy group, and unlike signs of the yin tribe, you can be indirect in your approach to life. When getting dressed, you prefer to be ladylike; overtly sexy looks are for women who need that sort of external boost. Your sensuality comes from within, and can merely be accentuated by your favorite organically shaped, cool-and-easy clothes in pure white, pale yellows, and misty greens. You can don a lace camisole just as easily as you can serve up a pair of leather pants, but prefer the former when it's time to really shine.

Take it from your notable Cancer siblings, award-snatcher Meryl Streep and the forever young Cyndi Lauper: Honoring your authentic self this birthday can only bring you closer to true happiness. This starts with what you wear as the party begins. For you, it might very well be a month of outfits, but do not fret—you can solve it by mixing up a few uncomplicated pieces.

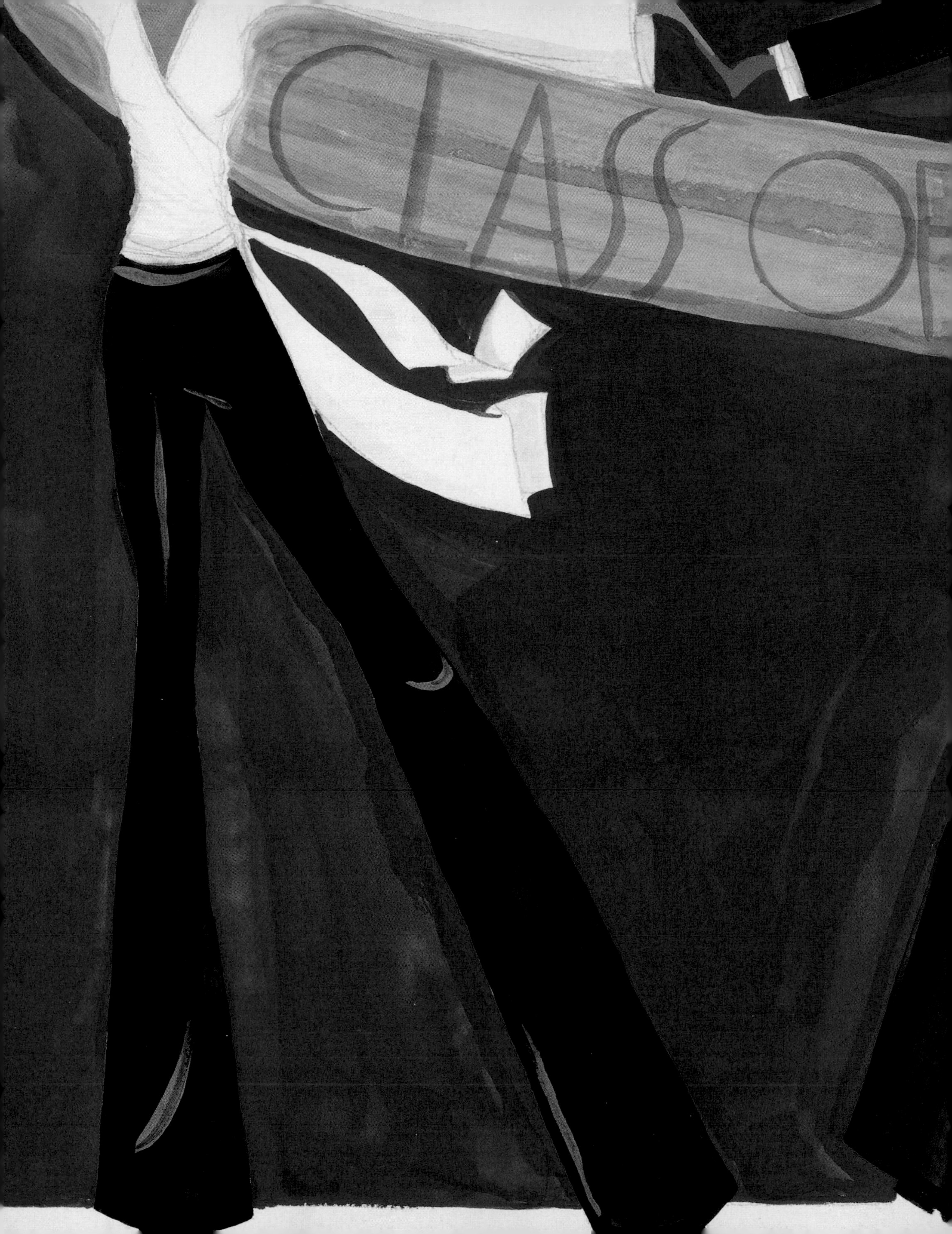
CLASS OF

JUNE 23 | TEN-MINUTE STYLE FOR A CLASS REUNION (OR ANY DAY YOU NEED TO LOSE TEN *VISUAL* POUNDS FAST).

It's that time of year again, when some celebrations can induce more stress than fun if you are not careful. Most women have witnessed the preplanning anxieties brought on by birthday parties full of friends you haven't seen in years, baby showers with all the women who can't wait to examine you from head to toe, and, my favorite, the class reunion!

Here is a great ten-minute style solution for shaving off ten visual pounds in a pinch:

Minutes 1:00–2:00:
Leather pants can be the best girdle you won't ever wear. The fitted skin has a mild suppression action that will lean out your bottom to the eye. Grab 'em!

Minutes 3:00–4:00:
Choose the highest heels you can stand in. Knee boots to match your pants will give you a high, thin, Catwoman feeling—and look very red carpet, too!

Minutes 5:00–6:00:
Wear bright white, or a bold, arresting color on top (a slimming coral wrap top). You want the top of you to sparkle and stand out in a room of little black dresses.

Minutes 7:00–8:00:
Hair should go up high, creating extra length to your body, minimizing the width. A fun high ponytail looks young and flirty, too, just like you used to pre-diploma.

Minutes 9:00–10:00:
Your makeup ought to be youthful-fresh. Do full coverage with an all-in-one foundation/powder, dust your eyes with pales, have natural, nude, or pink lips and barely a touch of blush—and get yourself to school, young lady!

JUNE 24 | GET THREE SUMMER LOOKS IN ONE BY CHOOSING THE RIGHT LAYERING PIECES.

Layering works! Go from a "fully loaded" outfit to "simply fab," and have three outfits in one. Busy women, with or without a confident sense of personal style, know what it is like to have to change in a flash—in a taxi, in a ladies' room, or even in the backseat of your own car. Space is limited, but you work with it, and you just hope for the best outcome.

Here are three-in-one ensembles that can provide you with very different looks:

Fully loaded: One-piece swimsuit + drawstring pants + nude sandals + linen shirt (open) + crushable straw hat
Completely Chic: One-piece swimsuit + linen shirt (front-tied) + drawstring pants + nude sandals + hair up in a twist
Simply Fab: One-piece swimsuit + crushable straw hat

JUNE 25 | MAKE A PACT WITH YOURSELF TO BUY YOUR NEW SHOES A HALF SIZE LARGER FOR MAXIMUM COMFORT, BETTER-LOOKING FEET, AND AN OVERALL MORE RELAXED SENSE OF BEING.

I used to work with a fabulous female fashion executive who always seemed so "together." You know what I mean: Traveled without a hint of stress. Handled her own responsibilities (and just about everyone else's). Had the look of money at all times. With the latest haircut that always seemed to complement her face perfectly.

I once got up the nerve to ask her, "How do you always manage to keep it so together?" She simply replied, "I eat right. Get my sleep. Drink plenty of water. And, oh! I always buy my shoes a half size larger!"

She explained that a woman's body is chameleon-like and swells and shrinks without notice. And that her traveling schedule is so demanding that she must be loose, free, and able to kick back at a moment's notice, whether on airplanes, trains, or in a solitary moment behind her closed office door.

Follow her lead and jump up one half size on your next shoe purchase. Be sure to walk around in the shoes in the store before you purchase them to make sure you don't walk out of them.

JUNE 26 | CLAIM YOUR FORTIES AND FEATURE STYLE THAT BEST SUITS YOU, OR PASS ALONG AN AGE-EMPOWERING TIP TO A WOMAN WHO REALLY NEEDS IT—OLDER OR YOUNGER.

Most women in their forties are simply trying to find a look that reflects how young they feel versus the maturation process that their bodies may be going through. Gravity has no favorites, everybody feels its effects. This is where style clarity becomes your best friend. This is also when you need to take your time-earned wisdom and discipline along to the mall. Select figure-flattering clothes that celebrate and work with the body you have now.

Start the reevaluation of your wardrobe with your undergarments. If you haven't seen a bra/intimate specialist, do it now.

When dressing up, pop neutral clothes with unexpected bright underpinnings. Grab fun, flirty handbags and shoes to accent or distract from your challenging areas. Identify your best feature and put it on a pedestal. Even if it's only your ankles, if you've still got 'em, flaunt 'em like they're the cat's meow!

STYLE QUICK LIST: THE TOP FIVE FORTYSOMETHING STYLE ESSENTIALS

Professionally fitted undergarments

Underpinnings in bold, unexpected colors

A flirty, conversational handbag

Sexy "five-hour" shoes

A timeless, reliable evening dress splurge

JUNE 27 | GIVE YOUR POWER SUIT A REST AND WEAR A SWEATER SET AND SKIRT COMBO.

The ladylike look isn't always the one that keeps you on the fast track and coworkers' eyes off you and on your skill set. However, even in the business world, there are days when you can place your strong suit on sabbatical and opt for the classic alternative. For this, the time-honored, solid knit sweater set is the ideal choice. It's a two-piece legend with a singular reputation of business with a dash of comfort and pleasure—if only for the woman wearing it.

Match your sweet sweater set with a more serious skirt or pants to really bring out the best in your corporate top. For instance, a black pinstriped pencil skirt opposite a cotton/Lycra camel sweater set is a little more Ginger than Mary Ann, but still keeps the afternoon meeting in your hands. Try a more colorful cotton sweater set coupled with an A-line skirt for days when you have to go straight from desk to dinner. And lastly, your pale suit pants can be taken even more seriously with a rich black cashmere sweater set, sporting the shell for desk time and adding the cardigan for unexpected powwows with the boss.

If you don't own a great sweater set, invest in the best quality you can afford in solid neutrals first—adding seasonal color as you see the power unfold. You will leave your place of work feeling a little lighter, and your suits will return to work even more refreshed because you've given them time to simply unplug.

JUNE 28 | TAKE AN EXPERT BEAUTY CUE FROM BOBBI BROWN, A TOP MAKEUP ARTIST AND BEAUTY GURU.

What is your best-kept personal beauty secret?
I don't have one. My job is to share and help women feel good about themselves. Personally, my most important beauty secrets are eating healthy, exercising, and getting just enough sun.

What female celebrity has kept global beauty moving forward? What is it about her that makes it happen?
Audrey Hepburn. Her simple and elegant style comes from her great confidence and individuality.

Why is it so easy for real women to look just as good as the stars on the red carpet these days?
Unfortunately, they don't. Stars have a minimum of three people helping them get ready—makeup artists, hairstylists, nutritionists, massage therapists, chefs, personal assistants, etc.

As a busy person, what one beauty tip would you love other busy people to know that always gets you by, looking fabulous?
Have a small, organized, makeup bag with you when you travel. This way you can do your makeup en route, anytime.

JUNE 29

INSTEAD OF CARRYING THE ACCESSORY OF THE MOMENT, MAKE A CHIC BOTTLE OF WATER YOUR FEATURED FASHION ACCOMPLICE, AND MAYBE EVEN LOSE A POUND OR TWO *WITHOUT* THE GYM.

One of the best-kept fashion secrets of well-dressed women today is the importance of drinking plenty of water all day long. It may sound simple, but it can be a challenge to actually pull off on any given busy day.

Unlike the silver screen images of the glamour goddesses who proudly carried spirit-filled flasks in their handbags, keeping a "toot handy" when moments of duress ensued, today, water is the oh-so-chic stylish mock-tail to pull out of your bag. Women today are stronger, just as stylish, but less melodramatic!

Did you know that your brain is 95 percent water, your blood is 82 percent water, and your lungs are close to 90 percent water? Simply put, we are nearly all water.

You may also notice some immediate changes in how you feel and ultimately how you look in your clothes, since studies have shown that mild dehydration is one of the most common reasons for daytime fatigue. A well-hydrated body allows your bodily functions to happen quickly and efficiently and even boosts your calorie burning by 3 percent.

Vainly speaking, if you are trying to lose weight to get into those dream pants, some studies have shown that hunger and thirst sensations are ignited in unison. If you are dehydrated, the thirst mechanism in your body may be mistaken for that of hunger, signaling you to snack when your body is actually craving fluid—so drinking lots of water can assist in preventing overeating. Add a chic sliver of cucumber or lime to get the spa taste. Invest in a stylish holder that makes you smile whenever you pull it out. And most important, know that with each sip, you are making everything you wear look just a bit better over time. Think of it as a little professional stylist and personal trainer in a bottle.

corner office

home office

JUNE 30 | CREATE YOUR OWN VERSION OF THIS SUREFIRE, STYLISH OUTFIT COMBINATION.

Dressing for work is especially difficult as the summer heat intensifies now. The perils of trying to remain fresh and dry between leaving your door and entering your place of work are the first challenge. Then there are the hot/cold flashes you experience throughout the day, going from the hot outdoors to chilly air-conditioned indoors. What you wear needs to be professional and comfortable.

Top: Crewneck summer sweater (short or cap sleeve)
Bottom: Flat-front dress trousers (cropped)
Shoes: Kitten heels
Accessories: Work tote; skinny belt; chunky bangles or cuffs; huggy earings
Flex piece: White or neutral-colored long-sleeve cardigan sweater kept at the ready to toss over anything

JULY

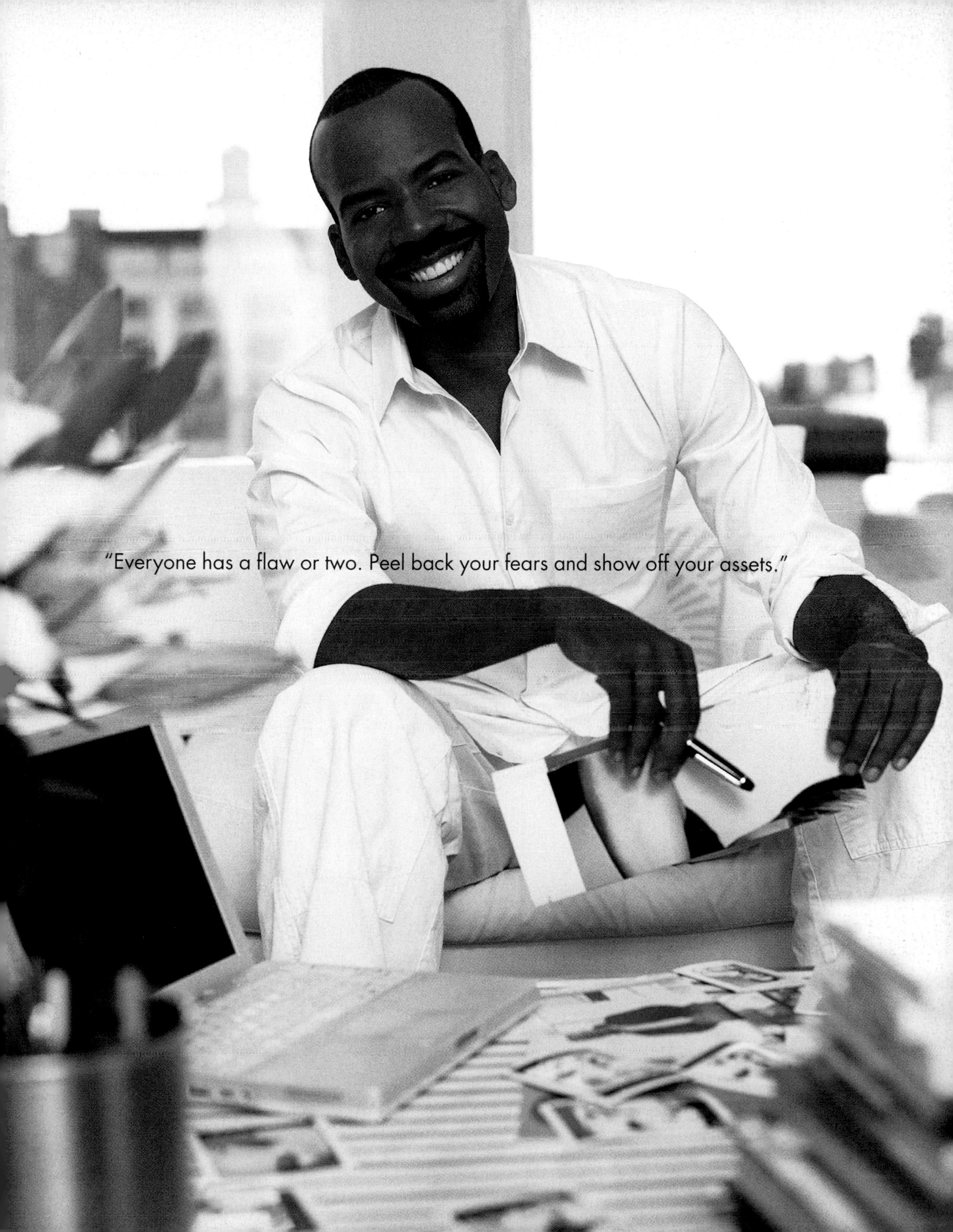
"Everyone has a flaw or two. Peel back your fears and show off your assets."

JULY 1 | PLAN AN EXCURSION INSPIRED BY CLOTHES THAT BRING OUT ANOTHER SIDE OF YOU.

Fashion is meant to inspire. A dress can arouse a mood that makes you think of a hot night of salsa dancing at an out-of-the-way nightspot. Standing in a certain pair of capri pants might stir up a notion to take in an outdoor play in the park. This response comes easily for some, but is more subconscious for others. Fashion designers use this instinct each season to create a theme and point of departure for their seasonal collections. You can do the same thing, and now is the time to try it.

Think out of the box at times and plan a trip based on an outfit. Summer madness? Yes. And oh, such fun.

Let's say you bought a Spanish-inspired lace skirt three years back, and ever since it has hung in the closet just waiting for you to wear it to a dance. Or maybe you have a pair of chandelier earrings that you always push aside for your sensible studs. You know, it's the kind of thing that makes people say, "Where would you ever wear these?" If the answer is Spain, that might be where you need to book your July vacation. If that's too extravagant, go for a great dinner at an authentic Spanish restaurant in town.

Use the start of this hot month to plot out your stylish getaway for the heart of summer, using clothes to take you there.

Affirmation:

I will live a little and plan a trip that is like none I've ever taken, using fashion as my trusted compass and international passport. With the right clothes and attitude, I can be anywhere I want to be.

JULY 2 | SLEEP.

Yes, this is an unlikely style tip. But at the core of every head-turning outfit is a woman's posture and carriage, much of which can be enhanced by a good night's sleep.

Your bed is where your body refreshes itself from life, and fashion is wear and tear. You may wear high heels for hours on end, which can add strain on the lower back, or wear stretch body shapers that suppress the flesh all day, creating tension and pressure, especially on the midsection. And working on your feet, specifically on floors without padding, can take a serious toll on your posture. This is why a full, restful night's sleep is something to plan for and maximize.

The top of July, the year's halfway mark, is the perfect day to turn your mattress. Take a few minutes (with the help of an extra set of hands if necessary). Your normal sleeping position can create a body impression in your mattress that over time can keep you from your best sleep. Most manufacturers say that every six months is fine, but you can also do it quarterly if you really want to be on top of things.

The mattress industry is heading toward nonflip mattresses, but most still need to be reversed occasionally. If you purchased your mattress and box spring before the turn of the new millennium, flip and rotate the mattress and rotate the box spring.

JULY 3 | TAKE AN EXPERT STYLE CUE FROM SANDRA DE NICOLAIS, A TOP NEW YORK STYLE-MAKER AND FASHION DIRECTOR OF *LIFE & STYLE WEEKLY.*

What is your best-kept personal style secret?

I never buy anything unless I can think of three things I already have in my closet to wear it with. If you can't get three great looks out of one item then it's not worth it.

What are the three fashion essentials every well-dressed woman should own?

1. A classic designer handbag. It will last for years and is worth the investment. Choose a style that works for every day, work, and weekends.
2. A pair of diamond studs, real or fake. You generally can't tell the difference. There's nothing like a luxurious-looking pair of earrings.
3. Chic high heels—sling-backs, pointy-toe pumps, or strappy high-heeled sandals. Whatever suits your lifestyle. A great pair of heels can make the outfit and eliminate potential frumpiness. Flats on anyone other than Nicole Kidman can be deadly.

What are the biggest mistakes women make when getting dressed?

Overaccessorizing and wearing clothes that don't fit properly. Avoid tricky shapes and anything that is too long, too small, or too tight.

(CONTINUED)

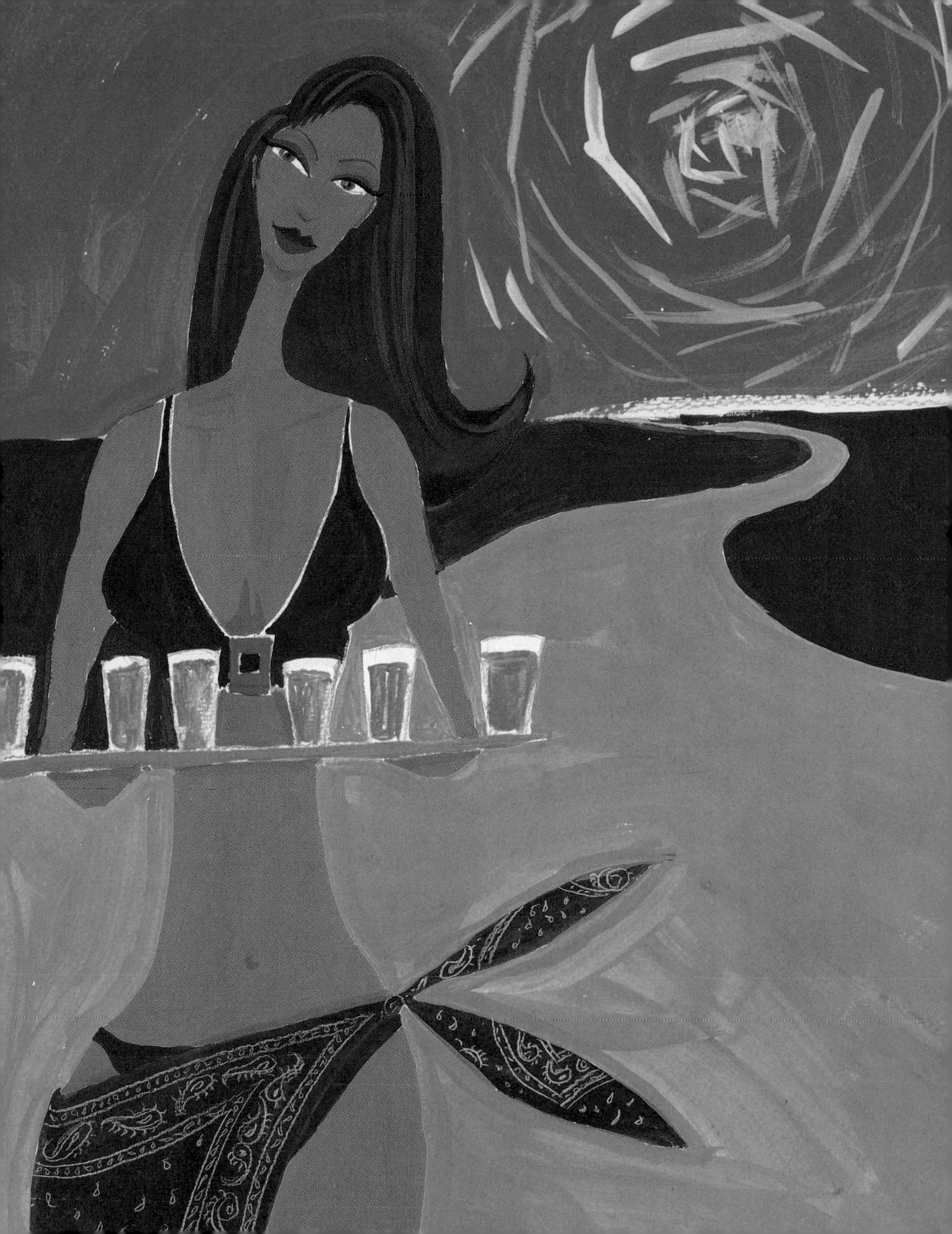

Who is the most stylish woman in existence, in your opinion? And what do you appreciate about her look?
Sarah Jessica Parker—she can wear retro, modern, or trendy styles and always look fabulous. Not everyone can pull off so many different kinds of looks and get it right every time.

If you could whisper a fail-safe style tip into the ears of women everywhere, without them feeling bad by hearing it, what would it be?
Avoid fashion fads and impulse buys. Not every trend is right for everybody. Make a list of what you already have and what you need each season. Then take your time and shop with a plan. Buy only what works in your budget. Great style is how you put it together, not how much you spend.

JULY 4 | CELEBRATE INDEPENDENCE DAY IN RED, WHITE, AND BLUE IN A WAY THAT PRODUCES FIREWORKS.

Summer is in full swing! You're like a big-city socialite with all the parties, fun three-day-weekend getaways, and lazy days lounging and sipping fresh lemonade with your closest friends. You wish, anyway!

Most Americans save the biggest and brightest cookout for Independence Day, or "The Fourth" as some of us say. You'll see the most family and friends, enjoy the most food, and hopefully serve up your best summer outfit. Whether poolside or on a picnic blanket, beachfront or backyard, the old red, white, and blue outfit of years gone by has changed. Stylish gals can do this patriotic ensemble in a way that will actually work—without looking like you stripped a flagpole bare. Here are some tips for sporting your independent style:

White Linen Sundress + Stack of Blue Bangles + Nude Sandals/Red Toes
= An American with an Accent

White Cotton Tank + White Capris + Red Scarf-as-Belt + Red Espadrilles
= A Hint of Holiday

Blue Wrap Top + Full White Palazzo Pants + Skinny Red Thong Sandals
= Red, White, and New!

Figure-Flattering Red Swimsuit + Blue and White Printed Sarong
= All-American Twirl

JULY 5 | DO YOU KNOW SARAH EMMA EDMONDS?

July 5, 1884: Congress awarded Sarah Emma Edmonds a pension for her service as a soldier in the Civil War, in which she fought dressed as a man.

Talk about a big-screen Civil War biopic just waiting to happen! Picture this: Sarah Emma Edmonds was a resident of Flint, Michigan, when the first call for Union enlistments was announced. She felt inspired to answer the call just like any other American. The difference was that she was not legally allowed. So she got clever and chopped off her hair, jumped into a traditional men's suit, answered only to the name of *Frank* Thompson, and attempted to enlist.

Her persevering spirit prevailed, although it took her four tries to get in. After being "sworn" in to the Union Army (without today's standard practice of a complete medical examination), Emma Edmonds alias Frank Thompson became a male nurse in the Second Volunteers of the U.S. Army on April 25, 1861.

Acting convincingly as Franklin Thompson, Emma successfully evaded detection for an entire year. She participated in the Battle of Blackburn's Ford, the Peninsular Campaign, Antietam, and Fredericksburg. Most interestingly, she sometimes served as a spy, ironically enough, "disguised" as a woman (Bridget O'Shea) or as a black man. It's a scene that just reeks of an Oscar nomination for the right actress!

In 1882 she started to petition for a pension as a veteran, and was granted one in 1884. Edmonds once said that she was "naturally fond of adventure, a little ambitious, and a good deal romantic—but patriotism was the true secret of my success."

So take your style cues from a woman who made history using "drag" to its best effect. Keep your patriotic spirit alive in her honor. By all means, don't jump into a men's-inspired suit and your red pumps! Simply splash on just a bit of red, white, *or* blue with whatever you wear today.

JULY 6 | PUT A DENIM SKIRT TO WORK.

When every other girl runs to jeans for a casual day at the office or a girls' night out, there is always one chic lady who steps out in a drop-dead denim skirt and leaves the party on pause.

Gone are the acid-wash miniskirts of the 1980s, and the long, ruffled-edged prairie skirts inspired by Western frontier times. Designers today have taken denim to the moon and back.

A knee-length denim skirt will never go out of style, if you choose one with a classic shape and updated details that aren't too trendy. This may sound like a difficult balance, so here's a guide. When shopping for your next version, or examining the one you already own, be sure that it features only one style attribute from each of the columns below.

SILHOUETTE	RINSE/TREATMENT	LENGTH
Box pleated	Garment dyed (super dark)	At the knee
A-line	Indigo	Just above the knee
Perfect pleated	Ring-spun (vintage look)	Just below the knee
Pencil	Crosshatch (crisscross texture)	Floor-length wrap or asymmetrical

If you choose a skirt with at least one of the attributes from each column, you have a better chance of it lasting for years to come.

JULY 7 | BABY ON THE WAY? BE MORE STYLISH THAN EVER.

•Never buy a garment without trying it on first. Take a fun moment and roll a stuffed, bulky sweater and shove it near your stomach. It will help you assess whether the dress is appropriate to take you well into your last trimester.

•Avoid pleats on pants and dresses, unless you are very thin at the start. In general, pleats are not flattering on a large stomach, pregnant or not.

•Whenever possible, use a tailor to lengthen the front of your dresses by a few inches ahead of time. As baby grows, dresses will become shorter in the back and hike up in the front. Leave the back alone.

JULY 8 | RELEASE PAST PATTERNS.

Ask yourself if you are holding on to any of these—and then let them go!

The hairstyle I wore when he proposed.
The suit silhouette I began wearing with my first big promotion.
The nail color and length I wore when I could finally afford professional manicures.
The hair color I chose when I first started going gray.
The skirt length I wore when my husband and I first started dating.
The makeup application I learned at the counter with my very first expensive designer lipstick purchase.
The comfortable shoes I started wearing after the birth of my first child.

JULY 9 | NO WHITE AT THE WEDDING—UNLESS YOU'RE THE BRIDE.

I am asked this question countless times a year, and it still baffles me. The desperation in the eyes of women when they ask it would lead this style guy to believe that all they had in their closet to wear to all weddings was, in fact, white clothing.

"Let's be honest. Who really wears pure white dresses anyway? Brides, that's who," says Carley Roney, cofounder of one of my favorite online wedding planning sites, TheKnot.com.

"To go out of your way to buy a white dress and wear it to someone's wedding just looks bad, even if you didn't do it on purpose. Wedding guests really shouldn't wear white if they can avoid it. Ivory is okay, but only if you really have nothing else to wear," adds Roney.

She offers a simple litmus test for you to do before you leave the house. "Look at yourself in the mirror and think, 'If I was standing next to the bride in this, would it be awkward?' If you think it might be or that it might upset her, it's a no-no." And back into the closet you go!

When you stop and think about it, with the scores of colors, prints, and patterns to choose from, is it really that hard to avoid the one single color worn by someone you care about on their special day? I think not.

JULY 10 | BUY PANTS IN MULTIPLES.

This is the time of year when most retailers are practically giving away their spring and summer merchandise. Remember, if you find an amazing deal (60 percent off or more) that you just cannot leave in the store, you may want to take home two.

Buy one pair and hem it at a length that's perfect for your typical high heels. The other can be taken up to a length that's just right for flats. No more jacking up waistbands or dragging pant legs. Now you are covered twice, for almost half the price.

Look for interesting and unique pants that speak to your event needs as well—for example, tuxedo pants for evenings and holidays; pretty, printed pants that go with conservative loafers or vampy heels for dinners; and jeans that always make you feel leggy.

JULY 11 | TAKE AN EXPERT STYLE CUE FROM CARMEN MARC VALVO, A TOP AMERICAN DESIGNER.

What is your best-kept personal style secret?
Never wear a new outfit head to toe, always wear something old and loved along with it.

What are the three fashion essentials every well-dressed woman should own?
A beautiful pair of black close-toe sling-backs because they go with everything; classic diamond stud earrings because they never go out of style; and, of course, a little black cocktail dress because, along with jeans and a T-shirt, it's a true staple of the modern wardrobe.

What are the biggest mistakes women make when getting dressed?
The biggest mistake most women make when selecting what to wear is to have too many preconceived notions of what's right and wrong for their bodies. Know what looks best on you but don't be afraid to try something new, you might just discover the next big thing that's good for your body.

Who is the most stylish woman in existence, in your opinion? And what do you appreciate about her look?
Audrey Hepburn, because she was the icon of my youth. She was, for me, the epitome of style.

If you could whisper a fail-safe style tip into the ears of women everywhere without them feeling bad by hearing it, what would it be?
Before you go out, look in the mirror and take off one accessory!

JULY 12 | GET THREE LOOKS IN ONE.

Choose the right layering pieces and peel your outfit down from "fully loaded" to "simply fab" in no time flat. Stylish women are ready for almost anything and they stay that way by having well-appointed outfits that never look too thought-out, yet always have enough versatility to be quickly shifted, peeled down, or built up to become a different look in a matter of minutes.

Fully Loaded: Fitted blazer + sweater set + white jeans + kitten heels + long slim neck scarf
Completely Chic: Fitted blazer + sweater set cardigan (over shoulders) + white jeans + kitten heels
Simply Fab: Sweater set shell + white jeans + kitten heels + neck scarf as *belt*

JULY 13 | LEARN A NEW FASHION TERM.

Guayabera shirt *(gwah-ya-bare-a) • 1. Lightweight overshirt made with convertible collar, short sleeves, and four large patch pockets. Has two sets of pin tucks in front and back running from shoulder to hem. Copied from shirts worn by the well-dressed businessmen in pre-Castro Havana. 2. Another style has embroidered stripes down the front instead of tucks and is styled for men and women. Shirt worn in Cuba by guava tree growers.*

Buy a traditional guayabera for your guy. You've seen them a million times, whether on footage of Cuba in its black-and-white heyday or on a sun-kissed concierge at your favorite island resort in the Caribbean. The loose-fitting, pastel or white short-sleeve dress shirt with pleats running down the front on each side is a staple of island men (and stylish women) to this very day.

The beauty is that any man can look just as dashing and feel instantly comfortable, while boasting relaxed elegance just by buttoning one on. And whether paired with jeans, linen pants, or khakis, the look says "Dance with me!" That would be after you shake me up a mojito, since you bought him that fabulous shirt.

JULY 14 | INVEST IN A CASHMERE SWEATER.

BEFORE WEARING THIS

Although the weather is still bubbling hot, packing a sweater in your travel bag is still a good idea. From frigid offices and workspaces to the movieplex in which you feel like you are actually living on the film set in the North Pole to shopping malls that are so cold you run in just to get away from the summer heat, keeping that extra layer around is key.

Beware of false bargains. There is that huge sign that reads "3 Sweaters for $30!" and lures you to buy cotton or, worse yet, synthetic. And off you go with your three, maybe even six frail sweaters that look amazing when folded on the store shelves, but can withstand about three washes before looking like the one you wore shopping.

Make a pact with yourself to change this habit with a simple solution.

(CONTINUED)

CONSIDER WEARING THIS

Instead of grabbing another cotton sweater of lesser quality, invest in *one* good cashmere sweater that may cost a bit more. You will have it longer, it will keep you warmer, and with the extended amount of wears it will pay for itself over time.

+

Match a great cashmere sweater with anything from jeans to tailored skirts and watch it adapt, making casual partners look more stately, and tailored pairings appear in good company.

+

(Tip: Since cashmere is knit of goat hair, hand washing with a bit of the same mild shampoo you use on your own hair will keep it looking like new.)

=

Casual cashmere that will serve you for years and years.

JULY 15 | SPRING/SUMMER CLEARANCE SALES SEASON. CHECK YOUR LOCAL MALLS AND BOUTIQUES.

From this day onward, prices will drop—so stock up if you can. What a great time to stock up on finds for next summer, or for the rest of this one if you really stop to think about it.

The smartest way to approach this opportunity is to take a deep breath, and call a salesperson to get a feel for what the reductions are, before bursting into the store. Many times, if you know what is ahead you can plan accordingly, or go at a later time when reductions really meet your pocketbook right where they should.

Be sure to get on your favorite store's mailing list, for select stores will cut prices in small reductions from now through the end of the month, and then hold a massive two-day clearance event, usually over a weekend or holiday weekend. You will know about it first. And whatever does not sell is sometimes shipped off to an outlet store owned by the same brand, so all is not lost. Find out where it is located, and get on its mailing list as well.

JULY 16 | GET A TEN-MINUTE STYLE FOR A LONG FLIGHT—ONE THAT IS COMFORTABLE AND ALSO LOOKS LIKE YOU SPENT HOURS PULLING IT TOGETHER.

Your summer travel schedule is like that of a rock star, even if many of your smaller jaunts simply take you to mountains up north, the local amusement park just off the highway, or out for a walk along a nearby waterfront.

Traveling in style is a toss-up. Many women say, "Why bother? No one will see me thirty thousand feet in the air. And I can always change when I land." Or so you hope.

I say getting fabulous for the friendly skies is a great way to take the edge off the work involved in traveling. Arrive at your destination knowing that you are ready for just about anything. You may even land an upgrade to first class if you aren't there already.

Here is a great ten-minute style solution that I call "plane and simple" for air travel style in a pinch:

Minutes 1:00–2:00:
Go for drawstring lounge pants in cashmere, merino wool, or velour. They're as comfy as sweats but look a bit more elegant. The longer the length the better.

Minutes 3:00–4:00:
Choose a fine-gauge sweater or sweater set. Surprisingly, thin turtlenecks are great on over-air-conditioned summer flights and look chic with lounge pants.

Minutes 5:00–6:00:
Ballet flats, slip-on slides or mules, and driving moccasins sans socks look rich, elegant, and feel as relaxing as first class, even if you're in coach.

Minutes 7:00–8:00:
Your carry-on bag is the style tip-off—whether a new, inexpensive canvas tote (note that I said "new"), or a luxe leather weekend bag. Bring the best bag you have.

Minutes 9:00–10:00:
Your makeup ought to be "barely there." It is dry in the sky, so focus on a great moisturizer, a bit of undereye concealer, a natural lip color or moisturizing gloss—ready for takeoff!

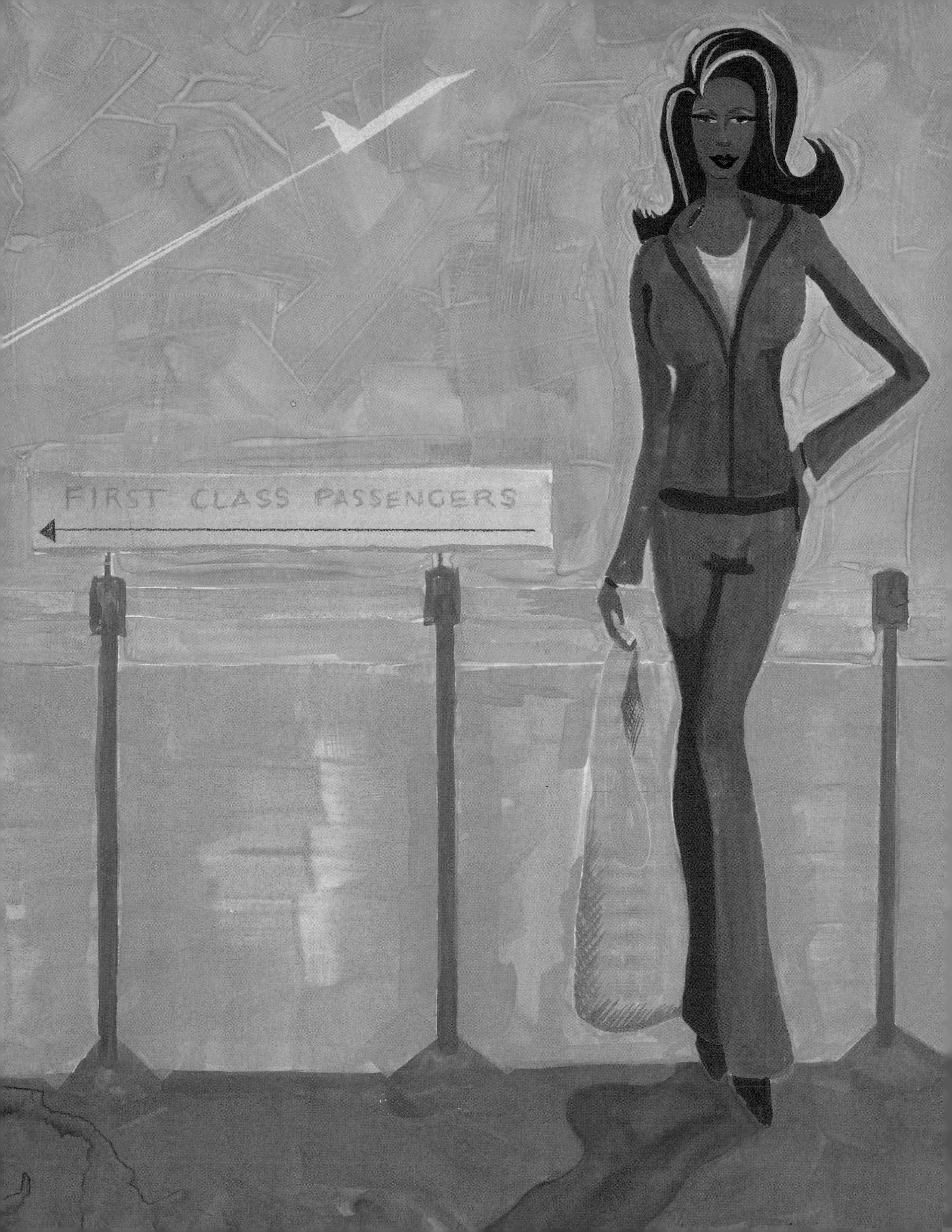
FIRST CLASS PASSENGERS

JULY 17

CLAIM YOUR FIFTIES AND FEATURE STYLE THAT BEST SUITS YOU, OR PASS ALONG AN AGE-EMPOWERING TIP TO A WOMAN WHO REALLY NEEDS IT—OLDER OR YOUNGER.

Designer Michael Kors says, "If you had great legs at twenty, you'll have them at fifty." He is so right. And aren't you lucky, as this applies for just about any of your great features!

Your fifties are about comfort and elegance. And contrary to many busy, sweatpanted moms and grand-moms, these two ideas *can* go hand in hand.

Fabrics like cashmere (you've earned it), merino wool (an inexpensive cousin to cashmere), and silks should be the holy trinity when looking for clothing for the cooler months. For instance, sweatpants can be plush, so that they are comfy and flattering. Look for those made in velour at the very least, so when worn with sparkly flats, you become a stylish host inside who can actually enjoy the party, or when out and about, your outfit actually deducts from your age.

This is the time to take heel heights down, while keeping them sassy. Kitten and Sabrina heels should be the key words when asking for assistance in your favorite shoe store. But keep one killer high-heeled pair for anniversary nights.

Know that your outfits shouldn't look like they did twenty years ago, and neither should your face or hair. Celebrating who you are today is when the real arresting beauty shines through. This means going a touch shorter on the hair, giving it a sporty edge and increased manageability. Ease up on the makeup. The flaws that come from maturity tend to be highlighted when masked with heavy products that claim to cover and conceal. Let your sensuality reveal itself in your posture and ladylike carriage, not necessarily a skin-bearing top or skirt. Allow clothes to closely skim the body's shape for the same effect.

STYLE QUICK LIST: THE TOP FIVE FIFTY-SOMETHING STYLE ESSENTIALS

A soft travel sweatsuit in a rich fabric

Sassy flat (or low-heel) shoes with sexy details

Youthful but age-appropriate jeans (slightly lower at the waist)

More skincare, less makeup

A trench coat with color, mystery, and glamour

JULY 18 | POP STYLE QUIZ.

1. Which design label struck fashion gold in the 1990s, is a favorite of Madonna and Sting, used the Medusa icon on many fabric prints, and is often mispronounced?

A. Comme des Garçons
B. Versace
C. Prada
D. Thierry Mugler

2. Which famous handbag costs upward of $10,000 at retail, is named after a famous English actress, and has a waiting list of several years just to buy one?

A. The Birkin bag
B. The Dunaway satchel
C. The Dench tote
D. The Satchel Page

3. Which sleeve is best for women with heavy arms?

A. Cap
B. Bracelet
C. Three-quarter
D. Dolman

4. Mismatched handbags and shoes are only okay if you . . .

A. Match the metal hardware on both
B. Pair versions proper for the same season and wear with confidence
C. Bring a spare pair of shoes that *do* match
D. Are admittedly and legally colorblind

(Answers: 1-B, 2-A, 3-C, 4-B)

JULY 19 | TAKE AN EXPERT STYLE CUE FROM JULIE CHAIKEN, A TOP NEW YORK DESIGNER.

What is your best-kept personal style secret?
Always wear a good demure watch, good shoes, and a good handbag. They'll make any outfit look pulled together.

What are the three fashion essentials every well-dressed woman should own?

1. A great black suit.
2. A great white suit
3. The perfect black dress

What are the biggest mistakes women make when getting dressed?
Not wearing proper undergarments. It is very important to wear the right pieces to complement the outfit. A wrong choice of underwear or bra can ruin an outfit.

Who is the most stylish woman in existence, in your opinion? And what do you appreciate about her look?
I have a soft spot for Liz Taylor in her early years. Again, simplicity.

If you could whisper a fail-safe style tip into the ears of women everywhere, without them feeling bad by hearing it, what would it be?
Stand with poise. Good posture makes your clothes look more expensive and adds polish.

JULY 20 | ADD AN AMERICANA PRINT TO YOUR LOOK.

I am a sucker for prints that celebrate Americana. Maybe it's my private school upbringing, or my time spent working alongside American design icon Tommy Hilfiger. Whatever the case, this month always brings to mind the preppy basics that make summer really feel real.

There is a certain youthful energy that will always go hand in hand with traditional Americana prints. The feeling of spending long days on the beach, riding a bicycle through the park with "no hands," or

(CONTINUED)

simply catching fireflies by night—the things young people do without thinking about it. And can't you just picture them all wearing those fun prints we all remember; especially patchwork and bandanna prints!

The sometimes goofy, checkerboard patchwork print—called "crazy" quilts—was designed to mimic a patchwork motif, very popular in America's postcolonial years, whereas the classic bandanna prints usually imitate a bandanna handkerchief, which was first made in East India with a method of tie-dying cloth called *bandhnu*, thus its name.

This time of year is when you will find prominently displayed (either new or vintage) wrap skirts, button-down shirts, sleeveless tops, shapely sheath dresses, and even capri pants—just to name a few—in either print. I say scoff one up to be instantly transported back to a simpler, more innocent summer. It is never too late. Just watch out for the countless ice cream cones, for they don't disappear from the hip area as quickly as they do from your hand.

TWO FOOLPROOF WAYS TO ALWAYS LOOK STYLISH IN AMERICANA PRINTS

•Americana prints in general are "conversational" and have a lot of elements to capture the eye. Remember this when choosing your silhouette: If you don't want eyes on your bottom, avoid skirts and pants—and go for a top that holds all the chitchat.

•Patchwork can be especially intense on the eye. Be careful not to become too "matchy matchy" with complementary clothing. For instance, a patchwork top in multiple bright colors may be best worn with a khaki skirt, or any other color bottom that is not in the top's color scheme.

JULY 21 | ADD PUNCHES OF BOLD COLOR.

Summer style is all about bold, intense color—worn in unexpected combinations. Think juicy tangerine, saturated magenta, and Caribbean azure just to start your palette. Yes, your clothing colors should sound and feel as yummy as your food.

The hottest and easiest way to start sporting this look at your next summer fete is with solid pieces, leaving colorful prints and patterns for when you are more confident. Combine fun layers in nontraditional pairings to make your host outfit sparkle from start to finish. Here are some of my favorite combinations:

Tangerine Orange Top + Popsicle Pink Bottom + Tan Shoes
= Palm Beach Chic
Powder Blue Top + Grass Green Bottom + Bleach White Sneaks
= Fresh Air Fun
Intense Lavender Top + Banana Yellow Bottom + Barely There Flip-flops
= Havana Nights

Don't panic if donning strong saturated color is a stretch when you usually stick to neutrals and dark colors. Another great way to stand tall wearing this motley summer trend is to start with one clothing item in your favorite bright color, and pair it with a bleach white item to cool it down.

Always remember that party clothes should inspire fun, evoke a festive mood, and invite compliments. Hey, you worked hard to put them at ease, so why not get a few "thank yous" *before* the party is over.

JULY 22 | NO ELECTRONIC TOOL BELTS, PLEASE. DO AN ELECTRONIC SPOT-CHECK BEFORE YOU WALK OUT THE DOOR.

We can hardly imagine our lives before cell phones and PDA devices. They've become must-haves in our professional and personal lives. Getting on the grid we call technology, the worldwide web, the matrix, or simply the global superhighway can ruin more than your quiet time and manners, it can also do a number on a great outfit. When they are not in use, don't wear them like an accessory. Do what I call a "technology spot-check" on your total look today.

Remove any device that is clipped to your waist unless you want a larger waist and imbalanced silhouette. Drop the PDA from your pockets, especially any interior jacket pocket near the bustline—not a good look for any woman. And whatever you do, never keep a wireless cell phone headpiece clipped to your ear unless you are going for that "Lieutenant Uhura" look from the original *Star Trek* series—cute for Halloween, frightening for an elegant woman of style.

Think about it. Is being reachable that important at every waking moment? Usually not. Women went decades without being on the grid 24/7, managed to get loads of things done in a day, and remained stylish in the process.

The only person in hosiery who should be keeping any electronic devices attached to the body is Batman. Key word: man. And even *his* red-hot Bat Phone was off in the corner, under glass.

JULY 23 | HAPPY BIRTHDAY, LEO GIRL.

No other astrological sign can accelerate from zero to sexy as quickly as the wily Leo woman. Growl! Sex appeal for you means feeling self-assured from the inside, wearing the best you can afford on the outside.

As a daughter of the sun, you always put yourself first, creating a world of beautiful things that you can enjoy daily—not keeping them on reserve for a special occasion as most other women would. Feeling feminine is like basking in the sun for most Leo gals, which often times means sacrificing a little bit of comfort and ease, for the clothing or accessory that makes you feel like a glamazon from any red carpet or runway. And the feeling is the key, for you are happy with your size, weight, and assets, knowing that when you are ready to strut your stuff, it is all good.

People around you see you as a daring dresser. You know that the best and brightest designers are the ones who really keep you standing tall—and that secret remains between you and your clothes, on their label. And while you favor the spicy colors found in an exotic, Eastern marketplace, like tamarind, curry, and ripe eggplant, you have been known to toss it all for a crisp white summer dress.

Madonna and Halle Berry are also Leos with a penchant for pulse-racing ensembles.

JULY 24

PLAN A CLOTHES-SWAPPING PARTY FOR ALL WHO NEED A THRIFTY WARDROBE BOOST. YOU'D BE SURPRISED HOW ONE WOMAN'S DISCARD CAN BE ANOTHER DIVA'S DAZZLER!

Clothes can be expensive and are not to be wasted. Recycling clothes that don't work for you anymore makes as much sense as recycling the tons of glass, plastic, and other materials we use. Especially after the fashion magazines have lined up all the trends for the season, giving you that itch for something new, even if it is only one little dress. Okay, and maybe just a handbag. And that adorable shoe that simply needs to meet your foot. Your pulse starts racing right there in the store, and there go the savings! Not to fret.

Smart, stylish women everywhere have been decoding the system and feeding the need to purchase an entirely new wardrobe each and every season by hosting fun, inexpensive clothes-swapping parties. They are simple, low prep, outrageously funny, and bond-building in a way you can never predict. Here are the four easy steps to your great first event, and possibly a whole new look from a second-chance wardrobe:

Step One: Invite a few friends with varied fashion tastes and similar figures. They don't all have to be your exact size.

Step Two: Decide on an equal amount of clean bottoms, tops, shoes, accessories, and unopened beauty products to bring along as well as a potluck dish and/or fun cocktail or mocktail.

Step Three: Let the party begin! Crank up the music and ask each guest to walk the group through their collection, as a designer would, sharing the history of each garment—the first-date dress, the major sale shoe, the job-winning interview blouse.

Step Four: Open the floor to bidding on each item, using your own items as currency to swap for the item of your choice. The owner makes the final decision as to the highest bid based on her personal preference.

At the end of the party, you will undoubtedly have at least one new item. What's left can then go to a charity. Do something proactive, productive, and fun!

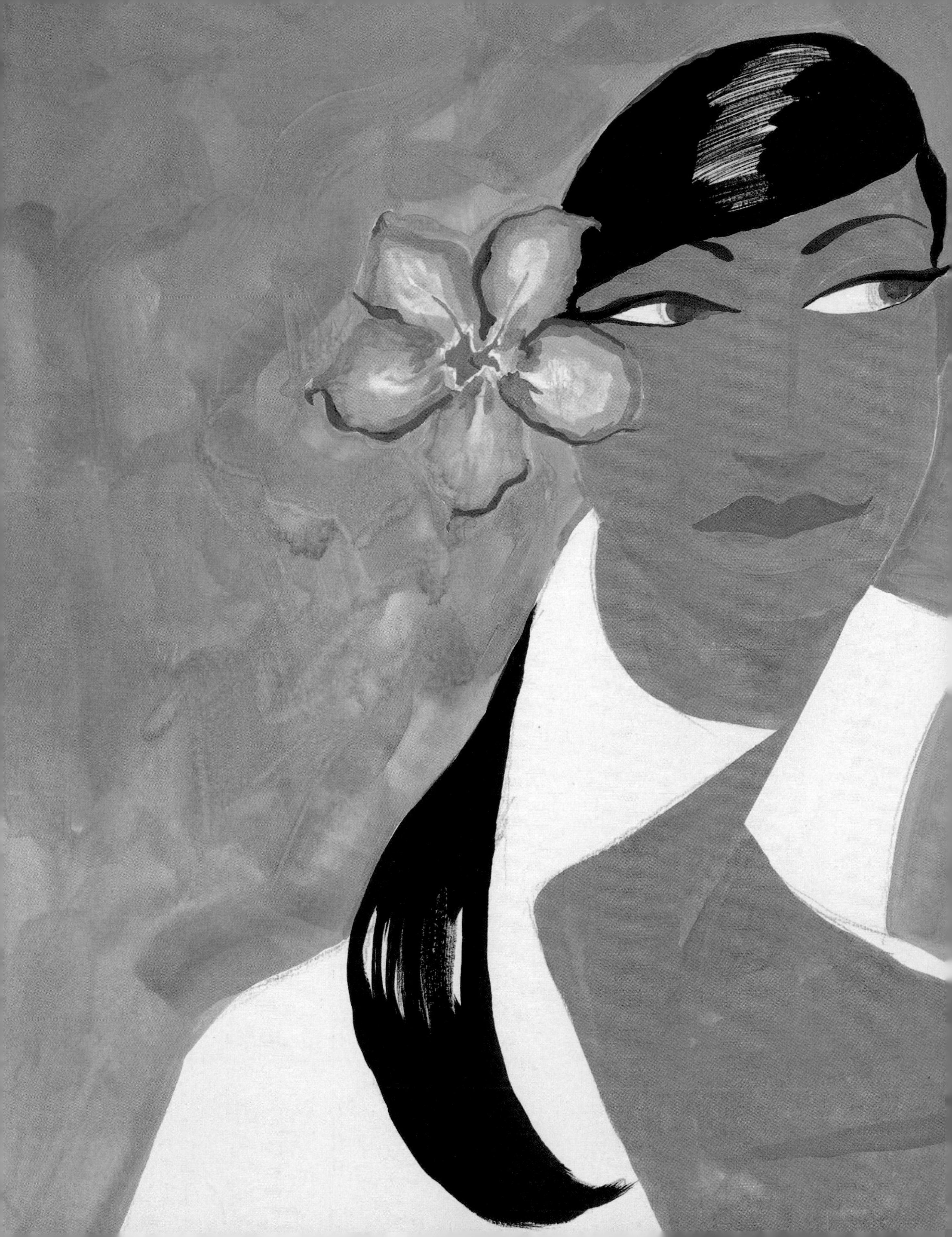

JULY 25 | ADD A FRESH FLOWER TO YOUR HAIR INSTEAD OF A TYPICAL HAIR ACCESSORY AND CELEBRATE THE WARM WEATHER, WITH ALL ITS ROMANTIC POSSIBILITIES.

Think back to the silver screen glamour goddesses of the 1930s and 1940s. The most notable flowered icon is jazz legend Billie Holiday. Her signature gardenia, always placed at her left ear, created a feminine look that made her a stage standout whether appearing at a smoky jazz club or making her groundbreaking debut at New York's Carnegie Hall. You can also fast-forward to today and see Hollywood darling Ashley Judd at just about any red carpet premiere or event, wearing what has become her signature as well, a row of moist, fresh flowers of different types, to complement her many different style moods.

You can take this theme into your life today by choosing a fresh flower that speaks to your mood and outfit. Flowers not only represent states and countries, they also have a nonverbal language and certain aromatherapeutic qualities that may send both an outward cue and a bit of inward therapy.

If you are in need of balance or love, choose a red rose or a red chrysanthemum for your hair. On the days you might be dressed modestly, a classic violet is the perfect accent of flora. And don't forget to rev up hot nights with the help of the exotic ylang-ylang flower or a traditional carnation, which are said to be aphrodisiacs.

The one flower you don't want in your hair for any reason is an artificial one, unless, of course, you are on a date with a sexy mannequin.

JULY 26 | BUILD AN OUTFIT AROUND A CRISP WHITE SHIRT FOR A CLEAN AND STATELY LOOK ALL DAY LONG.

Ah, the white shirt! Clean, fresh, pure. It's a simple measure that makes a powerful style statement. A bright, solid white shirt, regardless of the material, is like a blank canvas—it offers limitless possibilities.

When you put on a white shirt, whether it's a luxurious silk blouse, a perfectly pressed combed cotton button-down, or the simplest short-sleeved T-shirt, you are creating a well-lit stage for your face and hair. White attracts light and gently reflects brightness onto whatever is nearby. It also transmits a gentle glow that makes you a standout.

There are no bounds when selecting the perfect bottom to complement the perfect white top. Keep it simple and classic, à la Katharine Hepburn, by matching it with finely tailored pants in any color. Or strike a more feminine note by wearing it with a knee-length black pencil skirt or camel-colored A-line skirt. Use a white shirt to top off a sexy pair of dark jeans and don't forget to add a fun belt for a wink of personality. For an evening look with a chic twist, take red carpet wonder Sharon Stone's cue: pair a man-tailored white dress shirt, unbuttoned to your "sexy place," with a luxurious floor-length skirt that falls with dramatic flair. Now you are talking maximum impact with minimum effort!

Keep your white shirts impeccable by carefully following the cleaning instructions on the label. And don't rely on just one or two to get you through. Invest in several quality versions in different styles so you can pluck one from your closet as effortlessly as a Kleenex at any moment to help you shine a little brighter.

JULY 27 | MAKE THE BEST USE OF CANDLELIGHT.

Stuff happens, such as windstorms as you walk out your door in perfectly coiffed hair, bright lights that shine through your skirts offering a glimpse of your most private areas, and the ultimate, trendy black lights in hip establishments that reveal every microscopic fiber of lint on your person. However, stepping into candlelight can be a woman's best friend if you know how to work it.

DO A CANDLE SHIFT

When seated at a candlelit dinner table, shift the candle away to the table's center so that your face receives just a hint of an all-over glow! Never sit directly above a lit candle. When leaning in on smaller bistro tables, your chin can be positioned directly atop the candle's flame, creating a ghoulish glow to your eyes and cheekbones. Not sexy.

GET MOUTHY!

Choose lipstick or gloss that incorporates shimmer. Matte lips or Chap Stick may be your thing by day, but step out with a nighttime lip that has a glistened finish to maximize a candlelit glow.

BE SHEEN *AND* HEARD

Select a top that has a sexy sheen, not an overt shine. Don a matte satin blouse that has understated twinkle for the most elegant effect.

RIGHT TO BARE ARMS

If the room is warm enough, go with bare arms and rub an extra layer of light moisturizing oil on your arms so that the warm light has a place to reflect. For added impact, incorporate a touch of fine body shimmer. Be careful of large specks of glitter unless you are in Vegas. And even there less is more.

JULY 28 | TAKE AN EXPERT STYLE CUE FROM NAIMA TURNER, A NOTED NEW YORK PERSONAL SHOPPER/STYLIST.

Has a typical day of shopping changed over the years?

Today, women lack the time to really shop due to their busy careers, family demands, social obligations, charitable endeavors, workout commitments—you name it. The challenge is to find the time to do something that was once considered a luxury but has become a chore. This is where someone like myself comes in to help out. Most women shop today for one of two reasons: pure pleasure or necessity. For me, it is my first love and my career. And what a fun one at that!

What is the most interesting thing you've learned over the years about women shoppers?

There are distinctly different types of women shoppers. I counted four personas over the years:

Browsers: There are women who just browse, uncertain of what to purchase. They tend to be impulsive shoppers. Sometimes (not all the time) this woman's style comes off a bit thrown together and even bit unkempt, depending on the day.

Loyalists: Then there is the woman who is a hard-core brand loyalist and only shops and purchases "big labels" for a number of reasons. Possibly to define status, to keep up with the trends she reads about, etcetera. Women who purchase luxury items often do so with one of the best-kept secrets in mind when it comes to shopping and building a wardrobe: consignment shops. She often looks polished, or a bit overdone, and hasn't minded paying top dollar to do so.

Sharpshooters: There is also the woman who shops and knows exactly what she wants and often appears pulled together. Her style is well-defined. She is a woman who enjoys shopping alone, without her friends, and has developed her own style confidence. She's mentally focused before heading to any store and is not shopping on impulse.

Party shoppers: Ever hear of party shoppers? Well, women who shop with their friends because they want trusted opinions before making purchases are what I have come to call party shoppers. Sometimes their friends actually decide for them; they have yet to develop their own style and/or confidence to shop on their own.

JULY 29 | GO SILK.

Remember the look of the silk blouses worn by Oscar winner Faye Dunaway in the 1976 film *Network*, where she portrayed the driven and often amoral TV programmer Diane Christensen?

Even thirty years later, you'll see the silk blouse in jewel tones with a bowlike sash tie at the neck, or a gold or silver flared-collar stunner that fits the bustline on any given runway each season. Why? Because the idea of the tailored silk blouse offers a dose of power, balanced with the perfect hint of femininity and frailness in its fabric and languished posture.

Marry the top with pants or a skirt that has an obvious modernity such as slim cigarette pants, or pencil skirts—even slouchy, boyfriend-cut jeans keep the look in the here and now.

JULY 30 | SHOP BY STYLE, AND NOT ALWAYS BY NAME. LEARN HOW TO FIND YOUR FASHION FIX AT TIFFANY'S OR TARGET.

Smart shoppers know to take a garment at face value before ever looking inside to see the label.

Status shoppers might be shocked to know that top designers take the same approach when creating expensive clothes for any given season. They shop the vintage stores, thrift shops, swap meets, and even off-the-beaten-path yard sales to find great ideas that will inspire designs that are unique and fresh. On goes their label, and a new designer trend is born.

As an educated and stylish consumer, you can have the same power by reconditioning yourself to shop like a designer—high, low, and all in between—looking first at the idea of the garment, then at the quality (or condition if vintage), next at the price, and lastly at the label.

You will find yourself shopping in some of the most unlikely of places that lack the cachet of high-end stores, but don't be surprised if you bump into a few other stylish women browsing right along with you.

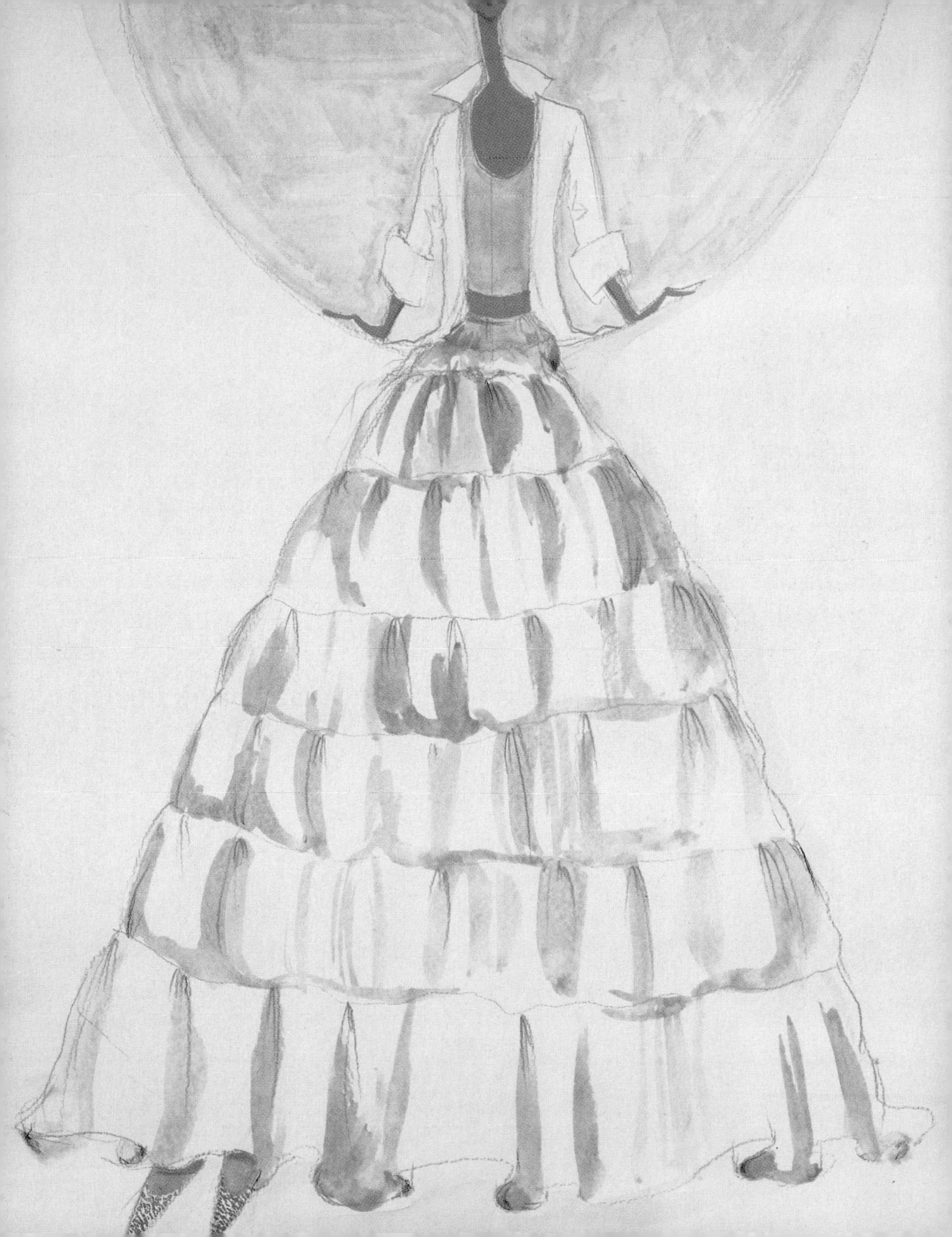

JULY 31 | CREATE YOUR OWN VERSION OF THIS SUREFIRE, STYLISH OUTFIT COMBINATION.

The beauty of what is traditionally the hottest month of the summer is the fact that everything (and everyone) is usually a bit more relaxed. So prim and proper clothes take a backseat and everyone seems to understand.

Gauzy cottons, naturally wrinkled linens, and crepelike silk chiffons are amazing fabric choices for fun bohemian tops and loose skirts that can just be rolled up into a suitcase—and look just as chic when you whip them out and toss them on sans pressing. All you need is a versatile swimsuit that can do double duty as clothing—and your look is created in no time flat.

Look in your closet and try to match this style equation as best as you can with what you have. Don't worry if the items you own aren't an exact match. Within this template, choose your own colors and details. Getting the look not so letter perfect gives it a hint of your personal style, which is always better than a carbon copy:

Top: Tankini swimsuit top
Bottom: Floor-length peasant skirt in a crinkled fabric; tankini swimsuit bottom
Shoes: Flat sandals with sparkle
Accessories: Colorful straw bag; festive dangling earrings; anklet
Flex Piece: White button-down shirt in cotton or linen (for cool nights)

AUGUST

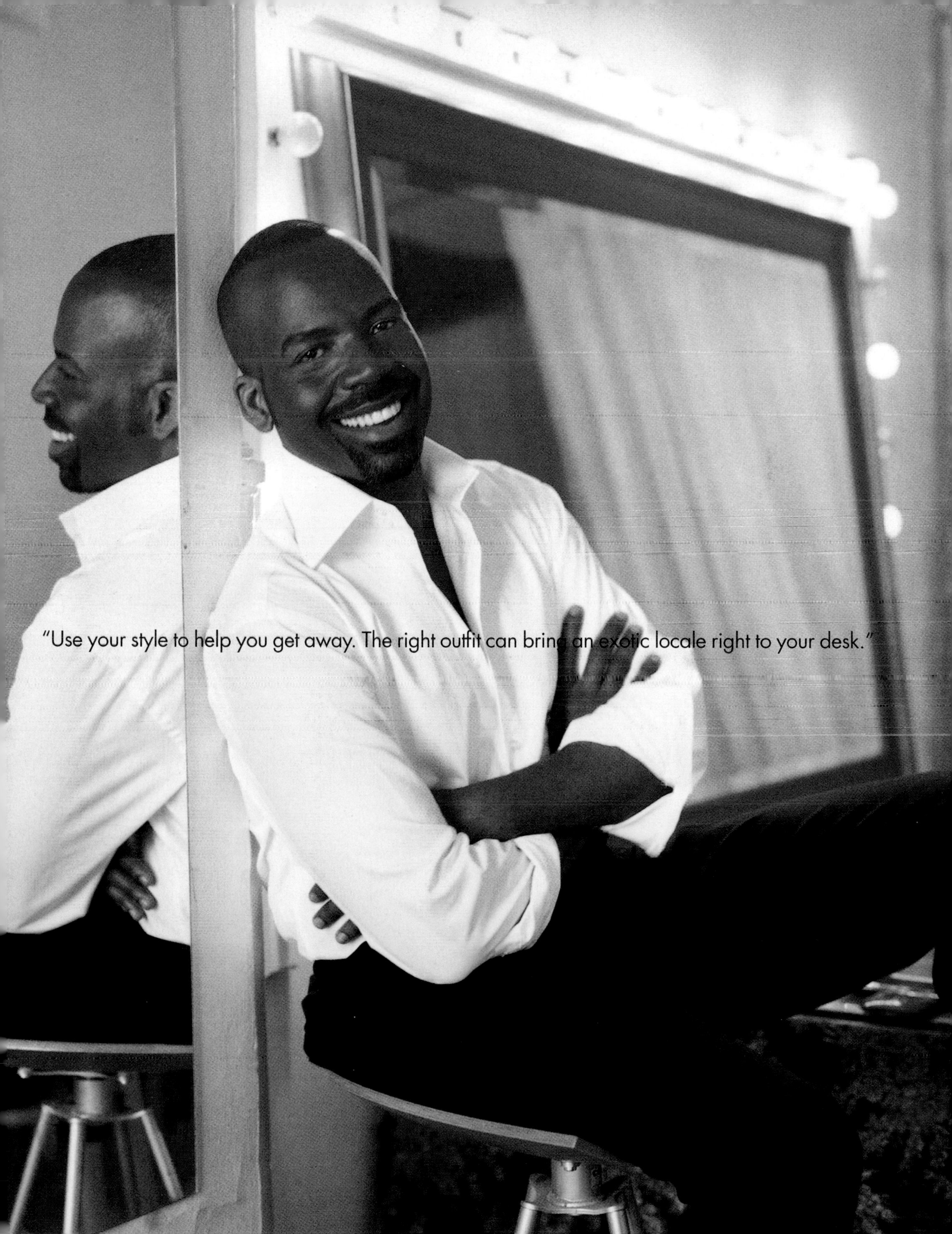
"Use your style to help you get away. The right outfit can bring an exotic locale right to your desk."

AUGUST 1 | BACK TO "COOL."

Remember back-to-school shopping trips?

The fact that everything you wore and carried as the school year began was brand spanking new somehow lessened the blow that the end of summer had come. What genius marketing all around!

Why not approach the fall feeling as fresh as you did with your new "school clothes," sharpened pencils, and crisp, blank composition notebooks? Think of it as getting geared up for business and going back to "cool."

Do an evaluation and edit of your fall clothes. Remove thirty "has-beens" from your closets and drawers. Get yourself in order. Toss out tattered undergarments, check for moth holes in your woolen wear, examine the soles of your business shoes, check whites under bright natural light for dullness, and, most important, try on tailored bottoms to ensure proper fit *before* you have to put them on in a hurry.

Affirmation:
In the spirit of back-to-school shopping excitement, I will edit my existing fall clothing each day and create fun outfits that make the coming season less of a downer.

AUGUST 2 | TAKE AN EXPERT STYLE CUE FROM KAREN KOZLOWSKI, A TOP NEW YORK STYLE-MAKER AND FASHION DIRECTOR OF *REAL SIMPLE* MAGAZINE.

What is your best-kept personal style secret?
I spend money on classic pieces that are good quality and breathe new life into them each season by styling them with more of-the-moment accessories such as belts, shoes, jewelry, handbags, and jackets.

What are the three fashion essentials every well-dressed woman should own?
The best-quality black suit you can afford, a neutral-colored cashmere sweater—turtle- or crewneck—and a simple black shift dress. All of these are timeless pieces that can be worn at least three seasons and can be dressed up or down, and updated with a simple switch of accessories.

What are the biggest mistakes women make when getting dressed?
Wearing clothes that don't fit properly. A size eight in one brand is not necessarily going to be the same in another. And different styles can fit differently as well. So try everything on and if you're between sizes, consider taking the garment to a tailor who can fit it correctly.

Who is the most stylish woman in existence, in your opinion? And what do you appreciate about her look?
Katharine Hepburn, because she made trousers fashionable, chic, and sexy for women, and like all truly stylish people she made getting dressed look effortless.

If you could whisper a fail-safe style tip into the ears of women everywhere, without them feeling bad by hearing it, what would it be?
Stop trying to cover perceived body flaws with ill-fitting clothing. Of course nothing looks good on everyone, but there are cuts and styles of clothing that work with everyone's particular body shapes. And it's all about using color, pattern, and proportion to give you the most streamlined, flattering silhouette. Don't hide under oversized clothing—embellish and embrace your shape!

AUGUST 3 | REMEMBER WHO YOU WERE *BEFORE* YOU BECAME A MOM.

Be among the moms out there who still care about looking stylish or encourage a friend or family member. So many women raising children just let them take over, allowing their style to quickly head south. Totally understandable. But you don't have to go out like that. Looking to vintage classics is a great way to get fresh head-to-toe style on a family budget.

WEEKEND (FOR AROUND $75)

Two contrasting colorful solid tank tops worn together + Thrift store 1970s dark rinse designer jeans + Large faux-gold hoop earrings and rubber thong sandals
= Sassy Soccer Mom

EVENING (FOR AROUND $125)

Basic white men's button-down dress shirt, tied at front, collar up + Pastel ball gown skirt (altered from that old bridesmaid's gown) + Authentic pink ballet flats (from a local dancewear store) + Vintage clutch, sparkly brooch, and earrings
= Mama Mia!

DATE NIGHT (FOR AROUND $200)

Vintage little black dress and a few alterations + Strappy high heels and bare legs + Single strand of faux pearls and classic red lips
= Madison Avenue Mommy

AUGUST 4 | TAKE JUST ABOUT ANY OUTFIT TO A HIGH GLAMOUR.

The smallest accessory can be the simplest style trick to turn your entire outfit around, making it appear more glamorous and sophisticated. Wear a quiet strand of pearls and make a little sheath dress speak louder. Toss on a sparkly, vintage brooch with jeans and a blazer and add a grown-up edge to a casual pairing. And greater than any of these, put on a pair of big, dark sunglasses. Most celebrities wear them for a bit of privacy and anonymity. (But they probably draw more attention to them than less.) What a pair of hip shades can do is make you look stylish.

Start sporting yours at this very moment with anything you plan on wearing today, the same way former first lady and style legend Jacqueline Onassis did. It was never about reserving them for glitzy outfits and fabulous events. She was known for simply walking into her post–first lady life as book editor wearing a simple cashmere sweater, trousers, and her signature big, dark sunglasses, which have come to be known as "Jackie O's." Those dark frames added a shot of unexpected elegance to her basic work clothes so she looked like a movie star.

If you are lucky enough to see a celebrity walking confidently past you in her well-appointed outfit, boasting beautifully styled hair, a perfect handbag, and her own big, dark sunglasses, just drop yours slightly and give her a wink. She'll be shocked to realize that you weren't who she thought you were either.

AUGUST 5 | TRY DRESSING FROM YOUR HEAD, NOT YOUR HEART.

Create a smart ensemble that you would want to see coming into a room. Some women are emotional dressers, point-blank. Their lives are marked by fashion in a way most men would never imagine. Many can tell you the color name of the lipstick they wore at their junior prom, the designer of the dress they donned on the night their husband proposed, and the first pair of work pumps they invested in—and the amount of hours they could wear them.

Yes, you may have worn those pants on your first date with the love of your life, but look at them now for what they are, and ask if they flatter your bottom half. Choose a top for its swooning factor—and not swoons from you because it reminds you of your sassy aunt's wardrobe from years gone by, but because it makes onlookers wonder if you were ever a model. And step into shoes that say "I have arrived." And this may mean passing over your most comfortable shoes and selecting the entrance-makers that look fierce for less time, but look like you've "arrived" in a limo versus mass transit and a hike. This is dressing from your *head*. Shelving what feels warm and fuzzy, and unearthing what registers as worldly and fabulous.

Here is a simple mantra for the moment of truth: Be still my beating heart. Be stunning my head-strong outfit!

AUGUST 6 | GO VINTAGE WITH YOUR BAG.

Thrift shops and vintage clothing stores are hotbeds for designers who are looking to get "inspired" to create new accessories. Why not grab an original as a designer would for a fraction of what a new status bag would cost (real or fake), and have a good chance of never seeing it on another woman's arm. Allow your new bag to really shine by pairing it with a simple solid outfit.

Since you probably will pay much less than you ever imagined, use some of the difference to have it refurbished at a shoe and bag repair shop. They can do almost anything. Seams and stitching can be reinforced, leather and suede can be cleaned, and beads can usually be replaced to perfection.

AUGUST 7 | GIVE YOUR CLOTHES THE "WHIFF TEST" FOR FRESHNESS.

One of my favorite Hollywood actors, Sidney Poitier, once told a story of how, in his humble family beginnings, his mother taught him very early on that "there is no shame in what you wear as long as it is clean." It is a simple but powerful lesson that applies to everyone, even the most stylish people with the finest of clothing. Appearing and, more important, smelling fresh and clean is a valuable statement of self-respect and respect to others—strangers or not.

Use this trick for any day you need extended freshness. Start by skipping your perfume. Instead, apply a fabric refresher spray directly to your clothing, especially the neck and shoulders (where embraces are received), and underarms, of course.

Clothes can be clean but still collect smells from simply hanging in the closet. And although refresher products are available in everything from citrus to lavender, the clean, just-laundered scent is always the best. When used as directed, you can spray generously and deep! Keep one in the office for unnerving power meetings and one at home for odors from pets, food, smoke, and plain old closet staleness.

AUGUST 8 | RETIRE YOUR BACKPACK.

Whether a mom, busy professional, or urban dweller, use your backpack only for hiking trips. This is the one accessory that does take me to the edge, especially when I see it on an adult woman who otherwise looks modern, stylish, and fresh: the academic backpack. You know the one. Two heavy padded straps constructed in what looks to be bulletproof nylon, anchored to a loaflike compartment boasting multiple zippers, and lumps that trace the outline of God knows what! Other strange adjustable straps dangle from the lower portion of the bag, and locker loops usually pop out of the top for when it is time to hang it up. Well, guess what, oh backpacked sisters out there. Today is the day to suspend it from a hook permanently! I beg of you.

Besides the unhealthy amount of stress, weight, and pressure on your spine, when heavily packed, the backpack is a heinous interruption to the drape of your clothing, casual or otherwise.

The straps wrinkle clothing and cause bunching right near the bustline, the bag portion blocks the majority of your back, and for some petite women it obstructs the view to an otherwise gorgeous derrière. They're also difficult to remove in a ladylike manner. A classic tote bag will do the same job and not compromise your look. Be sure not to overpack any bag you carry and alternate sides.

AUGUST 9 | TAKE AN EXPERT STYLE CUE FROM ANNA SUI, A TOP NEW YORK DESIGNER.

What is your best-kept personal style secret?
When you find what works for you, stick with it (bangs, red lipstick, etc.).

What are the three fashion essentials every well-dressed woman should own?
1. A great coat. During the winter, you don't remove your coat at a lot of the places that you go. So the only thing people see is your coat.
2. Great boots. They always make the outfit cooler.
3. A great handbag. It tells so much about you.

Who is the most stylish woman in existence, in your opinion? And what do you appreciate about her look?
Diana Vreeland and Marilyn Monroe. They both had their looks down.

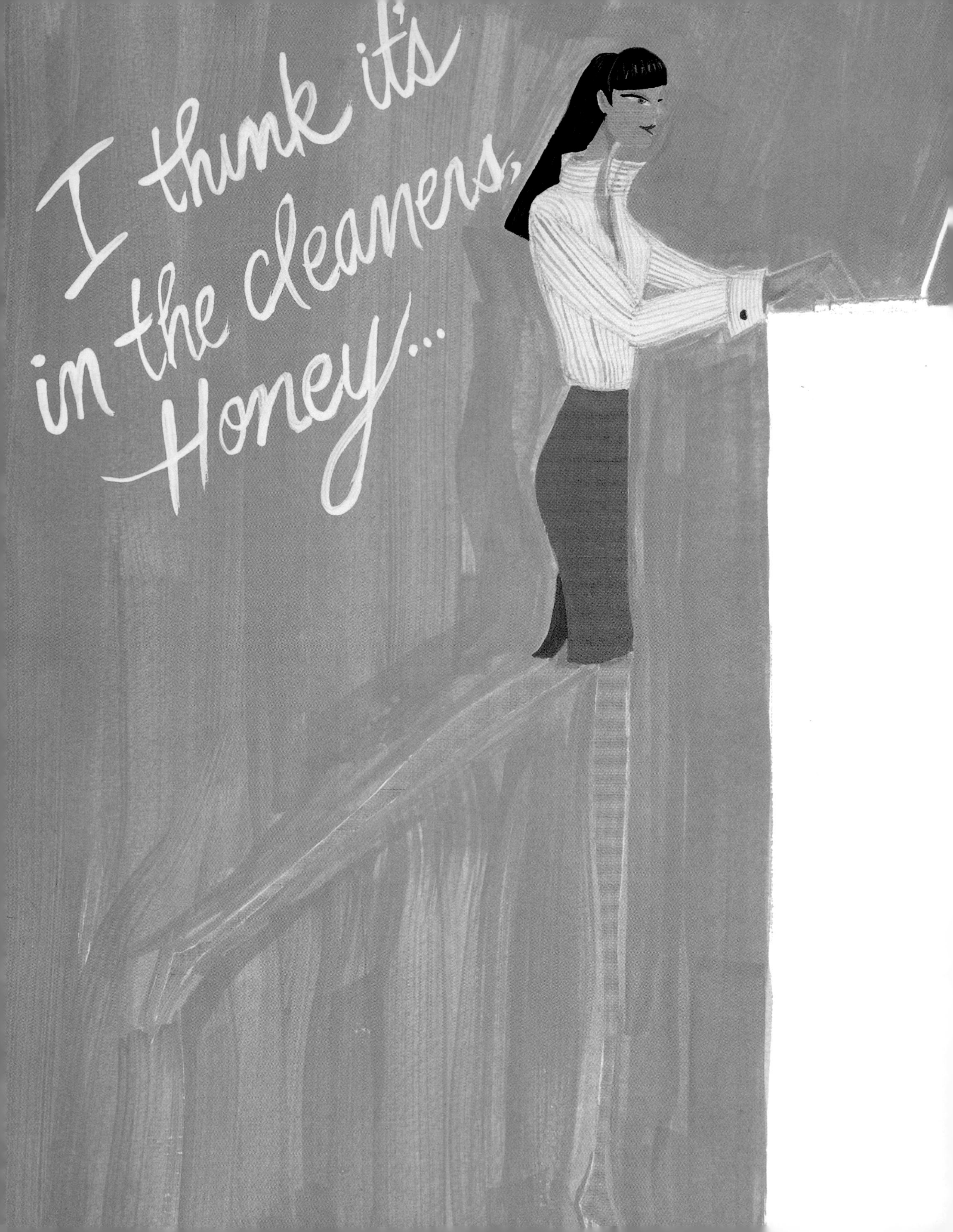

I think it's in the cleaners, Honey...

AUGUST 10 | GIVE YOURSELF A TOUCH OF MENSWEAR MIXED IN WITH YOUR LOOK TO CREATE A STRONGER AND SEXIER STYLE VIBE.

You don't have to look mannish when donning a bit of menswear. In fact, you can look your sexiest ever. You might have a man in your home who has a closet full of style treasures you can play with, or you may have to hit the stores, especially the vintage shops, to grab a few pieces to get started. Know that the mood can be achieved with the help of just a simple men's necktie. Even a thrift-store special.

Give a nod to man-tailored chic with one of the following easy-to-do style combinations and watch all the girls swoon:

Your Sexy Jeans + His Bold Necktie as Belt + Your Basic Tank + Your Hot Heels

= He's Always Around Me

His Striped Dress Shirt + Your Slim Solid Skirt + His Cuff Links + Your Sling-backs

= His Boss Lady

Your "Power" Suit Pants + His Suit Vest, Cinched + Your Fitted T-shirt + Your Flats

= She's Fully Vested

AUGUST 11 | LEARN A NEW FASHION TERM.

Lariat necklace • *Long strand of beads or metal, sometimes ending in tassels, that is not fastened by a clasp. Worn looped into a knot or with a slide so that the two ends hang free.*

Accessories speak volumes about your mood and desired style message, especially jewelry. Take necklaces for instance. Some nights an oftentimes matronly string of pearls won't have the sexy impact that you need atop a dress that celebrates your cleavage, your gold pendant looks like you've had it since your sweet sixteen, and that chunky jewelry of-the-moment is a little too island-chic for a night out on the town.

What you need is a necklace with vertical thrust to the eye that keeps all eyes on your curvy perfection. Enter the lariat necklace. I've heard it called the "bolo," "that snake necklace," or, my favorite, the "lasso." The lariat is a great way to complement a top or dress that features a V-neck, a plunging neckline, or a deep-cut wrap opening, as the shape of a traditional lariat falls along the same shape gently over the chest.

Although first made popular by 1920s flappers, this clasp-free necklace comes around every couple of years, sexily looping around the neck like a choker and draping down either your front or back. It is also the perfect accessory for a backless or strapless gown. The look most recently crested in the late 1990s with the rebirth of the Gucci label à la designer Tom Ford. And regardless of who designs the lariat you choose for your accessory collection, now you'll at least know what it's called when an admirer asks, and they will.

AUGUST 12 | NO PANTY HOSE WITH OPEN TOES.

The sidewalks are melting, summer is at a rapid boil, and you've got a dress-up occasion ahead. Your dress is light and effortless, your bag is sweet and charming, hair done, makeup perfectly applied, and your favorite open-toe heels await. Don't spoil them by wearing hose.

For some more mature women, wearing hosiery is linked to respect for select environments—for example, church. Many women wouldn't think of stepping barefoot into any house of worship, traditional business, or elegant restaurant.

The truth is, many houses of worship these days are just happy to have bodies present, in stockings or not. Some traditional businesses now bend the rules in favor of a woman's right to shoes without hose. And elegant restaurants, especially in big cities or hip downtown areas, are more concerned with their clients from the waist up, for that is all most other patrons will see between courses anyway.

AUGUST 13 | HAPPY BIRTHDAY, LUCY STONE.

Lucy Stone is known to women's "herstory" as a suffragist and women's rights activist in the 1800s and as a proud abolitionist. She was also the first woman to retain her own name after marriage.

By mutual agreement with her man, Henry Blackwell, she kept her maiden name when they married in 1855. Honor her tenacity by taking a look at the impact of your marriage, or your relationship. Look at photos of yourself before and after marriage. Do you like what you see? Have you continued to express the style that is authentic to you? Maybe there is something that you've gotten out of the habit of doing—such as wearing flirty dresses that could jazz up your appearance. You might find your mood and your partner's libido lifted by reaching inside to the woman you once were.

AUGUST 14 | TRY ADDING A PAISLEY PRINT WHILE POLICING YOURSELF ON THE PERFECT WAY TO DO IT.

Fall is ahead and there is one classic print that you should bring along when you meet it: paisley.

The 1980s were a heyday for this allover print featuring a motif shaped like the side of the curved hand with a curved little finger attached (similar to a teardrop with a curly, curved top). Most paisley prints feature rich, warm fall colors with bold shapes outlined in delicate tracery and swirls. The paisley print is of Persian origin, yet was popularized in Paisley, Scotland (thus the name), where the first paisley shawls were introduced two hundred years ago. The print has remained a cornerstone of traditional American sportswear, curving its way in and out of style every few seasons.

THREE WAYS TO ALWAYS LOOK STYLISH IN PAISLEY PRINTS

- Paisley prints don't have to be stiff and conservative. Take them to a "rock and roll" space by choosing them on velvet, velour, and satin items to add funk and edge.

- Because the print can be rigid and somewhat "busy" in its intricate and ornate design, keep the shapes of the clothes simple. For instance, avoid ruffle-front tops in paisley, unless you want to be Jimi Hendrix!

- Opt for accessories in paisley prints if you don't want to go full throttle. Satchels, boots with paisley trim, skinny belts, and even a pair of fashion gloves can be just enough to make the print pop. Less can mean more impact.

AUGUST 15 | GET TEN-MINUTE STYLE FOR A "GIRLS' NIGHT OUT."

There is something quite empowering about a group of women hanging in a pack, different flavors, all serving up major style!

Here is a great ten-minute style solution for any "girls' night out":

Minutes 1:00–2:00:
Pull out the top that makes you feel like shooting a music video. One shoulder, strapless, a fitted button-down, or even just a solid black tank.

Minutes 3:00–4:00:
Go fun on the bottom! Skirts with flair, cropped pants that show off your ankles, "skinny jeans" in dark blue or white, or even a quirky island print wrap skirt.

Minutes 5:00–6:00:
Girls notice shoes, so go for broke. Push that two-hour stiletto to four hours, just for the night. High-heeled wedges, metallics, barely there nude high-heeled sandals—you get it!

Minutes 7:00–8:00:
Ditch the work handbag without question. Dust off any sparkly evening bag that is normally too dressy for jeans—this is the one to put in the mix just for tonight.

Minutes 9:00–10:00:
Go for makeup that procures second looks. Think sixties sex kitten: nude, glossed lips; full bold lashes; smoky eyes; and faint baby doll blush—there will be no velvet ropes in your way!

AUGUST 16 | POP STYLE QUIZ.

1. Which accessories should never touch each other?

A. Watch and shoes
B. Necklace and earrings
C. Belt and hat
D. Shrug and leg warmers

2. Which designer is commonly known as the "master of the dress"?

A. John Lobb
B. Thomas Pink
C. Valentino
D. Brioni

3. Which versatile jean color will take you from day to night and casual to hip?

A. The darkest blue wash
B. A blue acid wash
C. Chic, "dirty" denim
D. Mango

4. Which trendy clothing item nickname is better off removed from every woman's fashion vernacular?

A. Wonderbra
B. Wife beater
C. My "skinny" jeans
D. None of the above

(Answers: 1-B, 2-A, 3-C, 4-B)

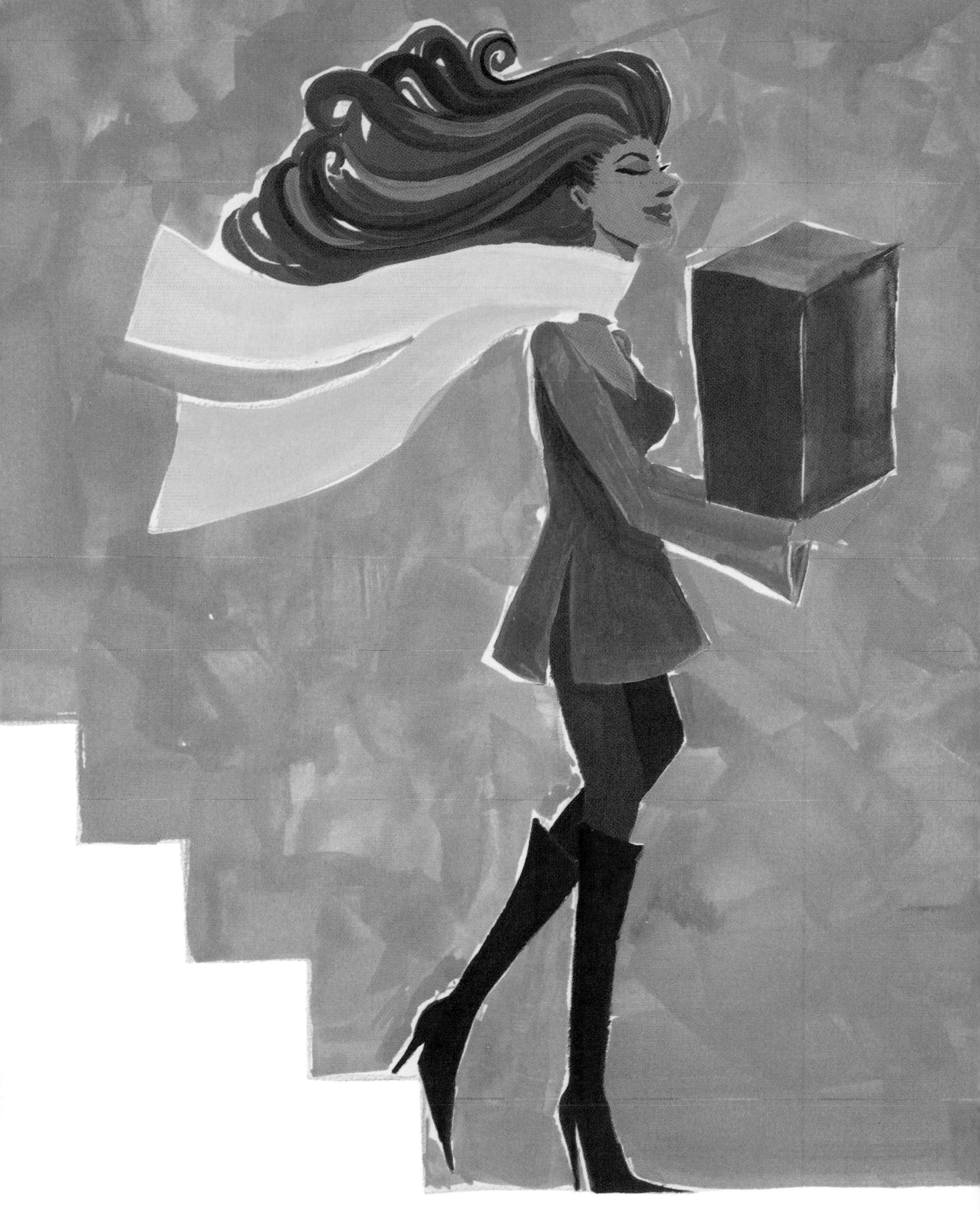

AUGUST 17

FILL AT LEAST ONE BOX WITH DONATIONS FOR A CLOTHING CHARITY—IT WILL FREE SPACE IN YOUR CLOSET AND HELP YOU CREATE EVEN STRONGER OUTFITS.

"Give and you shall receive" is what my mother always taught me. It may sound simple and silly to some, but the lesson is as essential to our existence as air, water, and of course, clothing. Some think of it as karma.

When looking at your closet today, choose one garment and ask yourself, "Have I worn this in the past year?" If your answer is no, let it go. You might just be opening up a new possibility for yourself and a person ready to work that garment now.

AUGUST 18 | SHOW OFF YOUR NATURAL SUN-KISSED GLOW BY WEARING WHITE.

High fashion in the late 1800s valued alabaster skin. A powdery white complexion denoted a woman of advantaged status, not that of a lowly sun-darkened field laborer. My, how times have changed.

A healthy, sun-kissed glow is de rigueur for the modern woman of style. The look speaks of wealth, travel, and exotic getaways whether you got the look in Tahiti or from a bottle at Target. Top designer Michael Kors believes that "a tan makes you feel skinnier, just like wearing dark clothes does." Make the most of it, especially this time of the year. Use these three tricks to maximize your sunny side.

SHOULDER UP

One of the most underrated sexy areas of a woman's body are the shoulders. They are the one area that usually looks great no matter what your size, height, or shape. Like your face, they catch the sun first and show off the results to the very end. So go strapless, or spaghetti-strapped, and let them glow!

WEAR WHITE

As much as you can, as long as you can, wear white. It reflects light onto your body and contrasts a (hopefully) lighter tone against your toasty one, making you appear even more bronzed.

EASED-UP MAKEUP

Sunny complexions can sometimes mean more even ones. Try to forgo heavy foundations and dark lip colors that can lessen your honey-dipped sheen. A moisturizer, a touch of lip gloss, lets you use the rest of that mirror time to show it off.

AUGUST 19 | INCORPORATE A DAZZLING EVENING SCARF INTO YOUR LOOK—EVEN IF IT'S THE MIDDLE OF THE DAY.

The house of Prada, the Italian label run by design genius Miucca Prada, has reinvented the way modern women dress by confidently mixing clothes and accessories traditionally kept back for evening with flirty, sporty daytime wear. And the characters on the hit series *Sex and the City* followed suit, wearing much of the actual Prada collection and matching the sensibility with the help of noted costume designer and New York style icon Patricia Field. Think of how Carrie Bradshaw had absolutely no qualms about hitting Gotham's busiest avenues, mid–business day, sporting a pink ballerina tutu on her way to lunch with her best friends.

The spirit of these characters and design label should inspire a certain freedom in you. Start small and grab your favorite evening scarf. Snatch it from behind your formal clothes and let it see daylight.

Use this moment to bring out your most fantastical evening scarves in metallic silk organza, pastel featherweight cashmere, beaded silk chiffon—you name it. Tie it atop a serious pinstriped business suit, knot it onto the handle of your work tote, make it a belt for your jeans and white button-down shirt combination. Think of it as a basic and incorporate it fully into your wardrobe.

The look speaks of style confidence that you cannot buy. It is not about *SIC* or Prada, it is all about living and expressing your mood whenever you want to, regardless of fashion dictates.

AUGUST 20 | STOCK YOUR TINY GLOVE COMPARTMENT WITH THESE TEN ITEMS TO GIVE YOU QUICK, BIG MAKEOVERS, FROM CLEAR POLISH TO BREATH MINTS.

License, registration, and insurance, ma'am? Sure, you have all three, but do you have style insurance handy?

You'd be amazed at how much makeover magic a tiny glove compartment can hold, helping you in a pinch better than AAA ever could. I rank a few travel-sized style and beauty basics that are essential when hitting the road. In this order, stock the following items in your car's locked glove compartment. They should all fit in one plastic sandwich bag.

Lipstick—A blushy nude shade that works with anything you have on.
$50 in cash—If you don't have the accessory you need, you can just whisk off and buy it.
Breath mints—Fresh breath is the international symbol of good manners and respect.
Hair band—Even when clothes fail, create a tight chignon and look instantly pulled together!
Earrings—A chunky pair of bold faux diamonds can give you instant sparkle.
Fragrance—Keep one that smells similar to a clean bar of soap, thus the hidden intent.
Nail polish remover towelettes—A clean bare nail look will always outshine a chipped coat of polish.
Clear nail polish—Hey, if you've got the time, strip all ten and shine them up. Killing time when arriving early never felt so productive!
Emery board—Shape is everything. Leave the "jagged edge" to Glenn Close.
Costume jewelry necklace—A fun, inexpensive one that you don't really care if you lose, from faux pearls to a cool pendant, if it makes you smile and feel better, you'll look better.

AUGUST 21 | DO THE *NEW* FASHION MATH.

Say you are longing for a power business skirt suit costing $750. The year-round fabric, shape, color, and pattern are classic and you'll wear it ten years from now with no concern. Simply take two years just to be modest and consider the number of wearings you'll get. Within the 104 weeks, you might wear it every other week together, and a few times as separates. Maybe 75 wears all-in-all. If you divide that whopping $750 quality suit by 75 wears, you are really only paying $10 per wear for a suit that may have the power to seal million-dollar deals. Basically, a little more than the cost of a take-out lunch.

Keep this equation tucked under your wig for the next time you are near tears over a price tag standing between you and a garment that is meant to go home with you. Sometimes you can't afford *not* to buy what you know will continue to get you by.

AUGUST 22 | MAKE SURE YOUR STATIONERY REFLECTS THE STYLISH WOMAN YOU ARE—OR WANT TO BE.

We live in a Post-it world. Who really has time to write and send a thank-you card when you can fire off an e-mail in a fraction of the time? Well, the choice is yours. And the message will be very clear on the receiving end with the decision you make.

Women spend so much time on their hair, nails, clothing, shoes, makeup, undergarments, accessories, and fragrance. Why not on personal stationery, too?

Fine stationery is a vestige of a time gone by, a day when people took the time and care to correspond with a bit of dignity, romance, and style. The paper you chose to write on, the pen you used to write out your thoughts, what you sealed your envelope with (maybe wax), even the stamp you chose to show your personal sensibilities and taste. Just ask your mother.

Style begins and ends with every expression you send out to the world, whether it's on your back, atop your head, on your feet, or from your desk. The treat begins in your quietest moment as you speak on pure linen paper and the texture takes you back, and it ends in the hands of your addressee, reading and *feeling* every word you intended to say. These are things a quick e-mail can never achieve.

AUGUST 23 | HAPPY BIRTHDAY, VIRGO GIRL.

Like the bullish Taurus, you are a true classic. You are the sign of sharing and responsibility, two characteristics that help to make your daily ensembles look accessible and ever appropriate to those around you.

You are not the woman who needs a constant dose of new clothing to be happy. Although sale racks may be tempting, your clear perspective on what really works for your body and budget will always lead you back to shopping for items that will last. For this, you oftentimes don't mind paying full price to ensure that you will get what you set out for to add to your well-organized closet, in your size.

Look at your stylish Virgo counterparts, Greta Garbo and Sophia Loren. Classic women who used the power of the silver screen to create and bolster a timelessly stylish image that still gets raves decades later.

AUGUST 24 | TAKE AN EXPERT STYLE CUE FROM TRACY TAYLOR, A TOP NEW YORK STYLE-MAKER AND FASHION DIRECTOR OF *MARIE CLAIRE*.

What is your best-kept style secret?
I always look in a full-length mirror before I walk out of the house. I'm also a huge fan of lint rollers and hand steamers.

What are the three fashion essentials every well-dressed woman should own?
Black turtleneck, black trousers, chic high-heeled black leather pumps à la Manolo Blahnik or Christian Louboutin. Wear these items together with subtle makeup, groomed hair, and simple classic earrings—diamond studs (not too big) or pearl studs (same) or medium-size hoops—and you will always look chic.

What are the biggest mistakes women make when getting dressed?
Looking like they forgot to take a look in the mirror. Look at your outfit in the mirror through the eyes of someone whose taste you admire. Look at the entire outfit from head to toe as if you were looking at a photograph of yourself from across the street. Proportion, balance, tailoring, cleanliness, and fit are so important! Sometimes it is the smallest and relatively inexpensive details that make a huge difference—like pressing your clothes, proper hems, and maintaining the appearance of leather shoes and handbags.

Who is the most stylish woman in existence, in your opinion? And what do you appreciate about her look?
Jacqueline Onassis was the embodiment of style and taste. Her style followed her throughout her life and always looked timeless. *That* is style. It was effortless. I think what also made her so chic was the way she carried herself—her grace and poise. She was gracious, charming, and had a global sense of what was appropriate without being too conservative. She picked classic pieces and made them her signatures. Those pieces live on today: the Bernardo sandal, white jean, black turtleneck, navy Henley sweater, and big black plastic glasses. These items live on as modern-day classics.

If you could whisper a fail-safe style tip into the ears of women everywhere, without them feeling bad by hearing it, what would it be?
If you look in the mirror and think too much jewelry, take a piece off. If you think an outfit makes you look bigger than you wish you were, it probably does. Wear it if you love it and walk out the door confidently, but don't wear clothes that are too tight, ever!

AUGUST 25 | GO FROM SOCCER MOM TO ROCKER MOM.

Whether it is your minivan, your convertible, or your commuter tote that acts as your mobile corner office, keep it stocked with a few essentials, which will keep you ready for any style crisis that may arise. Here is the short list to long-lasting style:

MAKEUP/BEAUTY

Premoistened face-cleansing pads for a fresh restart to your day

Concealer, lip gloss, mascara, pressed powder, a soft blush, nail polish remover, an emery board, cotton swabs, nude nail polish

ACCESSORIES

A basic jeweled stud or huggy, a dramatic pair of drops, your best pearls

A thin silk scarf in a solid bold color, a thin black belt, a thick belt with attitude

FRAGRANCE

A just-out-of-the-shower scent (think Rain, Cucumber, Lavender, Citrus)

TOTE ESSENTIALS

A knit jersey dress in black—or black pants and solid camel-colored shoulder wrap, rolled into tissue paper

A strapless bra

Nude or black high heels

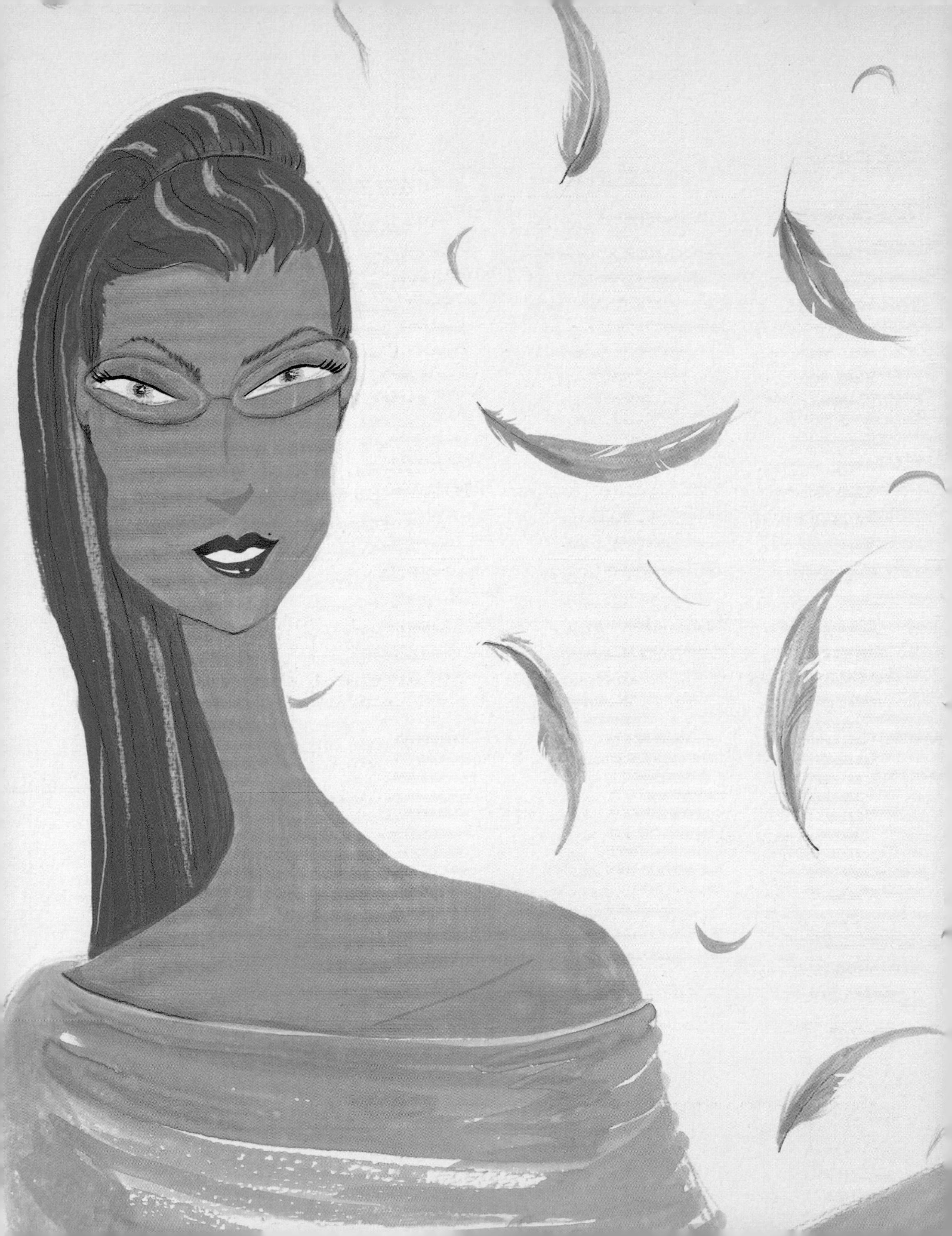

AUGUST 26

REASSESS YOUR EYEWEAR AND BE SURE THAT WHAT YOU ARE WEARING ALLOWS YOU TO PUT YOUR BEST FACE FORWARD.

Eyewear is sometimes the first accessory someone will notice on a woman. So kiss the days of just wearing eyewear for improved vision good-bye. Stylish women today select and feature their eyewear as easily and as consciously as they would a handbag, earrings, or any accessory of the moment.

If you are a woman who wears eyeglasses, either for correctional purposes, sun protection, or simply to mix up your look, keep in mind the proper way to match your frames to the shape of your face. Ten style commandments for choosing the perfect pair for your face:

•If your face is somewhat triangular, opt for frames featuring stronger tops than bottoms, adding the weight to the top of your face, balancing out the rest.

•Generally speaking, your frame size is best when in proportion to the size of your face.

•By and large, your frame shape should contrast with your shape.

•Square-faced women look strongest in frames that soften your angles. Your best choices are narrow frames in the oval family.

•If your face is round, choose narrow or rectangular frames to add the illusion of length to the face.

•If your face is somewhat like an inverted triangle, run to rimless frames in neutrals, which are wider on the bottom, extracting weight from the bottom of your face.

•If you are a diamond-faced girl, try frames that feature detailing or distinctive brow lines; classic cat shapes and rimless styles work as well.

•For impact, use a frame color or accent color to pull out your eye color.

•If your face is oblong, select frames with bold temples and enhanced depth to add the illusion of width to the face.

•Invest in several quality pairs. This is no style area to skimp on. If you are tired of looking at the same pair each day, just think how others might feel.

AUGUST 27 | WEAR AN ARRESTING AND UNLIKELY COLOR TO BRING OUT YOUR COLOR.

Color can evoke distinct moods from a passerby or simply from within. Have you ever taken the time to notice how you feel when you wear a drab color? Or the reaction you have to your favorite color on someone else? The feeling is visceral and sometimes hard to capture and describe, but it definitely exists.

For instance, pink signifies romance, love, and friendship, whereas red-based orange corresponds to desire, romantic passion, pleasure, a little domination, pointed aggression, and a hunger for action—you determine the type.

Light yellow is associated with intellect, freshness, and joy. Aqua is associated with emotional healing and protection, and its little cousin light blue is also associated with healing, as well as health, tranquillity, understanding, and softness.

Be careful when wearing pale purples, for they can evoke romantic and nostalgic feelings—not the best break-up outfit idea.

Stick a toe in the water and pick a color you might never imagine yourself wearing today. One you forgot you had, or maybe a new piece you grabbed on sale just to justify the experiment. Gauge both your internal reactions and those around you. You'll be amazed at how a simple adjustment of your color knob might bring the day's picture into astonishing clarity.

AUGUST 28 | BRING OUT YOUR CURVY FIGURE; GET TO KNOW THE CLASSIC WRAP DRESS.

Resurrect that classic Diane von Furstenberg wrap dress, a timeless silhouette.

Most real women have curves. Beautiful hips. Breasts that actually have volume. Butts that show more flesh than bone. And legs that may not be a mile high but have character and lines that say "woman."

If you are one of those real women who never quite knew what the perfect dress was for her body, your answer may have been under your nose for decades in the wrap dress—a garment that has continually enjoyed its fifteen minutes of fame since the 1970s, in fabrics such as matte jersey and even good old polyester.

Full-busted women should try wrapping one on today. This silhouette can separate your breasts, while giving the illusion of a smaller waist with its tie function that defines it to the eye, thus visually pulling it inward. Another joy is in its adjustability. You can actually enjoy dinner tonight and have an escape hatch if you really can't resist dessert. Also, in the future, if said desserts begin to add up, this is the dress that won't betray you. It will roll with the punches, expanding and decreasing as your body evolves from season to season, year to year—unlike your supermodel counterparts.

AUGUST 29 | TAKE A MOMENT TO LUXURIATE IN A "POWER BATH."

Who has that kind of time? You do! Bathing in relaxed luxury, versus a pounding shower, is the first step to any stylish night on the town, or power day for that matter.

A recent study conducted at Pennsylvania State University found that most people take a shower for an average of nearly eighteen minutes. Imagine how much longer that feels in a warm bath filled with your favorite scented bath gel, natural sponge, and soothing music? Probably more like an hour!

Think about it. You have the bathtub. You keep passing by those bath salts and special soaps that have been wrapped in plastic since this time last year. Why not give them a quick whirl, using just about the exact same time you would to shower. This is how you can pull if off with or without children, a significant other, or a grand Jacuzzi bathtub.

The time it takes to close the drain, turn on the faucet, and add your product of choice is about thirty seconds more than turning on the shower. Do this step before handling another piece of typical preparation for the day, like putting on your coffee. Once you return, your liquid queendom awaits and your average eighteen minutes looks better than ever.

Shut off the phone and step in, knowing that the time spent bathing will help you to mentally unearth the outfit that got you all those compliments in the past. You can prioritize the three most important tasks you'd like to accomplish during the day ahead—and not a single task more. And unlike the dodging water spray of a shower, the gentle waters of your quiet bath caress your entire body all at once, almost doing some of the active legwork of washing for you—thus a little more energy reserved for your entire day.

Taking a shower will never be the same once you know the bath's calming effect is just as easy to come by.

Another bonus: You don't have to wear a shower cap.

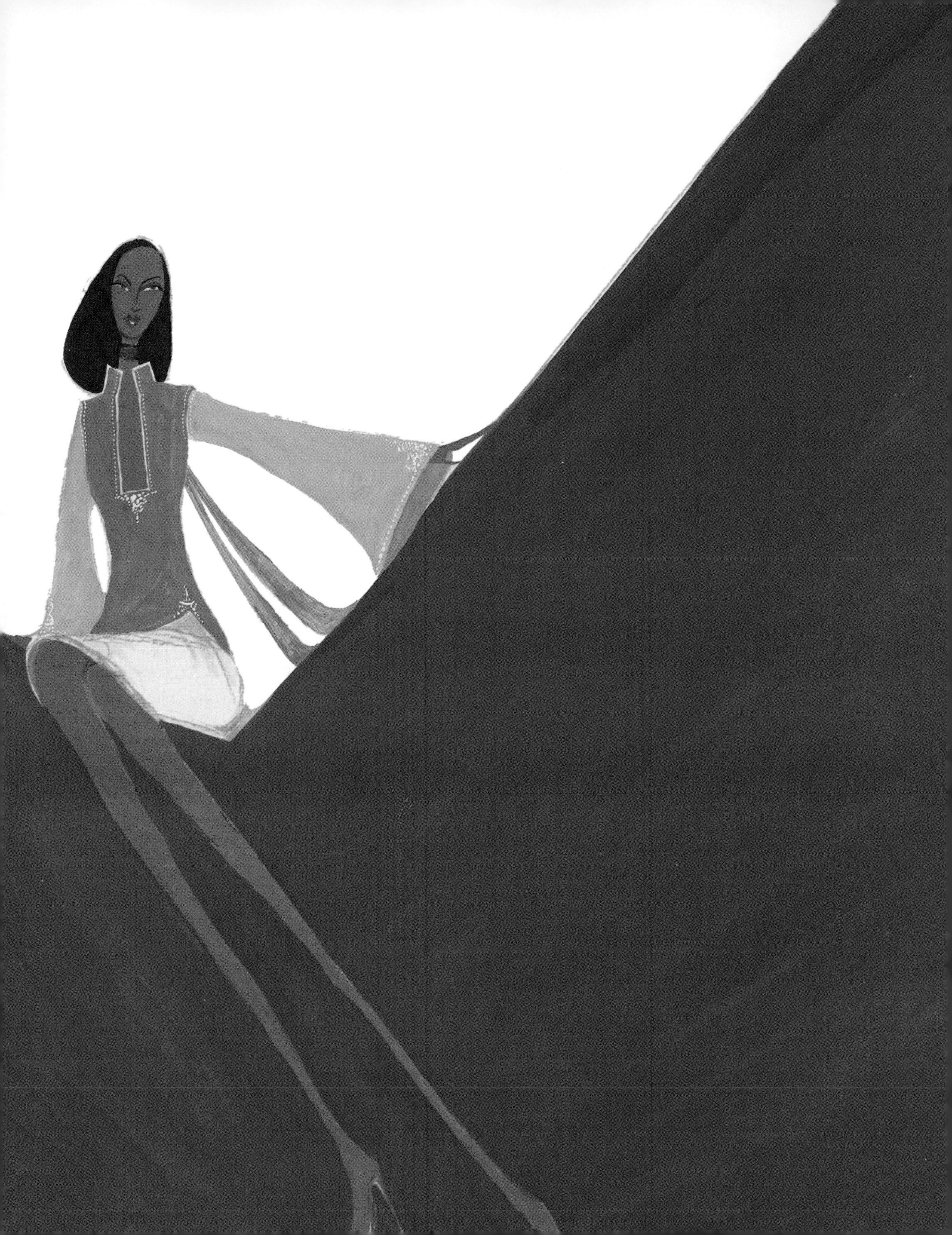

AUGUST 30 | IF YOU ARE A SIZE 8 WHO REALLY FITS BEST IN A SIZE 10—CHOOSE THE SIZE 10.

Ill-fitted garments are one of the biggest, most frequently committed style faux pas. That's because most women instinctively believe in, and shop by, standard sizing numbers. What they don't realize is that these standards are anything but universal when comparing designers, mass brands, and specialty boutique clothing. For instance, you may fit perfectly into a size 8 from the Donna Karan Collection, while it seems you may need a crowbar to slide into the same-sized garment from Banana Republic.

It takes a bit of courage to actually shop for your true size and figure and not by manufacturer numbers. Women have been trained to find validation and pride in remaining a certain size throughout their lives. Try to just let it go!

At the end of the day, your size should remain between you and your clothes. There's a reason those silly little labels are inside. But if you can't bear to see that number at all, just know that you can always cut it out!

AUGUST 31 | CREATE YOUR OWN VERSION OF THIS SUREFIRE, STYLISH OUTFIT COMBINATION AND RUN WITH IT!

Summer is winding down, but your glow is still in effect. Celebrating style diversity can be a fun way to play up your sun goddess hues, yet it can also be tricky if you wear too much from any old faraway land.

The way to balance out the look is by pairing a bold ethnic separate with one that is clearly more conservative, stately, or downright sexy. Each unique piece will play up the other. And it is a quick way to high style, without looking like you are in a costume.

Top: An ethnic print top (Asian, African, Moroccan)
Bottom: Your sexiest dark, fitted skirt
Shoes: A classic high-heeled sandal in a bright color
Accessories: Just diamond studs—stop there!
Flex piece: An extralong thin scarf

SEPTEMBER

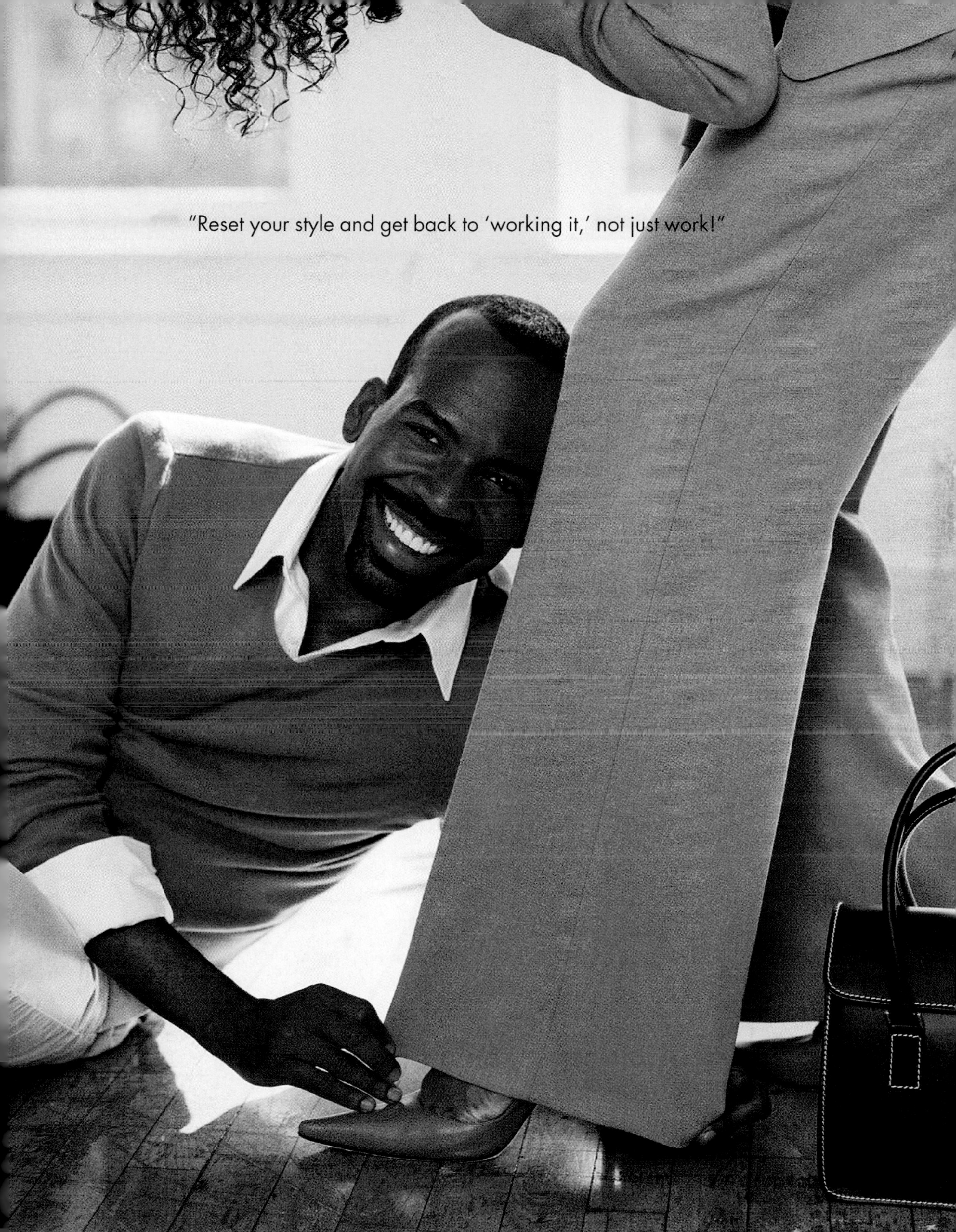

"Reset your style and get back to 'working it,' not just work!"

SEPTEMBER 1

MAKE A FRESH START TO BEAUTY BY EMPTYING YOUR MAKEUP DRAWER, TOSSING THE EXPIRED PRODUCTS, AND ORGANIZING WHAT'S STILL WORTHY OF MEETING YOUR FACE.

Your skin is holding on to the last touches of your summer glow, the cooler weather inspires you to layer and accessorize—unlike those dauntingly hot days of summer when all you wanted to wear where three easy pieces. This time of year is also when a bit more makeup can really unify a fall ensemble.

Most makeup has a shelf life—like other perishables. You may not know it from the packaging or the product itself—changing color and odor as old food would—but the dangers of germ life lurking beneath the surface can spread to your eyes, pores, and mouth, sometimes causing infection.

Pull out every makeup product you own. Try your best to recall when you purchased each item and eliminate the old according to the "freshness dates" below. If you can't recall, look at how worn the packaging is for a hint. If that trick doesn't help, you may as well be on the safe side and simply toss it. Sometimes a lost $10 eye pencil is better than a found $100 eye infection. Time to give your basic makeup areas a face-lift using the this guideline for disposal:

PRODUCT	LIFESPAN
Powder	8 months for a compact; 8 to 12 months for loose powder
Eyeliner	3 to 6 months for liquid; 6 to 12 months for pencil
Eye shadow	3 to 6 months for liquid; 6 to 12 months for powder and cream
Mascara	3 months
Concealer	4 to 6 months for water-based; 6 to 8 months for wax-based
Lipstick	1 year
Foundation	6 to12 months

Affirmation:

I will honor my skin and only apply to it what is good for it.

SEPTEMBER 2 | WEAR YOUR WHITE CLOTHES AND CONTINUE TO DO SO STRAIGHT THROUGH UNTIL NEXT LABOR DAY!

The style dictate that says "never wear white after Labor Day" is a dated notion of old Southern society.

Wearing white was seen as a sign of bad manners because it placed the wearer out of the fold of society's approved standards of dress. There are many reasons why this mandate may have come about—possibly from the idea that white reflects light, making it best for summer.

The late nineteenth century through the 1950s was a time when more people were entering the middle class. When striving, we tend to try harder than those who have already arrived at success. Today, there really are no rules like this for fearless, modern women of style.

So, keep your white clothes in heavy rotation throughout the year if the fabric is appropriate. A crisp white cotton poplin shirt or blouse, a pair of pure white trousers in cotton twill (similar to the weight of a khaki), or the classic bright white jeans can be worn year-round paired with darker colored winter clothes. But cotton voile won't keep you warm enough in most places in America in winter.

A great navy blazer or tweed jacket from your favorite winter suit, paired with eye-popping bleach white pants is a fabulous look. Or, imagine your pristine white shirt, worn beneath your favorite solid autumnal sweater, matched with a great white jean. The white collar, cuffs, and pants create a fresh frame around a shot of rich color. This is graphic simplicity at its best.

Any way you spin it, white has the same modern power of black—just in reverse. It is still a great base color for almost any outfit and evokes a clean wink to even the stuffiest of ensembles.

SEPTEMBER 3

TAKE AN EXPERT STYLE CUE FROM MANDI NORWOOD, A TOP NEW YORK STYLE-MAKER AND EDITOR IN CHIEF OF *SHOP ETC.*

What is your best-kept personal style secret?

Have a closet full of white shirts! A crisp white shirt always looks expensive and makes everything you wear with it look expensive. It's also a fabulous fallback. If you tumble out of bed ten minutes before you're due in a meeting, you can throw on a white shirt and three things will happen: (1) you'll look as though you carefully planned and primed your outfit; (2) you'll look fresh and clean—and rich; (3) your skin will be illuminated by the bright white shirt, thus reducing the need for an emergency layer of Clarins' Beauty Flash!

What are the three fashion essentials every well-dressed woman should own?

1. A crisp white shirt, see above.
2. A pair of navy pants—they're less predictable and stuffy than black pants, and still go with absolutely every other color on the planet, like chocolate brown, pink, lavender, camel, or red. Also, they tend not to lose their color as quickly from dry cleaning.
3. A trench coat—after searching for forty-one years and finally finding the perfect one, I now know what all the fuss is about.

What are the biggest mistakes women make when getting dressed?

Wearing too much perfume. Standing next to a woman who is drenched in perfume makes me gag. It's horribly unsocial, disrespectful, and just downright bad taste. It's like bad breath—just because you can't smell it, doesn't mean it doesn't exist.

Who is the most stylish woman in existence, in your opinion, and what do you appreciate about her look?

Audrey Hepburn. In one of my favorite photographs of her, she's simply wearing a pair of cropped pants and a T-shirt, but I swear she looked drop-dead stylish.

If you could whisper a fail-safe style tip into the ears of women everywhere, without them feeling bad by hearing it, what would it be?

Smile! It's stylish, contagious, and free! Looking foul-tempered never looks stylish.

SEPTEMBER 4 | IN THE FITTING ROOM, IF IT'S HARD TO TAKE OFF, LEAVE IT.

For example, pants that fit perfectly everywhere but are slightly snug in the waist, a shoe that feels tight around the toes, and a dress that accentuates your best features and then some won't look or feel any better on you three months or three years from now.

Take a deep breath in front of that three-way mirror and make certain that what you are wearing looks and feels absolutely amazing right then and there. The future is now.

SEPTEMBER 5 | KEEP YOUR MAKEUP WHERE IT BELONGS—ON YOUR FACE!

Getting dressed in a hurry, especially when slipping on tops, can lead to a makeup stain that can destroy a total look in a nanosecond. Most women have been there too many times to count.

Why not purchase an inexpensive silk scarf to be your protector? Nothing fabulous, just a silk scarf large enough to cover your entire head when draped, and sheer enough to allow you to breathe when using it as a quick makeup shield for pull-on tops.

This may very well be one of the oldest "backstage" tricks in the book. Actresses, models, dancers, and TV hosts do it as a rule, whereas most women in the real world simply risk it and hope for the best.

It is also a great reason to retire an old scarf that no longer helps your outfits, or purchase a new one and reserve it only for this purpose. Either way, you are covered.

SEPTEMBER 6

LOOK BACK AT WOMEN'S HISTORY AND USE THE STRENGTH AND STYLE OF YOUR FOREMOTHERS TO INSPIRE TOTAL CONFIDENCE IN YOUR CLOTHES—AND IN YOUR CHARACTER.

New Jersey was the last state to eliminate women's suffrage after the Revolutionary War. Women in New Jersey actually voted until 1807 as a matter of course, without complaint from men in office, until a very close election was clearly decided by the female vote. The male legislators nastily revised the laws to then banish women from the voting process. Wyoming was the pioneering U.S. state or territory to then grant women suffrage in December 1869. Louisa Ann Swain of Laramie, Wyoming, was the first woman to legally cast a ballot in a U.S. national election.

Pay homage to the spirit of Swain and the many women who fought for this right by sharing her story.

SEPTEMBER 7

DON'T MATCH YOUR CLOTHING WITH YOUR MAKEUP.

When I was a teen, I remember a night when my beautiful, chocolate-brown mother left for a night out with friends wearing bright blue eye shadow. She looked to one of her gal pals for confirmation and said, "Blue top, blue eye shadow, right?" She meant well.

Matching your clothes with your makeup is actually *not* a good idea. But complementing or artfully coordinating your clothing with makeup colors is ideal. And it is not as difficult as you may think, according to celebrity makeup artist Sam Fine, who has consistently created amazing looks for such stylish women as Vanessa Williams and supermodel Iman for over a decade. Fine explains, "This is totally a myth! There are no rules and regulations to makeup. If you are good at applying makeup, and you have a wonderful top, and you can pinpoint the perfect shade of makeup to complement it—go for it! But don't feel obligated to match the color of a dress with your lipstick or any makeup.

"The best way to think of makeup is as a tool to enhance your natural beauty. Use neutral shades on the face and they will go with any color clothes."

The makeup should complement your complexion and enhance your features. Notable style is about creating a look that has a visual unity. The clothes, accessories, hair, and makeup all connect because all the components give a nod to one another—not mimic one another.

Everything in one color is boring. Introduce varied textures, like glossy lips and smoky eyes with a tweed jacket and slick leather pants. Mixed combos such as this make for a gorgeous, harmonious look!

SEPTEMBER 8 | HIT A DESIGNER OUTLET STORE AND FIND HIDDEN TREASURES.

Outlet shopping doesn't always mean that you are getting the best deal. But it can be a source of great savings for value.

A phenomenon that gained major steam in the 1980s, the outlet shopping experience was originally a less-than-glamorous, off-the-beaten path, deal-hunting experience that select shoppers would hear of and keep to themselves. Warehouses in off areas held truly inexpensive treasures, ranging from clothing from a season gone by to housewares and accessories that, upon digging through, proved to be in perfect condition yet at a fraction of the original cost.

The outlet concept was a win/win both for companies with piece goods that had to be cleared from inventory and slightly irregular items that were still usable, and consumers looking for a way to cut corners. It takes some wherewithal to dig a little and forgo the usual fancy retail environments, though. Decades later, the outlet stores have become a fact of life.

A word to the wise for women who shop when the outlet store racks are fully loaded: Often, if an item is present, fully stocked, in a multitude of colors, your deal won't be as great as if you found it twisted in a bin with dozens of other unmatched separates.

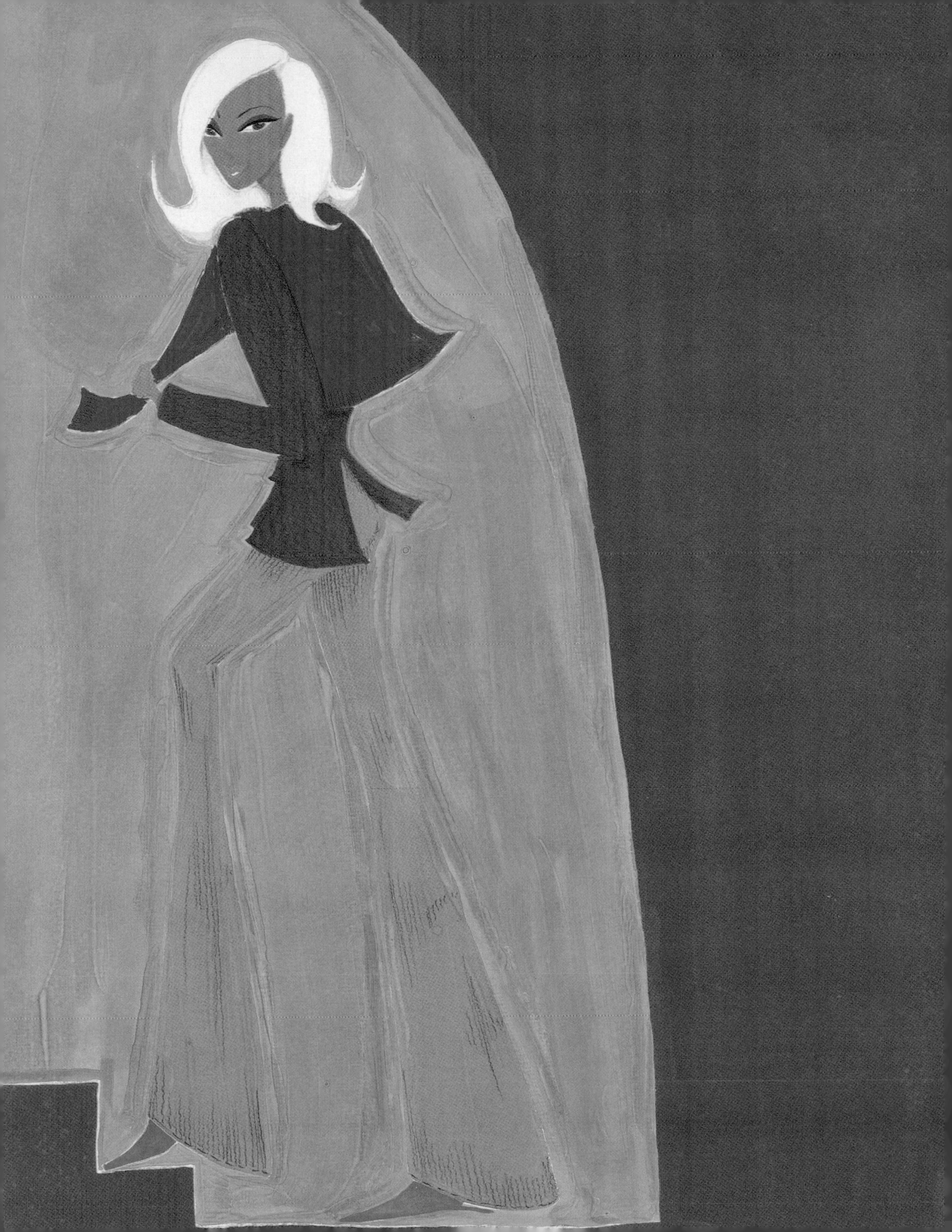

SEPTEMBER 9 | A TEN-MINUTE STYLE FOR A DAY IN THE COUNTRYSIDE.

Many women hate to see the supple days of summer come to an end. I, on the other hand, see it as an opportunity to strike up real fashion!

Off with that special person to the countryside this month for a wine-tasting, day of antiquing, or the start of a weekend at a bed and breakfast, make the send-off as stylish and cozy as possible.

Here is a great ten-minute style solution for any day in the countryside:

Minutes 1:00–2:00:
Start with a tailored blazer that speaks of early autumn (think tweed or herringbone), and wear the collar up! Break half a suit if you need to.

Minutes 3:00–4:00:
Go corduroy on the bottom, from knee-length skirts to flare-leg cords. Select a top that's girlier than the pants. Colorful silk camis work if it's warm enough.

Minutes 5:00–6:00:
Grab your brightest sweater to wear as an accessory (over the shoulders, or around the waist) and to wear if it gets chilly. Orange, corn, or pink are tops!

Minutes 7:00–8:00:
Lay low in suede loafers or flats that have something feminine on them, not your work flats. Imagine what Audrey Hepburn would wear.

Minutes 9:00–10:00:
If you have freckles, show them today! Give your skin and your makeup bag a break. Groom your brows and lashes with clear mascara, a touch of lip gloss, and run to the hills!

SEPTEMBER 10 | DESIGN A POWER-LUNCH ENSEMBLE MEANT FOR SEALING THE DEAL.

Focus on understanding and managing your wardrobe as artfully as you would any other aspect of a well-run business, investment, or career.

Consider what's most important as far as projecting your image and achieving the goal you're after. Break the concerns down into percentages and plan your outfit accordingly.

Think about the room in which you'll be conducting the important business meeting and the people you'll be with. You might be going in to apply for a loan, negotiate the best deal on a car, have an extended client lunch to promote a new service, or simply vying for a second date.

After any of these pursuits, the majority of the time you will spend presenting yourself and your ideas will be spent seated, with your top half doing most of the negotiating.

Have some distinct wink of uniqueness—a brooch, textured shirt, a jacket collar with pronounced stitched edges, or even a perfectly folded silk pocket square. One simple accent can make you a standout.

This does not mean abandoning your lower half either, just make sure your top half has *more* impact. Business is business and your style can be a silent partner that really makes a big statement.

SEPTEMBER 11

BE READY FOR ANYTHING WHEN WORKING FROM HOME. KEEP STYLISH FAIL-SAFES RIGHT NEXT TO YOUR COMPUTER AND YOUR REMOTE!

According to the IRS, 23.6 million Americans worked from home at the start of the new millennium. In the process, many of the dress requirements that came with being in a corporate environment said good-bye.

Working from home, freelancing and running your own firm may not be as relaxed as you may think. Some people find the need to dress to get in the proper state of mind. You need to feel (and appear) even more alert and professional if only in your phone voice, e-mail composition, and maybe even video conferencing posture. Those who are cooped in an office dealing with you already imagine your feet being propped up and your favorite soap opera on mute while you correspond with them. So you sometimes have to be even more conscious than they are to keep things smooth. And your clothing still plays a role, even if it is only used for spontaneous meetings. You certainly need to be prepared for running into colleagues, clients, and potential clients even when you've opted for a quiet table in a neighborhood café to get some work done.

Here are five great style tips for the woman who works from home, just to keep her in a style that meets the rest of the world:

• Always keep a blazer clean and pressed: Even if you are in casual pants and a tank, a blazer can pull you all together if you are asked to report to lunch or a meeting with no time to create a total look.

• Keep your hair clean and pulled back: Add a touch of "seriousness" to even a quick-fix outfit. Add a white blouse, and your best video conference look is complete in no time!

• Use downtime for online shopping: Use your downtime to really search out killer sales online. This is downtime well spent.

• Make sure your voice mail greeting is ultraprofessional: So even if you are speed-showering, cooking dinner, and painting your nails all at the same time just to make a client event, it will sound as if you just stepped away to the copier. This comes across stylish, smart, and in complete control.

• When in doubt, wear all one color: Monochromatic dressing from head to toe can move easily from casual to professional. Keep it classic and solid and you'll fit into any new workplace style tone, at least for the day.

SEPTEMBER 12 | TAKE AN EXPERT STYLE CUE FROM DANA BUCHMAN, A TOP AMERICAN DESIGNER.

What is your best-kept personal style secret?

Whether you're dressing for day, evening, or weekend, clothing should make a woman feel strong, sexy, glamorous, chic, and comfortable. Let the mirror be your guide. Look at yourself, like yourself, and find the positive. All women are beautiful and we need to change the way we see beauty and be happy for all that we have.

What are the biggest mistakes women make when getting dressed?

Every woman has issues with her body whether she's a size 2 or a size 12. Embrace your flaws, like yourself, and your inner beauty will shine through no matter what you are wearing.

If you could whisper a fail-safe style tip into the ears of women everywhere, without them feeling bad by hearing it, what would it be?

Always go shopping with the proper shoes—don't try on evening clothes with loafers or sneakers on your feet. If you are trying on cropped pants, pair them with mules or shoes you would actually wear.

Let go of all your fashion fears. Try pieces you may think you could never wear. You will be completely surprised.

SEPTEMBER 13 | NIGHTTIME IS THE RIGHT TIME FOR BROWN.

Years ago, brown shoes were considered appropriate for daytime affairs. Think about the sporty chocolate brown and white, perforated spectator pumps from the 1920s that women wore with their perfect pleated skirts and cloche hats to an afternoon game of tennis, or the espresso brown, round-toe Mary Jane shoes of the 1940s that paired perfectly with pretty cotton dresses for strolls along storefront-lined streets.

Black ruled the evening. But now brown is just as gorgeous as black. So now your dressy brown heels are, in fact, appropriate for nighttime affairs, as long as the event isn't super formal. But even then, a pair of classic brown, strappy high-heeled sandals worn to ground an elegant floor-length, ivory evening gown with gold detailing would be spot-on appropriate!

Just remember that dressy, formal shoes, regardless of the color, can be worn all the time if you walk in with your head held high, like you mean it! Night or day!

SEPTEMBER 14 | LEARN A NEW FASHION TERM.

***Froufrou** (froofroo) • Fluffy trimmings such as ruffles, ribbons, and laces. Derived from French, "rustle" or "swish." From the name of the play* Froufrou *written by Henri Meilhac and Ludovic Halévy in 1869.*

Certain fashion descriptions can be pure onomatopoeias. Froufrou is hands down one of my favorites.

Can't you just see hands flying around in circles as one describes a garment or the interior of one's home as "froufrou"? You instantly see fussy fabrics, romantic and decorative details, and disproportionate embellishments that have no beginning and no seeming end.

There are times when froufrou is exactly what the style doctor ordered, such as gala events that call for a masquerade theme, like Mardi Gras celebrations, and, of course, the garden party that requests a look that honors "Southern elegance." And why not?

Froufrou is all about excess and excitement, fantasy and fashion escapism! Taking a step out of what is functional and minimal, and enjoying the romantic details of a ruffled gown that dusts the floor, a blouse that has lace, ribbons, beading, and bows—and that is only on the collar! The point is going all the way over the top, or leaving it alone.

Women who attempt the in-between are the ones who get into trouble when a stylish affair calls for froufrou, or one of the aforementioned themes. Load it on ad nauseam like a queen who wants to display her treasures. And when in doubt, add one more brooch just to be safe.

SEPTEMBER 15 | USE YOUR ANIMAL PRINT INSTINCTS.

One thing that always makes me chuckle about the fashion world is our tendency to announce what is "in" and what should be thrown "out." For some reason, every few seasons the ubiquitous animal print hits the top of everybody's "in" list as if it were just introduced for the first time. This is the month we begin our tirades. So heads up.

This is all to say that animal prints will always have fashion validity—so never toss them "out." They are considered an oxymoronic "trendy classic."

THREE WAYS TO ALWAYS LOOK STYLISH IN ANIMAL PRINTS

•Pairing animal prints with neutrals is always a safe bet. For more growl, partner them with classic red separates—or colors in the same warm family.

•Animal prints can be tricky on really curvy areas of the body. If you have any pronounced zone that may be mistaken for that of an animal costume when wearing said prints—think twice.

•Look for animal prints on textured fabrics for a really authentic feeling—without being cruel to the wild. Velvet, boiled wool, and even corduroy have a great hand that pops animal prints right off their surfaces. This adds a bit of intrigue and allure to an otherwise ordinary top, skirt, or jacket.

SEPTEMBER 16 | PUCKER UP WITH A NATURAL LIP.

Consider a nude or flesh-tone-based lip color that has a hint of pink or peach to warm it up. To find your best shade, look at the natural color of your bare lips—that is the base tone you should try to match in a modern, fresh lipstick. In a pinch, ask the salesperson who looks the least made up on your next trip to the makeup counter. She (or he) will help you along.

Add a touch of gloss atop your new lip color to give it a youthful glow. Don't overdo it, just a fine coating that seals it onto your lips and slightly magnifies the color.

When pulling back on your lips, you can play up another area of your face, such as a more dramatic eye treatment for nights out, or warmer cheeks to really pop your smile.

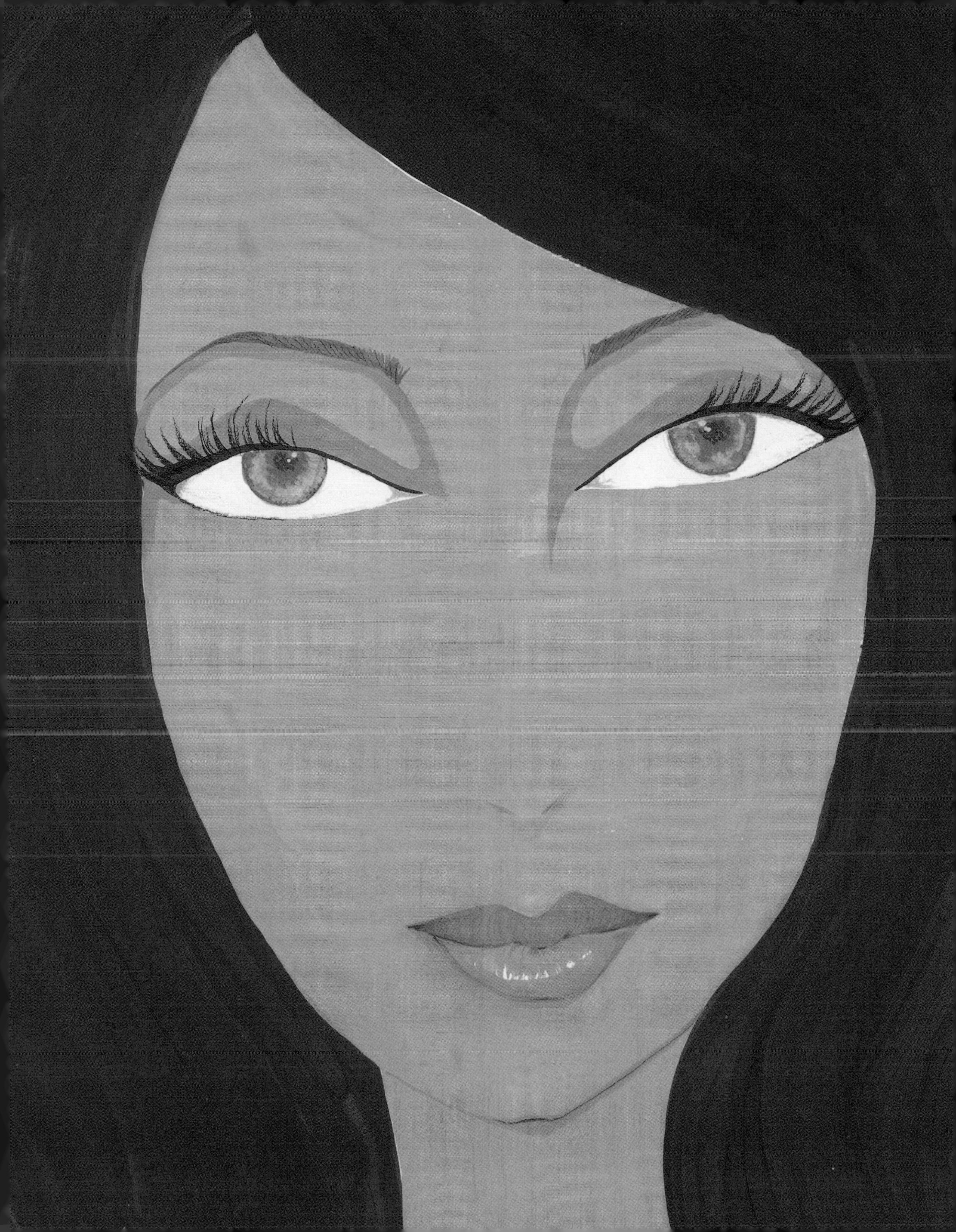

SEPTEMBER 17

TAKE AN EXPERT BEAUTY CUE FROM NADINE LUKE, A TOP NEW YORK MAKEUP ARTIST, M·A·C DIRECTOR OF MAKEUP ARTISTRY INTERNATIONAL.

What is your best-kept personal beauty secret?
I use lip gloss on my eyes. And I use cream colors for eyes, cheeks, *and* lips.

What are the three beauty essentials every woman should own?
1. Foundation that is a perfect match. This is the base on which to build your beauty. If this is too dark, too light, too heavy, or not enough, your entire look is off. How many times have we seen women with the wrong foundation! It's the first thing you notice and what you always remember.
2. Brushes are an essential key to any makeup. If you wanted to paint your house you would not use a toothbrush, the same idea applies to makeup. If you want the best results you need the right tools. At M·A·C we do not have a set of brushes because everyone's needs are different, therefore we want our clients to select brushes with an artist and this way they can create their own brush set to suit their eye shape and lifestyle.
3. Mascara is as critical as wearing the right undergarments. Imagine a supersexy skintight dress and showing a panty line. Your mascara is the push-up bra for your lashes. It gives you what you may not have naturally. Victoria is not the only one who has a secret, so does M·A·C. It's Zoom Lash!

What are the biggest mistakes women make when applying makeup?
Not updating or changing your makeup look. So much has changed. We have new formulas, new textures, new products, and new trends. There is nothing like getting your makeup done by someone who sees you with an objective eye. You can always adapt new products into your current makeup regime. When you change your hair color you also have to change your makeup colors.

Who is the most stylish woman in existence, in your opinion? What do you appreciate about her look?
Iman. She has a presence that cannot be denied. Her beauty is timeless, natural, and flawless. I appreciate that she has a beauty anyone can identify with no matter what his or her background.

If you could whisper a fail-safe beauty tip into the ears of women everywhere, without them feeling bad by hearing it, what would it be?
Less is more. Don't use makeup to cover, use it to accent. Keep the innocence—remember the transition stage from teenager to woman. Don't make it obvious.

SEPTEMBER 18 | POP STYLE QUIZ.

1. Which is the best bra color to create a true disappearing act?

A. Classic black
B. Soft pink
C. Any color in sheer lace
D. Nude to match your skin

2. Which successful designer first made a name for herself as the head designer for the house of Chloé, now has her own label, and is the daughter of a famous pop music legend?

A. Tracee Ellis Ross
B. Stella McCartney
C. Chastity Bono
D. Jennifer Nicholson

3. Which time of year has been traditionally most appropriate for white clothes?

A. Between Memorial Day and Labor Day
B. Between Labor Day and Memorial Day
C. Between January 1 and December 31
D. Between Christmas Day and New Year's Day

4. Next to shipping casual clothing ahead via FedEx, what is the best space-saving technique when packing for a long vacation?

A. Laying garments flat and gently rolling into logs
B. Laying garments upside down and folding into quarters
C. Layering garments inside of each other to create outfits, and folding
D. Folding each garment and placing each in an alternate direction

(Answers: 1-D, 2-B, 3-A, 4-A)

SEPTEMBER 19 | WORK SMARTER, NOT HARDER, BY HAVING A WORK TOTE BAG THAT ACTS AS A VIRTUAL CORNER OFFICE.

As fashion legend has it, the tote-bag design was originally based on the simple, functional design shape of the common paper shopping bag. Utility at its very best, and stylish to boot!

I always look for these top five tote traits for function and fashion:

One: The top of most work totes should offer you the option of remaining cleanly open for quick access, or zipper securely in an instant, looking just as good either way.
Two: Your handle straps should have padding where they rest on your shoulders, and be long enough to do this atop anything from a thin top to a bulky coat and layers of clothes.
Three: Before investing in a new tote, inspect the inner and outer pockets to make sure they are a mix of sizes, welcoming anything from a slim writing pen and PDA device, to your cell phone and mini makeup bag. Also, outer pockets should have zippers or patch pockets for added security.
Four: The color of your most used work tote should be super-versatile and rich, almost like you really don't need to work at all. The look of a promotion is what I like to call it. Choose black, and invest the most you can afford on a skin or fabric that speaks of upper management (and avoid resting it on concrete and soiled surfaces to keep it looking that way).
Five: Weigh it before you stuff it. If it feels heavy when empty, just imagine how it will feel on your busiest days. Go for the lightest version you can find that offers the above details. And remember to switch off arms when carrying for long periods of time.

SEPTEMBER 20 | JUMP INTO A CLASSIC TAN AND NAVY ENSEMBLE.

The quiet elegance of classic tan (or camel) and navy are two defining colors of traditional American sportswear. The cornerstone of a casual and smart elegance perfected by such design legends as Bill Blass in the 1960s and 1970s, American staple Ralph Lauren in the 1980s, and young design hero Tommy Hilfiger in the 1990s and beyond.

Wearing these stately partners now does not mean limiting your look to Muffy's blue blazer and wool gabardine camel pants. You can funk it up while remaining appropriate for just about any room you enter. And as an aside, swap black for navy if you are feeling a bit edgier. How's that for compromise? Consider these benchmark matches:

Navy Chiffon Skirt + Tan Wrap Top + Nude Kitten Heels + Faux Crocodile Belt
= After-Work Flirt

Long Tan Overcoat + Navy Sleeveless Mock Neck + Tan Trousers + Tan Flats
= Cubicle to Corner Office

Navy Sailor Pants + Gray T-Shirt + Tan Eisenhower Jacket + White Sneakers
= A Sporty Retort

SEPTEMBER 21 | WELCOME AUTUMN.

There is almost nothing like the palette of fall when foliage bursts into flames and embers right before your eyes. New England towns and their winding roads are aflame in crimson and ochre tones, which can mimic that of splattered oil paint.

We learn early on how to distinguish and identify the colors of the changing seasons. Tracing leaves as elementary school art projects, decorating pumpkins, and making construction paper turkeys to celebrate the joy of giving thanks. Let's guess, pumpkin, chocolate brown, amber, forest green, and maybe a touch of red.

Don't look like you took a roll in the autumn leaves and neglected to dust off. Give a nod to the season by switching up the predictable and tossing in fun, seasonless colors and clothes that will set you apart.

Bold Pink Turtleneck + Tan Tweed Skirt + Chocolate Knee Boots + Gold Bangles
= Sweet November

Orange Cords + Navy Blazer + Blue-and-White Striped Shirt + Tan Driving Moc
= Frost on the Pumpkin

Tan Overcoat + White Turtleneck + Red A-line Skirt + Black Rubber Wellies
= Awestruck Autumnal

SEPTEMBER 22 | TOSS ON A BLUE BLAZER BEFORE ANYTHING ELSE.

Ever wonder if the ubiquitous Brooks Brothers had *sisters?* If so, they would have never left the house without their navy blazers or a sports jacket. Well, actually, I doubt you'd see a proper lady of the mid-1800s sporting a sports coat, as this trend didn't even come alive for men until the 1920s, and women soon followed in the 1950s with the help of legends like Katharine Hepburn, one of the first Hollywood stars to don trousers and the classic navy blazer both on-screen and off. Retail legend has it that she always headed straight to Brooks Brothers for her tailoring, of course.

Some winning combinations:

Blue Blazer with Gold Buttons + Knee-Length Chino Skirt + Brown Sling-backs
= Updated Preppy

Blue Blazer in Cotton + Bleach White Trousers + Red-and-White-Striped T-shirt
= Nantucket Natty

Blue Blazer with Matching Buttons + Matching Trousers + Black Top (Yes, Black)
= European Chic

SEPTEMBER 23 | HAPPY BIRTHDAY, LIBRA GIRL.

Air signs don't mean airheaded, especially when it comes to the Libra woman. As a sign symbolized by the scales of balance, your fashion sense is spot-on indicative of what the stars have created you to be. This is never truer than when it is time to stand and face your closet and re-create who you are for this day. There is never a shortage of ideas, for your benchmark balance brings boundless options.

Most Libra women will take a moment to shop, even when totally inconvenient—during lunch breaks, on the way home (even though you are late), or between important deskwork—flipping through catalogs and online shopping sites. This is exactly why your eye is keen, your take on trends is laser sharp, and your closet is an amalgam of all your constant "research."

You crave trendy looks but know when enough is enough. Accessories can be flirty and feminine (dazzling handbags, exotic dangling earrings), yet you know exactly what clothes to pair them with to help them "chill" out a smidge. Other women in your life know you have this gift and often look to you for advice on how to do the same.

You will see a mirror of your style balance when you stop to assess your well-known Libra counterparts—like actresses Gwen Stefani and Gwyneth Paltrow. Like you, these stars are eclectic one day, überappropriate the next—with no apologies or explanations betwixt. An even and measured expression of self through clothes is a Libra's forte. This is always executed with artful honesty—something other signs need more of, for we all have many moods. Keep claiming them.

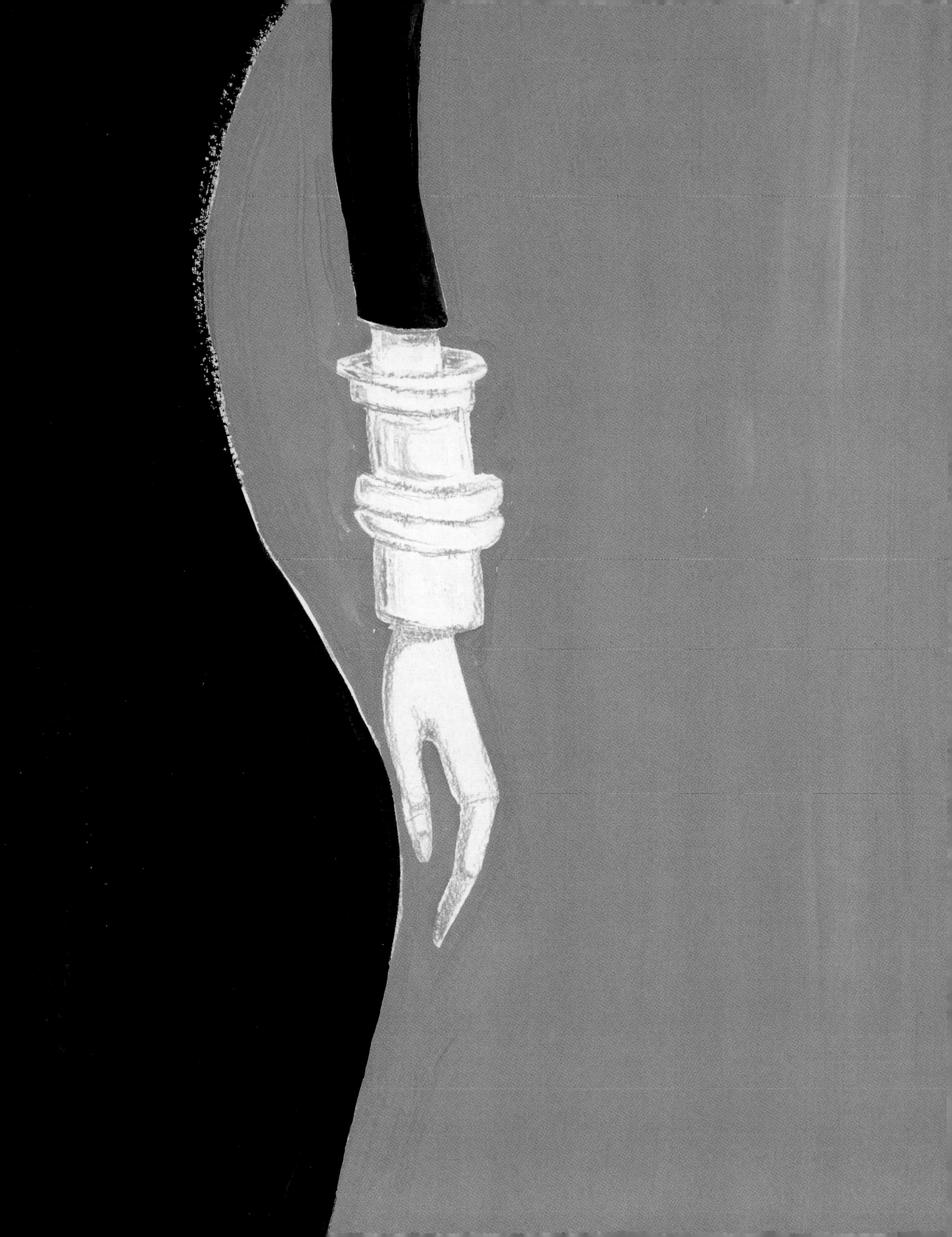

SEPTEMBER 24

ACCESSORIZE LIKE A FASHION MODEL AND STACK MULTIPLE BRACELETS OR BANGLES ON ONE ARM FOR A LOOK THAT HAS IMPACT AND A HIGH-STYLE EDGE.

Don't put on just one, unless the one speaks loudly.

Wear a short-sleeve, sleeveless, or fitted three-quarter-bracelet-sleeve top. Accentuate your fashionable side by leaving off all the meek, lightweight jewelry and stacking on chunky, substantial bangles and bracelets all around the same size. Go ethnic—African, carved, burnished copper, turquoise, or clear Lucite, or sterling silver, beaded, or a shelled variety. Stack the amount you love only on one arm, and just when you think you're finished, add one to two more to get the real look hot off any high fashion runway. Tip: choose the arm you don't use to handle the telephone.

SEPTEMBER 25 | CHOOSE PERFECT, FLOOR-LENGTH PANTS FOR YOUR PETITE FRAME.

Petite princess, short and sassy gal, and my favorite, vertically challenged diva—whatever the nickname, proudly standing on shorter legs does not mean having a shortage of style.

Finding perfect pants seems to be the number-one issue petite women face when shopping. They can never find as many options as their taller counterparts, which fit into the trends of the season—and honor the classics.

Avoid cropped or capri-style pants. Simply put, short pants that cut the leg at any point atop your ankle will actually make your legs look shorter. The eye is easy to fool, but even easier to get on your side. Capri pants are a surefire way to come across "short" with just about everyone you deal with.

Floor-length or floor-skimming pants with a slightly wider leg have an amazing ability to visually lengthen the leg. By nearly touching the floor they offer one long, clean line that adds a vertical thrust to your frame, registering as long, lean, and sexy. You can maximize this by wearing shoes in a similar color to add a few more inches—similar to the illusion of professional figure skaters and their signature nude tights and flesh-toned skates, creating the longest legs possible.

The one advantage petite women have over the Peggy Leggies of the world is their ability to choose sweet or sexy at any time. Sometimes having "miles of legs" does nothing but entice when you simply want to be heard.

SEPTEMBER 26 | TAKE A STYLE TIME-OUT DAY.

You might need a style sick day, so go ahead and take it! Contrary to what our current climate of makeover mania may have led you to believe, looking like you just stepped off a fashion photo shoot in New York City or the Hollywood red carpet is virtually impossible. And who would want to?

The idea of a "makeover" is a self-improvement concept created and fueled by mass media—television, magazines, books, and film. Who could ever forget that classic scene in the movie *Pretty Woman* when Julia Roberts's lady of the evening gets a new, high-class designer look after a dream shopping spree with the debonair Richard Gere. Women in theaters around the world had heart palpitations at the idea of a makeover and a man, all wrapped up in a blue Tiffany box.

Television talk shows swear by the power of the before and after, glamorous red carpet events show our favorite celebrities effortlessly strolling as if they simply threw on a gown and tossed their hair up; popular women's magazines devote entire issues to makeovers with step-by-step instructions showing women how to get the look of their favorite stars—with the products advertised between each story, of course.

The truth is, ladies, that not even the biggest and most fashionable celebrity women look the way you would imagine them to when they are not in front of a camera. Every woman needs a balanced blend of style and comfort to feel great. And when this perfect mix is found, looking great is simply a bonus.

You've seen those women who try really hard to look perfect every day. Maybe they are working behind the beauty counter at your favorite department store, donning a hair, face, and clothing combo better suited for a nighttime gala. You may have witnessed a flight attendant trying to conceal her frequent-flyer mileage with a bit too much makeup. Or the classic, the woman who has her perfect look down to a uniform that's so figured out, she doesn't realize that hosiery isn't really necessary in the summer sun.

When you aim for high style each day by simplifying your style statement, you are on the road to real comfort and creating another side to your style signature. Less is so much more, especially when attempting to create 365 looks that you are happy with, and sends your intended message to the world. Enjoy taking your days off, for they will make the days you do dress up that much sweeter and more inventive.

SEPTEMBER 27 | HIS CARGO PANTS DON'T HAVE TO BE YOURS.

Military-inspired cargo pants have been around for decades. Originally, it was an army-issued men's pant idea that was always more about function than fashion. Today's casual, civilian versions are definitely more about fun fashion. And for women, who prefer to carry their cargo in a sweet little handbag, they can be worn in cool ways without looking fad-attacked—today or ten years from now.

Try pairing army green cargos with a neutral, hooded sweater and a bright, bold T-shirt or camisole for a touch of what I call the weekend warrior. I also love a woman in classic tan cargo pants worn below a fitted black button-down shirt and sexy, slim knee boots—a great day-to-night option if you have little time to change.

White cargos in warmer months look amazing with a crisp bleach white, untucked dress shirt and nude-colored strappy sandals. Or, stately navy cargo bottoms in cotton or even satin, married with a

(CONTINUED)

form-fitting, navy ribbed turtleneck, a chunky black belt, and boots for a mysterious marine-inspired look for a night on the town.

Notice that the outfit ideas are boiled down to solids and simple pieces that bring most of the attention back to the cool details on your cargo pants. This is the stylish technique that brings out their best, as most cargo styles say a lot without saying much at all. The goal is to feature your cargo pants with easy tops, slick shoes, and bold accessories, so people will think you knew about them well *before* they were super trendy.

SEPTEMBER 28 | DRESS FOR THE CORNER OFFICE—WITH THE SAME EXCITEMENT YOU HAD FOR THE INTERVIEW THAT GOT YOU THERE.

Your résumé is letter-perfect. Your sharp pressed skirt falls just around the knee. And your manicure, makeup, and hair look as if you spent an entire day in the salon. You were so ready for the job interview that you had absolutely no fear of the outcome, for you knew that you gave it your absolute all. Because of this energy and excitement in putting yourself together, here you sit today, many months later, looking like you are the "before" makeover mug shot of the woman who came in for the interview. Believe me, it happens to the best of us.

At what juncture does all the interest in looking your absolute best end, and simply reporting to work begin? I don't believe there is a hard-and-fast start date. Like any other poor habit, it accumulates into a real issue bit by bit, day by day, meeting by meeting, deadline by deadline, missed promotion by missed promotion, and the list of stressors is nearly endless. Sometimes looking the part can be a real job!

Use today to think back to the way you wanted to be perceived when you walked through the door of the company for the interview, or even the very first week reporting to work. Was it authority you wanted to convey? Did you hope to transmit a vibe of maturity and sage wisdom? Or, like most of us, a look that speaks of contentment, as if you really didn't need the job—leaving no scent of desperation. Clothes deliver messages. A power suit that fits well means business. Your most sophisticated pair of work heels will lift you physically and emotionally. Tops that reveal your amazing taste help you to appear competent at any meeting you preside over. This is the look you want to recapture today using the clothes you may have let slip to the back of your closet, or worse, never bought more of after purchasing the winning interview outfit. If the latter is your story, time to go shopping for the corner office!

Take a good look at what you are saying when you walk into your place of business each and every day. Not just your words, e-mails, memos, and reports, but your nonverbal messages, too, which often speak just as loudly. Simply put, instead of dressing for the job you are in, always dress for the position you're striving for.

SEPTEMBER 29 | DRESS TONALLY IN SHADES OF ONE COLOR FROM HEAD TO TOE.

Some call it minimalist. Some call it boring. But you will be calling it your secret style weapon by day's end.

Tonal, or monochromatic, dressing means creating a complete clothing ensemble either by using one color or similar shades of a chosen color. It's a straightforward approach to dressing that's easy to pull off, and the result is a neat and elegant look that gives the illusion of a taller, leaner, and more proportioned you.

This is certainly not a figure-concealing style strategy, but more of a figure-enhancing trick. Imagine dipping yourself into your favorite, wearable color. Think of the sleek monochromatic attire worn by Olympic speed skaters, or a svelte modern dancer in matching leotards and tights. I'm not suggesting you suit up in that manner to tackle your day, but it's always okay to dream in the extreme for inspiration, especially when getting dressed!

Start by selecting a color you love and that looks great on you. Feeling a little apprehensive? Ease into this new look with dark hues like black, midnight blue, or deep espresso. Or you may want to make your monochromatic debut in stereo! Do this by choosing a more vivid color that looks equally good on your lower half as it does on your top. If you want to minimize the appearance of your bust, hips, thighs, or buttocks, go for rich earthy tones that make a bold rather than loud statement. Colors like eggplant, pumpkin, and cinnamon might just be your style trifecta.

Beyond picking your colors, there are few hard-and-fast rules besides making sure the fabrics of your tops and bottoms are similar or at least complementary in weight and appearance. If you're combining separates that may not be exact color matches, be sure to check their compatibility in daylight before facing the world. And last, but certainly not least, you may want to stop the color parade at your shoes—you don't want to look like a uniformed flight attendant between trips. Choose a solid dark or neutral shoe that's in harmony with your ensemble.

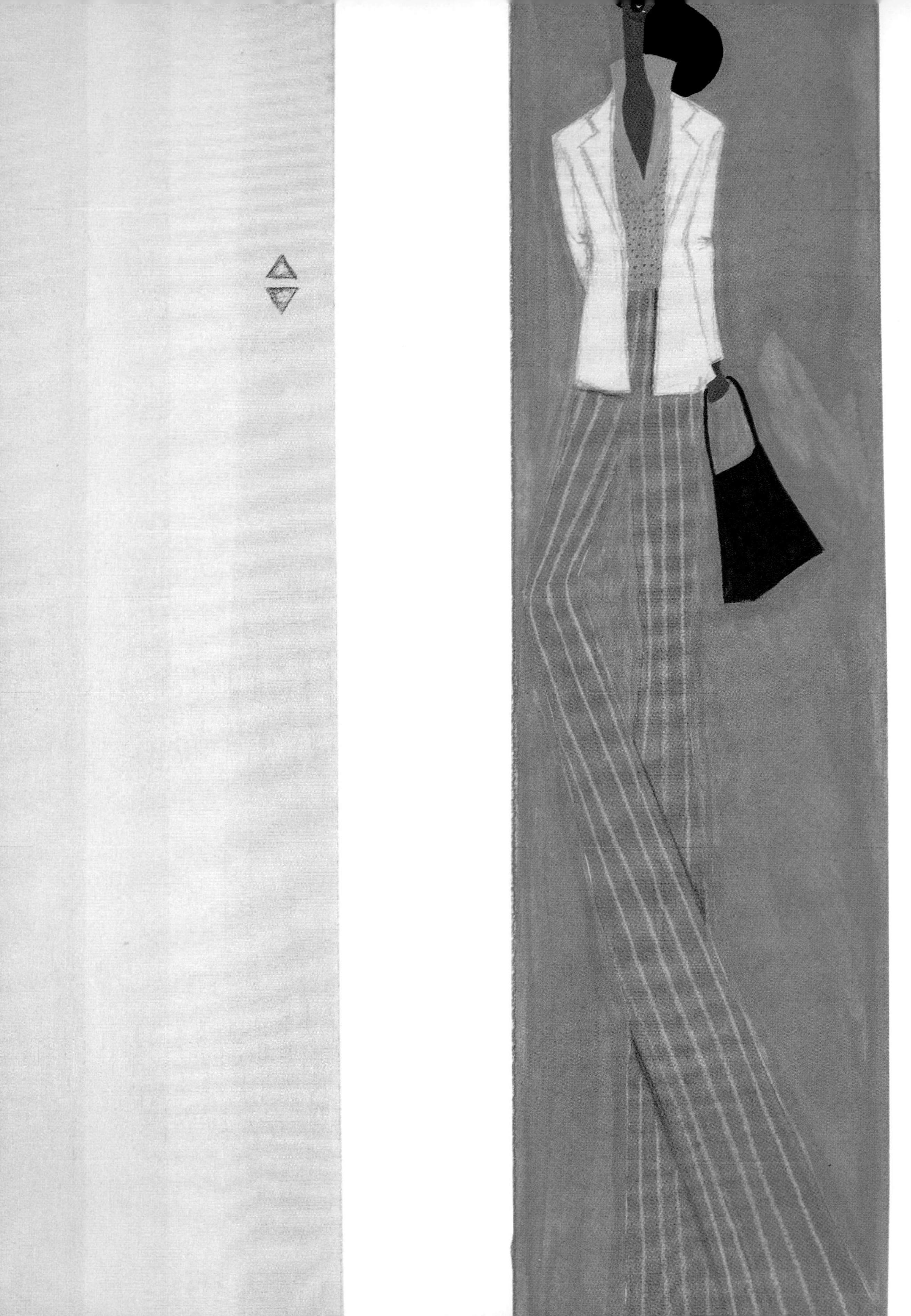

SEPTEMBER 30 | AN OUTFIT IDEA CHEAT SHEET. TAKE IT AND RUN!

Time to get serious. Work and school replace waves and sand. And I believe that smart clothes equal smart responses when getting back to business. It's similar to choosing to have a messy home or a neat one.

Ever notice that when people enter a messy home, they care little about where they drop their belongings—mess welcomes more mess. But when entering a clean, well-appointed home, they are usually a bit more conscious about where they toss their keys.

The same holds true for clothing; when the look means business, the response from those around you is usually quickly postured to offer the same.

Get a block of time back right now. Look in your closet and try to match this style equation as best as you can with what you have. Don't worry if the items you own aren't an exact match. Within this template, choose your own colors and details. Getting the look not so letter perfect gives a hint of your personal style, which is always better than a carbon copy:

Top: Solid tailored blazer or jacket; blouse with small print
Bottom: Pinstriped pants
Shoes: Classic pumps
Accessories: A satchel or handbag in a skin or faux-skin print
Flex piece: A shimmery camisole to transition into night!

OCTOBER

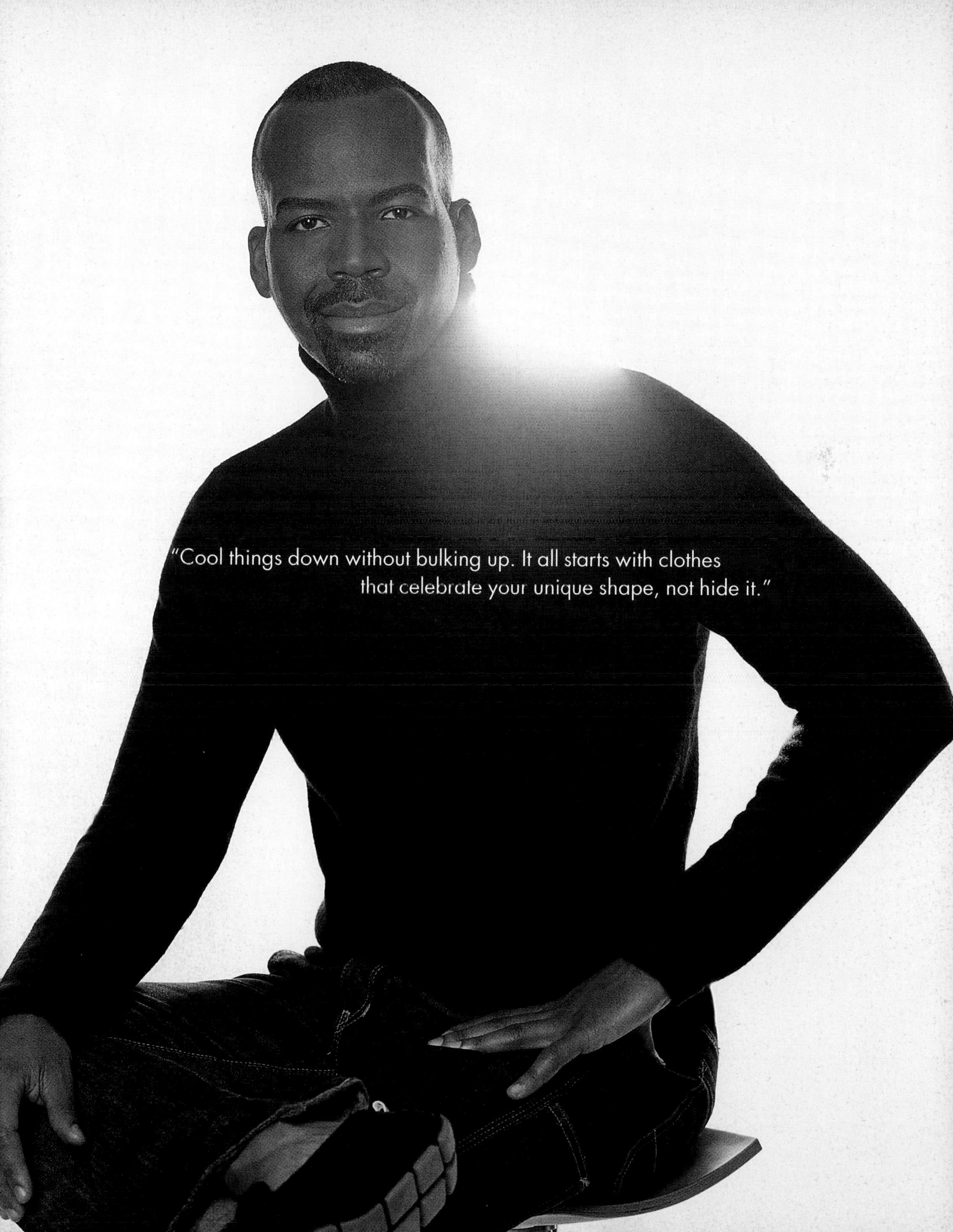
"Cool things down without bulking up. It all starts with clothes
that celebrate your unique shape, not hide it."

OCTOBER 1 | JEAN MAINTENANCE.

A perfectly fitted pair of jeans is to a modern woman's casual wardrobe what a little black dress is to her cocktail attire—the style epicenter. Sexy, fitted jeans in a super-dark indigo rinse speak to women looking to turn up the heat. Some gals prefer a slouchy, square boyfriend-cut jean that looks as if you snatched them from the dryer before your man did—also very hot.

Fall is the ideal time to find a pair of jeans that look made for you—traffic-stopping, head-turning, entrance-stealing denim that lifts you where you need it and minimizes areas where you need forgiveness.

Use the first day of October to assess your favorite jeans and make sure they are still your fail-safe casual basic that makes you shine whether just throwing them on with a tank or dressing them up with a lace blouse. If you don't have this pair, it is time to go shopping so you are casually prepared for the cooler months ahead. As you probably know, the scavenger hunt called jean shopping can take all day if you do it right. But before you hit the stores, arduously looking though the hundreds of styles that always crop up this time of year, remember these ten rules so you can find your most fabulous fit without feeling frustrated:

Stretch is best for curvy girls.
Bring an honest girlfriend to tell you how you *really* look.
Pronounced bleaching can create a spotlight where you need it (or don't).
Want more J-Lo, look for smaller back pockets.
Want less J-Lo, avoid puffy cargo pockets, especially on the rear.
Petite princesses should go for maximum length, and rarely capri styles.
Make a day of jean shopping, take your time, and try on at least ten pairs.
If you find a pair you *love,* grab it in a few different colors.
You can always bring them back—buy them and try on again at home.
Disregard the size, get the pair that flatters best.

OCTOBER 2

TAKE AN EXPERT STYLE CUE FROM LOIS JOY JOHNSON, A TOP NEW YORK STYLE-MAKER AND FASHION AND BEAUTY EDITOR OF *MORE* MAGAZINE.

What is your best-kept style secret?

My secret vice: a huge stash of Dolce & Gabbana underwire camisoles and Le Mystere microfiber thongs, which make everything and anything look better. I buy the D & G camisoles in leopard to make me smile to myself every morning. They never leave bra bulge and give a smooth base under sheer sweaters, cardigans, and tees. Pricey but I stock up whenever I see them in fear of not finding them anymore. Also the Le Mystere thongs in nude and black completely disappear under clothes and are truly comfortable.

What are the three fashion essentials every well-dressed woman should own?

These three items always make you look slim, chic, and work in just about any situation: (1) a pair of beautifully cut, slim black trousers that are lean through the hips and thighs, sit just at the top of the hip like those by Helmut Lang, Dolce & Gabbana, and Theory, and look equally good with boots and heels; (2) a perfect black cashmere turtleneck that fits like a second skin in a good three-ply quality like those by Tse or Loro Piana or J. Crew; and (3) a trench coat in classic beige like the signature Burberry looks amazing over everything from a pencil skirt to jeans to a little black dress. It's seasonless with a removable liner and adds a casual kind of sophistication.

What are the biggest mistakes women make when getting dressed?

Putting the idea of this-minute style and status before taste. Your clothes should always make you the star, not the other way around. Sometimes women try too hard to look fashionable without asking the "does this make me look great" question. Also the head-to-toe logo look makes women walking billboards. Stick to one or two at a time, puh-leeeze.

Who is the most stylish woman, in your opinion? What do you appreciate about her look?

I'd still say Coco Chanel for her instinctive style and imaginative accessorizing. She's the designer who put comfort and confidence in fashion, giving women pants, sweaters, and the casual chic that's become the wardrobe template for every woman today.

If you could whisper a fail-safe tip into the ears of women everywhere, without them feeling bad by hearing it, what would it be?

Real style is all about grooming whether you're in jeans, a tailored suit, or an evening dress. Don't leave the house without delinting, glancing at the rear view in a full-length mirror, checking your makeup in a magnifying mirror, and adding your signature perfume.

OCTOBER 3 | INVEST IN A VERSATILE QUILTED JACKET THAT FLOATS ON THE BODY.

Some call it a barn jacket. Many women think of it as a preppy staple, and others mistake it for something a man would only wear while hunting wild game.

Well, there is nothing wild about the quilted jacket. A classic cornerstone of American outerwear, inspired by English hunting jackets, they are slightly boxy, unfitted, and usually waist-length or longer. And although the short coat hit its legendary style stride with American women in the 1940s and 1950s, most authentic versions are still made across the pond. The jacket's versatility is just as legendary.

With the collar down, and buttons fastened, you are ready for a walk along a foliage-lined brook, and just by whipping the collar up high and slightly cuffing the sleeve, your look becomes less "harvest" and more heart-pounding, ready for a casual night of live jazz on the town.

Companies like Barbour and Orvis have perfected the lightweight quilted jacket. You can find it reversible in a soft, ladylike insulative silk that contrasts the traditional diamond quilting pattern that is said to provide extra warmth for outdoor treks. Classic navy, tan, or loden green are legends, but why not bright orange just to bring it into the fashionable side of your closet—away from the basics!

I love it on a woman for travel: the quilting is warming in colder spots, cool and instantly breathable in the heat.

From suits to weekend wear, the quilted jacket will complement almost anything short of an evening dress. And sometimes a certain woman will try it—and pull it off just by confidence alone.

Don it atop slim pants and festive flats, or toss it on over a more organic and earthy wrap skirt. The nearly weightless quilted jacket is known to recover from wrinkles with ease and quickly reduce in size for traveling. Look for versions that are light enough to pack in your carry-on case for chilly, first-class cabins.

OCTOBER 4

EDIT DOWN YOUR SNEAKERS TO THE ONLY TWO PAIRS ANY WOMAN REALLY NEEDS: A PERFORMANCE PAIR FOR EXERCISE AND A CUTE PAIR FOR FASHION ALONE.

Many women have multiple pairs of sneakers, most of which look a bit run over.

Truth is, a woman of style and efficiency really only needs two pairs. One really good performance pair that is designed especially for your chosen exercise, or a cross-trainer that allows you to participate in varied exercises with proper support.

The second pair should just simply be cute! Maybe canvas in a bright color, a retro chic pair with a nod to a 1950s bowling shoe, or a hip-hop Adidas from the eighties. Choose a pair with personality to match, or contrast yours and keep them fresh for simply relaxing, not running.

OCTOBER 5

SHIMMER AND SHINE. NOT JUST FOR THE NIGHT! SHIMMER AND SHINE BY DAY.

Sequins, sparkly beads, metallic mesh, shimmering embroideries, jewel-encrusted shoes, and even lamé tops, once reserved for more formal evening affairs, have edged their way into the sunlight on the most stylish women who like to push the envelope.

Here is the bottom line to this recent fashion myth. Designers, stylists, and trendsetters alike are always looking to be different each season. They strive to have newness, originality, and a look that mirrors nothing else around them.

Enter the mixing of traditional eveningwear with everything from sporty daytime clothes to serious suits. And I must give credit where credit is due: from costume designers like Patricia Field, who made the women of HBO's *Sex and the City* fashion superheroines, to European designers like Giorgio Ar-

(CONTINUED)

mani and Karl Lagerfeld who first told women it was okay to toss on a sequin tank beneath a power suit and be ready for evening all day long.

Now, whether you're a soccer mom or an expecting mom, evening separates that sparkle can enhance your mood—and the mood of those around you—if they're incorporated into your look with a wink of fun. A shimmering satin blouse with jeans and high-heeled sandals with crystals is as appropriate for a lunch with the ladies as it is for a day at the art museum with him—just don't do it from tip to toe. Measured doses of dazzle always work best.

OCTOBER 6 | CASH IN ON YOUR GREAT SENSE OF STYLE OR SELL SOMETHING ON AN ONLINE AUCTION SITE.

A few years ago we would have frowned at the possibility of auctioning off our personal items to people around the country and the world. But in the age of eBay it happens every minute. It is as simple as logging on, registering, uploading a photo and description of your goods, and launching the bidding.

Constance White, noted fashion journalist and eBay style director, explains, "It's a great way for a woman to make extra money, pare down her wardrobe, to cycle out last year's clothes, and make room for this season's. There's a psychic bonus to selling. It's great to know that the red satin shirt that you bought in a moment of uncharacteristic exuberance is making someone else very happy."

"Buyers benefit in two ways. First, on eBay, you usually win your item at a great price well below retail. Second, women love that eBay gives them access to fashions they might not otherwise be able to get. Not everyone lives near a great fashion store where they can run out and buy Seven Jeans or a Marc Jacobs handbag. Yet women are so savvy and knowledgeable about fashion these days. They want to have a wide choice."

OCTOBER 7

TAKE AN EXPERT STYLE CUE FROM JOAN KANER, A TOP NEW YORK STYLE-MAKER AND SVP FASHION DIRECTOR OF NEIMAN MARCUS.

What is your best-kept personal style secret?
Think black—as a career woman I've found building my wardrobe around one color works. Black takes you from morning to evening—leave the office, go to dinner—it's sophisticated, elegant, timeless, and always appropriate.

What are the three fashion essentials every well-dressed woman should own?
A great quality handbag and a good pair of simple expensive pumps. The third would be an important watch, because being on time matters.

What are the biggest mistakes women make when getting dressed?
Being slaves to fashion trends. It's important to know what works for you—for your figure and your lifestyle. Full skirts may be trendy, but if you're too large, skip them and try a simple A-line or pencil skirt instead.

Who is the most stylish woman in existence, in your opinion? And what do you appreciate about her look?
That's difficult. I have several:

1. Audrey Hepburn. In a class by herself, especially when dressed by Givenchy for her films.
2. Katharine Hepburn. Talk about self-knowledge! She was sophisticated but wanted comfort in her clothes, they suited her no-nonsense style.
3. For sheer elegance, the late Babe Paley and Gloria Guinness. Polished, refined, and classy.
4. Jackie Kennedy. During her White House years she brought grace and elegance to the role of first lady.

If you could whisper a fail-safe style tip into the ears of women everywhere, without them feeling bad by hearing it, what would it be?
The old adage "less is more." Before you leave the house take a good look in the mirror; if you're unsure, take something off. Also, remember the outfit that you felt best in whenever you are out shopping; look to replace it.

OCTOBER 8 | GET THREE AUTUMN LOOKS IN ONE.

Fully Loaded: Fitted velvet blazer + turtleneck atop camisole + dark denim A-line skirt + knee boots
Completely Chic: Turtleneck (push-up sleeves) + dark denim A-line skirt + knee boots
Simply Fab: Fitted velvet blazer (turtleneck over shoulders) + camisole + A-line dark denim skirt + knee boots

OCTOBER 9 | TIE ONE ON FOR STYLE.

Leave it to the classic American brand J. Crew to show women that there is, in fact, more than one way to tie a scarf in cool weather.

Your scarf may be the last item you toss on before facing the cold, but it is usually the first thing to block the wind from your neck and chest, and an eye-level focal point for those around you. Tying it on with slovenly and reckless abandon can leave you chillier than you'd like, and questionably chic in the eyes of others. And you know how frustrating it is to try to retie a scarf when out in the cold. It just never seems to work properly!

Take thirty extra seconds before dashing out into the tundra, and try wrapping your scarf, any scarf, with a totally new twist. Choose a knot that really speaks to your outfit for the day, and the level of warmth you really desire. Take a look at these four stylish tying tips—courtesy of J. Crew—to tie on one:

European Wrap: With one end hanging loose at front, throw one end over the shoulder and let hang loose at back.
Hacking Knot: Fold scarf in half. Put around neck and slip loose ends through loop to adjust. This is a great in- or out-of-office look.
Classic Choker: For a dressier look, simply wrap around neck once and let ends hang loose at front.
Simple Ascot: Start with the classic choker. Then cross one end over the other, loop that end under, pull up through the hole. Adjust accordingly. Tucks perfectly into a jacket.

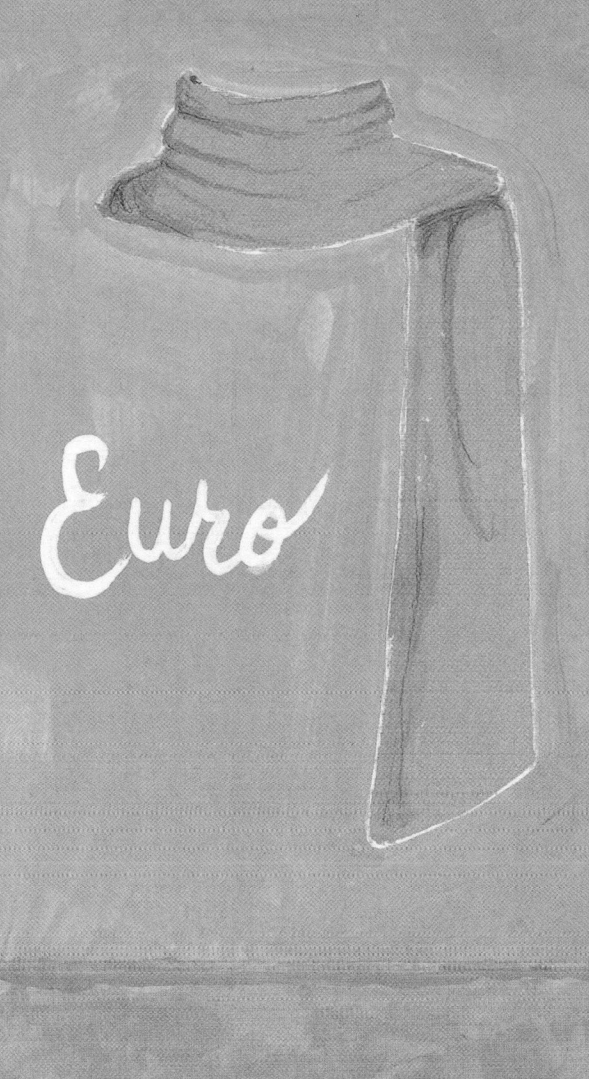
Euro

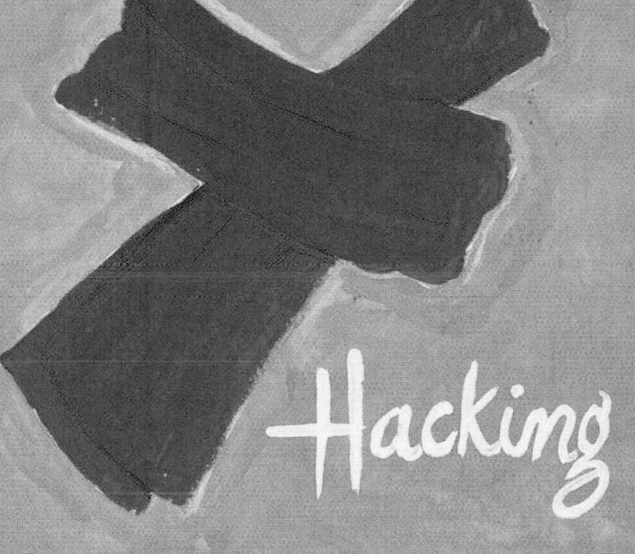
Hacking

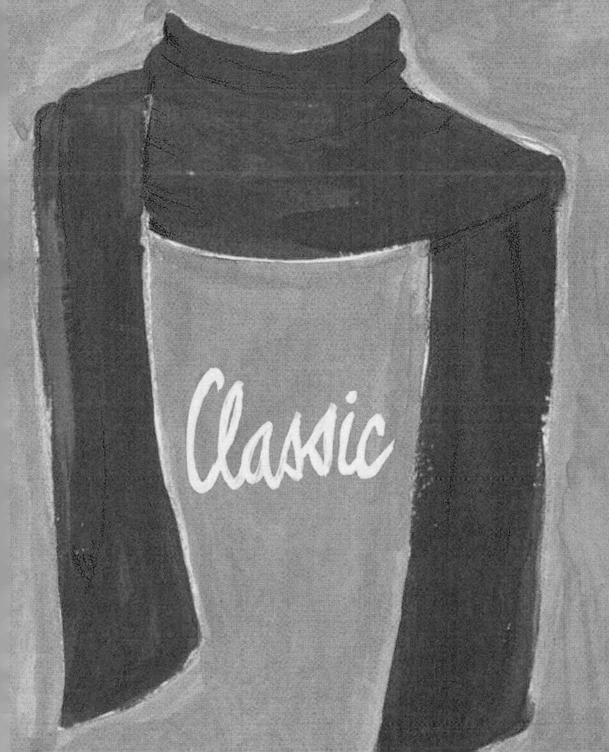
Classic

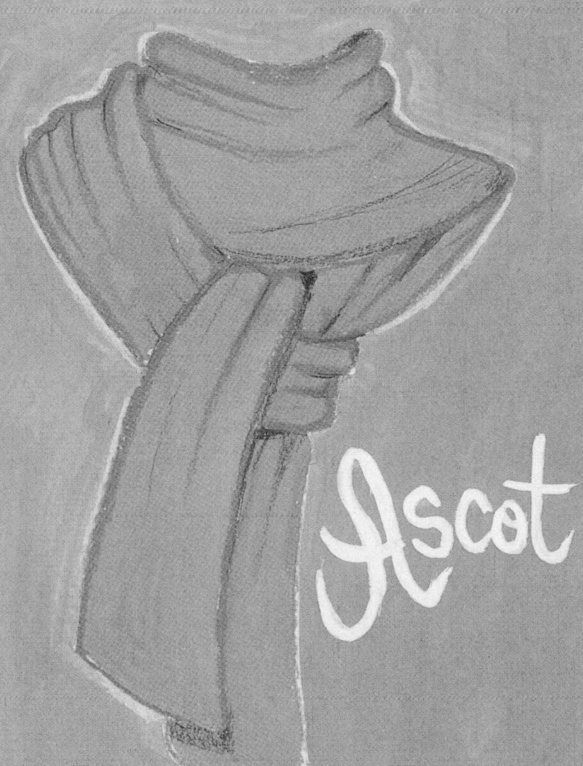
Ascot

OCTOBER 10 | WEAR A PAIR OF GLOVES FOR STYLE, NOT JUST FOR WARMTH.

One of the most interesting trademarks of a well-dressed woman in a classic Hollywood film, especially those of the 1940s, were gloves: lace gloves, embroidered cotton gloves, and chic satin versions reserved for evening.

Nowadays most women only slip into gloves out of sheer necessity, unless you are a high-paid hand model who will wear gloves even during summer months to protect your moneymaking assets.

Just as you would remove a clip-on earring before picking up the telephone, be sure to remove your gloves one finger at a time for maximum style impact.

SIZE MATTERS

Your glove length is what is most important and should complement the dress you are wearing. Purchasing gloves with button closures can be an easy measuring stick for your perfect outfit match.

Drama: Single-button–closure gloves (short, to the wrist bone) look amazing with three-quarter-length or long-sleeve dresses. Think of this choice as just a screen test.
Melodrama: Six-button-closure gloves (medium, just short of the arm crease) stand out best with flutter- or cap-sleeve dresses.
High Drama: Eight-button-closure gloves (long, just above the arm crease) are the best friend to a chic sleeveless number.
Drama Queen: Sixteen-button-closure gloves (formal length, on the biceps) are an elegant choice for strapless gowns and dresses. Think Grace Kelly.

OCTOBER 11 | HAPPY BIRTHDAY, ELEANOR.

Eleanor Roosevelt was fabulous without being classically beautiful. What did her dress style say about her?

Married to Franklin Delano Roosevelt in 1905, Eleanor Roosevelt worked in settlement houses before focusing on supporting her husband's political career after he contracted poliomyelitis in 1921.

Through the Depression and New Deal and then World War II, Eleanor Roosevelt traveled when her husband was less able to. Her daily column "My Day" in the newspaper broke with precedent, as did her press conferences and lectures. After FDR's death, Eleanor Roosevelt continued her political career, serving in the United Nations and helping create the Universal Declaration of Human Rights.

Two of my favorite quotes from this great lady actually set the tone for a style edict as well. Roosevelt once said, "Remember always that you not only have the right to be an individual, you have an obligation to be one." And she was also quoted as saying, "Do what you feel in your heart to be right—for you'll be criticized anyway. You'll be damned if you do, and damned if you don't."

Glean an example for your own posture and pride today when getting dressed, even if you are just heading to the grocery store. There is so much about you that no other woman can ever claim. Think about this and own one of your uniquely individual attributes.

It might be the persistent freckles you hated as a teen, your curvaceous bottom inherited from your mom, or just your naturally curly hair that never seems to get the hint that stick-straight hair is in. Use this opportunity to claim something, one thing, about you with confidence and pride, channeling the resilient strength of Eleanor Roosevelt, for as she said, "you'll be damned if you do, and damned if you don't." I say take the former.

OCTOBER 12 | TAGS AND LABELS BEGONE!

THE FOUR MAJOR OFFENSES

Winter coats: Using a small manicure scissor or a seam ripper, carefully remove any and all woven labels that may be stitched to the sleeve.
Eyeglasses/sunglasses: Simply peel off any clear plastic stickers that are affixed to the lens.
Suits: Again, using a small manicure scissor or a seam ripper, carefully remove any and all woven labels that may be stitched to the sleeve.
Leather handbags: Remove any exterior tags that are created of the same material of the handbag. Most are usually attached with a small beaded metal cord that pops off with ease.

OCTOBER 13 | TAKE AN EXPERT SKIN-CARE CUE FROM SONYA DAKAR, A TOP CELEBRITY SKIN-CARE SPECIALIST.

What is your best-kept personal beauty secret?

Stay away from the sun!! That is the number-one cause of premature aging, discoloration, and irritation. If I had to choose a second it would be to never go to bed without washing my face and applying my night regimen—regardless how long or short that regimen is. Since I was a little girl I practiced these two good habits.

What are three skin-care essentials every woman should own? Why?

1. Good cleanser with no harsh detergents like sodium laurel sulphate or acids. Just a gentle cleanser you can use morning and night that will wash away excess oil, dirt, makeup, and impurities.
2. Great eye cream—it is never too soon or too late to start using eye creams. This is the part of your face with no oil glands, and so it shows the signs of aging first. I recommend my clients start using it as early as age nineteen or twenty!
3. Amazing moisturizer, whether you have oily, acne-prone skin, combination skin, or dehydrated skin. There is the perfect moisturizer out there for you and your skin.
4. And if I can add one more—an SPF 30 sunblock.

What are the biggest mistakes women make when caring for their skin?

Women overprocess their skin. They overdo it with exfoliation, peels, scrubs, and products. They become their own chemists and aestheticians. They end up with thin, sensitized, cracked, discolored skin that will prematurely age! No one would dare do their own dental work, why would they do their own skin?

Who is the most stylish woman in existence, in your opinion? And what do you appreciate about her look?

Brigitte Bardot in her early days. When she was young she was a natural beauty. She looked natural, young, and sexy all at the same time.

If you could whisper a fail-safe skin-care tip into the ears of women everywhere, without them feeling bad by hearing it, what would it be?

That all women are beautiful because every woman is born beautiful with beautiful skin. We all start with clear, smooth, gorgeous skin, we just need to be sure to maximize, maintain, and appreciate it. And it is *never* too late to start.

OCTOBER 14 | INVEST IN A SWEATER SHAVER.

Look under the arms of your most-used sweaters, near the elbows, and where your arms brush against your midsection. These are the friction zones that create pilling, where nubs or bunches of fibers form on the surface of knitwear during washing and normal wear. Loose yarns and sweater fibers unwind and interlock with each other.

Invest in an electric sweater shaver or sweater stone to alleviate your best sweaters from this disorder. They are sold at most drugstores or mass bargain stores like Target and Kmart.

With the electric version, simply turn on and move the shaver over clothing in slow strokes and you're ready to go. The sweater stone is actually a gentle pumice stone that carefully removes unwanted fabric debris. It should come complete with a protective box when not in use.

Either of these will clean and refresh your sweaters in minutes, giving them a longer life and a new look.

OCTOBER 15 | GET TEN-MINUTE STYLE FOR HARVEST-INSPIRED OUTDOOR EVENTS.

Not every woman would be caught chugging a stein of beer at the local Oktoberfest, or be seen rummaging through baskets of new and used treasures at a fall outdoor vintage craft fair, but you'd be surprised how many stylish-cum-fun women would.

This month is all about taking in the last few breaths of weather that is mild and crisp. And right up to Halloween, why not be out and about wherever you can find a window of last-minute outdoor fun? Autumnal outdoor festivals abound this month.

Here is a great ten-minute style solution for any harvest-inspired outdoor event:

Minutes 1:00–2:00:
Begin with boots that make you *feel* ten feet tall. Leather or suede chocolate knee boots, riding boots, mukluks, or jodhpur ankle boots are chic and sporty.

Minutes 3:00–4:00:
Reach for fitted blue jeans you can cuff with big folds just above the top of the boots. Your belt should be chunky and hip, with fun details (Western is fun)!

Minutes 5:00–6:00:
Instead of a jacket, layer a down vest atop a V-neck sweater and button-down shirt. Choose all three in different fun fall colors (e.g., chocolate, rust, and pine).

Minutes 7:00–8:00:
A fun hat can seal the deal and hide bad hair days. Natty camel driving caps, tweedy Rasta applejacks, and corduroy bucket hats conceal and complement.

Minutes 9:00–10:00:
For hair think "windblown chic," a few strands should dangle. For face, go with an all-over moisturizer that has bronze highlights, a warm autumn lip, and get to steppin'!

OCTOBER 16 | LEARN A NEW FASHION TERM.

Diamanté *(dee-a-mont-ay) • Term used to indicate a sparkling effect as that of the reflection of gemstones. Der. French, "made of diamonds." Diamanté headbands were worn around the head, low on the forehead during the Edwardian period (1890–1910) and in the late 1920s. Dresses made almost entirely of sparkling beads, sequins, or paillettes giving a glittering effect were very popular in the mid-1980s.*

In the new millennium, many simply call it "bling." The shimmer and dazzle of a glittery top, dress, or accessory that is jewel-encrusted (be they faux or real) all fall under the look designers know as diamanté.

In the past, the look was all about formal or semiformal dressing. Most notably, legendary designer Norman Norell's diamanté mermaid evening gowns that graced such icons as Marilyn Monroe (he also created the infamous "Happy Birthday, Mr. President" dress).

Thanks to the stars of this new generation, from Halle Berry and Sharon Stone to Beyoncé and Gwen Stefani, the look has crystallized on everything from simple tops worn beneath stately blazers, to jeans and halters that shine like evening gowns. These visible icons have given real women the license to sparkle whenever they need a lift, dressy or not. The rules of when to shine are now best broken.

Caution when sporting a diamanté look, for it can bring light to areas where you may not want loads of attention. Celebrities are just the opposite and seek the flash of the cameras, and the eyes of the masses. If this is not your intent, save your head-to-toe diamond moments for when you desire the room's full attention. Otherwise, a diamond pin should suffice.

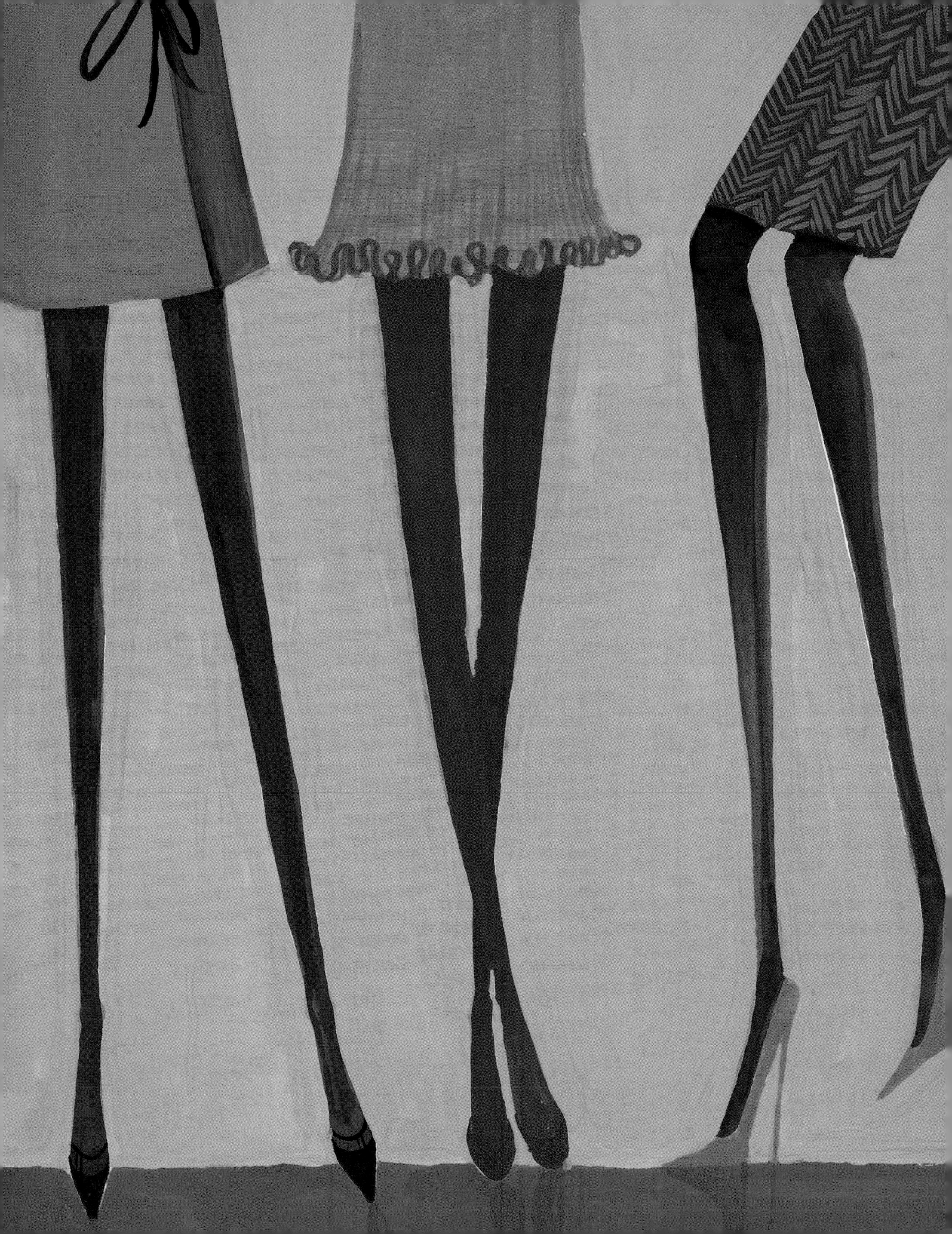

OCTOBER 17

EXPERIMENT WITH FUN, BOLD, SOLID-COLORED TIGHTS WITH YOUR SKIRT, ADDING DRAMA AND WHIMSY—AND MAYBE EVEN A LITTLE LENGTH TO YOUR LEGS.

Taffy. Banana. Tangerine. Plum. Berries. No, this is not a shopping list of snacks to get you through the day. These are some of the most flattering bold color choices in opaque hosiery—just to name a few.

You may remember images of the 1960s Mod fashion craze, where models such as Twiggy donned opaque tights that looked as if their legs had been dipped in a vat of bright Crayolas. And it seemed as if the more shocking the color of the tights, the better. Well, that was then and this is now.

The opaque hosiery of today has taken on a level of sophistication that welcomes women of just about any shape or size to look as fabulous as crime-fighter Emma Peel did on television's popular 1960s hit *The Avengers*. Whether you're a size 12 or 22, there are a few choice colors to try—and a few rules on what shoes and clothes to pair them with so you won't feel the need to peel them off before day's end.

TANGERINE

This color always rings in the early fall like a scene from a perfect New England postcard. Avoid wearing with black shoes and clothes, as not to look like a Jackie-O-Lantern. Chocolate to espresso brown shoes and clothing are much better.

PLUM

The perfect choice for your first baby step into this arena, this rich tone can be slimming and elongating to the eye—and artsy all at once. I like to think of purple tones as a very grown-up way to paint the leg in color. Try not to wear clothes that match in hue, unless you are aiming for a 1980s redux. As for shoes, go paper-bag brown to neutral tan to conjure up the feeling of wealth and status. Herringbones and chunky wool clothes in camel and sepia have a similar, to-the-manner-born air.

LIPSTICK RED OR BERRY

Depending on your berry of choice, this color could range from magenta pink to classic raspberry sorbet. Its natural partners to keep you looking like a lady, and not a teenager, are good old black shoes and clothes. From your favorite black A-line skirt and matching black sweater set, to a timeless black sheath dress matched with a killer, slightly pointed-toe pump. Berry good!

OCTOBER 18 | ADD AN AMERICAN INDIAN PRINT.

From fun ponchos to trimmed mukluk boots, these prints are alive and well today, giving a "bohemian chic" look to anything you pair them with. The zigzag print icon has stood the test of time and many a moon. And although the high-fashion set deems it cool every few seasons, the truly modern fashionista knows different—and never makes the mistake of feeling as though she is *discovering* American Indian prints for the first time. They've always been here.

THREE WAYS TO ALWAYS LOOK STYLISH IN AMERICAN INDIAN PRINTS

•American Indian prints hark back to a simple time yet are intricate and very identifiable. Use their strength in doses, and choose them on authentic silhouettes that honor their heritage. Avoid the zip-front leather biker jacket done Cherokee style.

•Geometric prints in general can read rigid and masculine. Look for the most feminine shapes you can find when looking to American Indian prints. Show a little shoulder, reveal the back—think the sexier side of Pocahontas.

•Classic versions have gorgeously woven patterns. Newer interpretations have literal, cartoonlike images of faces, feathers, wolves, and animals. Go for the former for the most fashionable feel.

OCTOBER 19 | TRY FOOTLESS HOSE. TRY MULES.

CONSIDER WEARING THIS

Major department stores carry footless panty hose by brands such as Spanx. If you need it, they provide the support of a full-fledged, control-top panty yet are only as long as capri pants. This way, you can achieve the youthful, modern bare leg look, and have a grip on your mules.

+

Choose a mule that has a slim heel for the longest, leanest look. Chunky heels can make the leg appear stumpy and thick.

+

Keep your heels exposed for as long as you can. Think about the actual amount of time you spend out in the cold. You probably have more mule days ahead than you thought.

=

Finally, a mule that's not so stubborn!

OCTOBER 20 | POP STYLE QUIZ.

1. Which shoes are the best choice to wear with cropped pants?

A. Gladiator sandals
B. A range from stilettos to stacked wedge heels
C. Chunky, square heels
D. A range from sassy flats to sweet medium heels

2. Which skirt detail should be avoided if your tummy can't be?

A. A skirt with a side slit
B. A skirt with a kick pleat
C. A skirt with a waistband
D. A skirt with a ruffled hem

3. Which jacket is best for women with fuller bustlines?

A. Double-breasted, pardon the pun
B. Single-breasted, let's not go there
C. Mandarin jackets, straight from the East
D. None of the above

4. Which of the following celebrities does *not* have her very own clothing line?

A. Jennifer Lopez
B. Eve
C. Gwen Stefani
D. Erykah Badu

(Answers: 1-D, 2-C, 3-B, 4-D)

OCTOBER 21 | STUDS REQUIRED.

"Our life is frittered away by detail. Simplicity, simplicity, simplicity," said Henry David Thoreau.

Whether authentic or faux, the look is the look, for there is nothing more elegant and versatile than a round, brilliant diamond that appears to be close to half a carat, set in platinum. They are simple, elegant, and timeless.

OCTOBER 22 | MEAN *BUSINESS* IN YOUR CAMEL HAIR OVERCOAT.

She steps confidently onto the busy street from her towering office building, hair whipping in the wind and creating a gorgeous storm cloud of its own. This is the feeling of a quality camel hair coat every time you decide to toss it on. Doesn't matter if you're heading to the grocery store in jeans, picking up the kids from band camp in sweats, or wrapping up a meeting with your most important clients—with a camel hair overcoat flowing behind you, somehow you begin to feel like Sigourney Weaver in *Working Girl*.

Traditional American stores like Brooks Brothers and Paul Stuart have mastered this wool/cashmere blend coat. Wherever you decide to buy, know that it should have a double-breasted design, hit you well beneath the knee, and feature pronounced cuffs and a peak lapel if it is a classic.

OCTOBER 23 | HAPPY BIRTHDAY, SCORPIO GIRL.

As a water sign, you flow in and out of clothes and allow your supple sexuality to guide the intent. You embody a confidence that allows you to not seek approval on what you wear and how you come across. This also allows you to vacillate among fashion extremes. Your maxi coat and stilettos feel just as sexy as your flats and baggy linen pants, because you know that your power to allure starts from way inside. When women around you are all following the magazine trend of the moment, you can try it, or trash it with no hesitation. Heck, you might even wear a vintage version that started it all years ago.

Although you are linked to other daringly stylish Scorpio celebs, namely Lisa Bonet and Winona Ryder, you couldn't care less. You know that you, too, are a style star. Adornment and clothing are passions for you that seem to incite passion in others. Some see it as sexy, others as simply hot, as for you, it's just another day in the skin you call home.

OCTOBER 24 | GO FOR A PROFESSIONAL LEG WAXING.

It doesn't seem to matter how many times you've done it, shaving your legs is one of the tasks that most women would probably forfeit as quickly as wearing a bra if our critically observant world would be so kind and allow it. The creams, the water temperature, the "just right" leg positioning, the dull blade that's handy and the new, sharp one that's across the room mid-shower, and the darn nicks—this is just the first thirty seconds. Thank God for pants, the get-out-of-shaving-free card of a woman's closet.

On the other leg, most modern women have experienced the love/hate relationship with professional leg waxing. The technician who looks like she should be off baking rustic bread in the old country somewhere, the open feeling of being tabled and dressed with a warm wax product like a large sheet cake heading toward the table, and the quick, delayed-sting RIIIIIIIPS, always followed by the advice to breathe. Yeah, that takes away all the pain! Breathing.

Of the two, the latter is far more of a "finished" look on a woman's legs. A quality professional waxing lasts for anywhere from 3 to 6 weeks, removes hair completely from the root, and makes your hair grow back finer (if at all). So besides the visual benefits, why not just treat yourself to a beauty break from work today and clock in some self-improvement time.

OCTOBER 25

TURN A STYLE TRAGEDY INTO A TRIUMPH! LEFT THE HOUSE WEARING TOO MUCH FRAGRANCE? FIX IT BY SIMPLY BLOTTING COLD WATER ON YOUR SKIN THE MOMENT YOU NOTICE—AND HOPEFULLY BEFORE SOMEONE ELSE DOES.

There is a quick fix based on the principles of fragrance and scent distribution. Research shows that fragrance lasts longer on dry skin, thus any scent specialist's first tip is to never apply your perfume or cologne on just-showered, wet skin. But the opposite applies when you are in need of a quick fix. Find the nearest source of cold water, splash your hands and firmly press the excess cool water where you applied your scent. The water will soften the blow without killing the entire top note, whereas warm water (similar to perspiration) may strike it up more intensely. Fire out!

Also, keep in mind that it may not be your trigger finger, but the *strength* of your chosen fragrance. Some intensities and aromas such as sandlewoods, musks, and deep florals require one spritz at the very most, whereas you can virtually load on (within reason) cucumber and citrus-based scents. You may want to consider downshifting to a lighter choice so you can spray away and not be "scent" any more dirty looks.

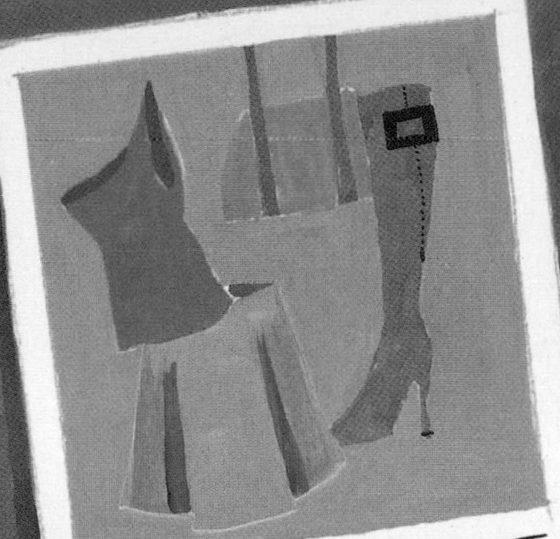
MY "GET PAST THE VELVET ROPE" OUTFIT (ADD SHADES)

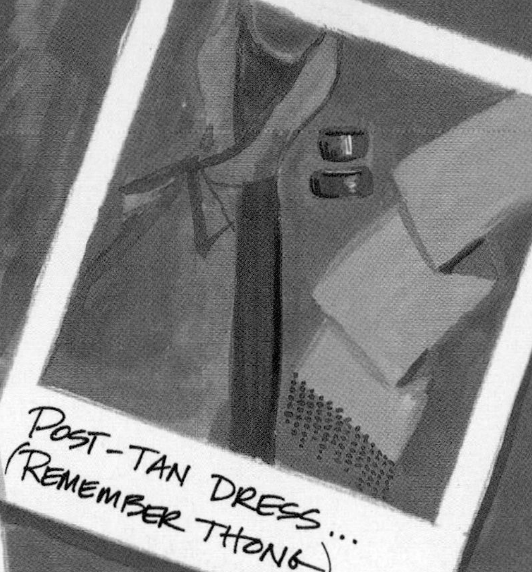
POST-TAN DRESS... (REMEMBER THONG)

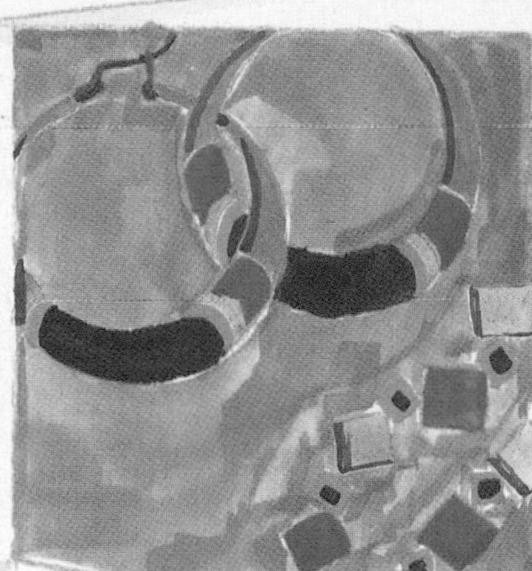
FROM RIO!

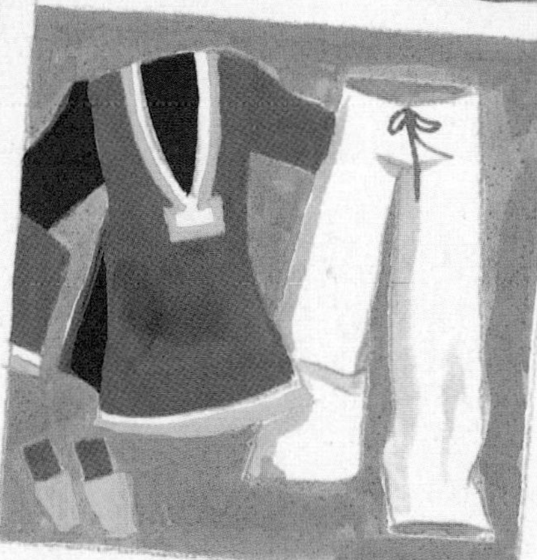
WINE TASTING OR BRUNCH WITH TERRY & LYNELL

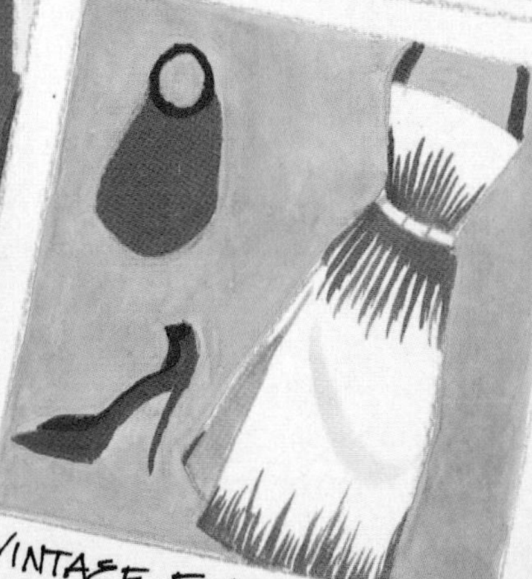
VINTAGE 50's SUNDRESS (SAVE FOR OUTDOOR WEDDINGS)

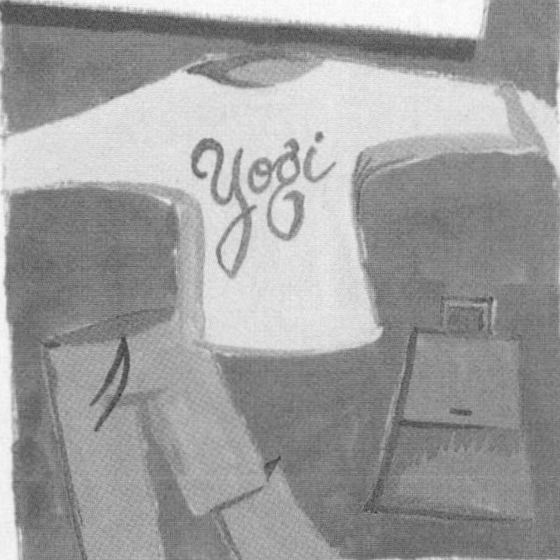
Yogi
FOR YOGA WITH THAT CUTE INSTRUCTOR

OCTOBER 26 | SNAP A PHOTO FOR THE NEXT TIME YOU NEED A STUNNING LOOK, BUT ARE STUMPED AND SHORT ON TIME.

Eliminate the guesswork from your compliment-winning outfits.

One thing I have learned in my years creating fashion presentations and reporting trends on national television is the art of never wearing the same outfit twice—or at least looking as if you are. I do it. The television hosts and personalities I have shared the stage with do it. But sometimes mixing and matching can only take you so far. There is an art to the process of looking fresh and new each day.

Enter the real world, where it is tough for some busy women to even remember what they wore yesterday without looking through the dry-cleaning pile or hamper. There is a simple solution that can help you keep track of your outfits, especially your compliment-winning outfits. Particularly the unexpectedly gorgeous ones you wish you could remember for the days when you have no time to spare.

First, be careful not to disassemble and discard too quickly winning outfits that can translate into winning ideas for the future. Take a moment and shoot a quick Polaroid or digital photo of your most compliment-winning outfits at the end of your day, either while wearing it or as it's draped across your bed—or hung on a hanger. Note the date it was worn, and a shorthand description of the actual elements (just in case the image isn't the clearest).

After a few weeks, you'll look up and have an instant road map, or look-book, of your best style when you have little or no time to dream up yet another outfit combination. You'll also avoid repeating them when some around you might be keeping track. And smart women know tha,mt this is the case most of the time.

OCTOBER 27 | WEAR ALL BLACK AND BE READY FOR JUST ABOUT ANY EVENT.

No, it is not just for funerals anymore. And where beatniks may have made the look famous in the 1950s, this day's all-black outfit idea is based on all things chic, minimal, mysterious, and, most of all, practical.

New York women have made the look famous, or infamous, depending on whom you are asking. They dip themselves in a figurative well of rich black ink, translated through clothing, creating one long, slimming line that forces the eye to look right into theirs.

Done casual, tailored, elegant for evening, or even with gym clothes, the idea is so simple, yet so many women forget to use this get-out-of-matching-clothes-free card, and run right back to the conundrum of doing so. Use this opportunity to try it just once, or save the solution for your next super-stacked busy day where you go from work to after-work cocktails, a quick dinner with clients, to a theater date and late-night dancing—whew! Exhausting just to think about it, but your all-black look will be wide awake and serving you stylishly at each and every turn, fitting in to every occasion if you create it properly. And this means just making it disappear so that it honors any room's level of formality.

Most important, make sure all your black garments match as closely as possible by testing them in the brightest daylight you have access to when getting dressed. There is nothing worse than seeing a woman in many shades of what she thinks is black.

WINNING COMBINATIONS

Black A-line Skirt + Black Knee Boots + Black Blazer + Black Blouse

= Power Meetings to PTA

Black Sweater Set + Black Leather Pants + Black Mules + Black Satin Scarf

= Desk to First Date

Black Jeans + Black Velvet Blazer + Black Turtleneck + Black Patent Pumps

= Gallery Opening to Nightclub Closing

OCTOBER 28 | RECAPTURE THE YOUTHFUL FUN AND FANTASY OF DRESSING UP FOR HALLOWEEN.

Remember the joy of laying out your Halloween costume the night before the big day at school? Maybe you took the time to sew it with your mom. You might have pieced together a character made up of great vintage things from your grandma's attic, and were finally allowed to wear a little more lipstick without being scolded. The possibilities were endless! And little did you know, the fantasy was the most innocent and pure form or escapism that you might have ever experienced. So why did you ever stop?

If you are the kind of woman who sneered at other adults in Halloween costumes in recent years, thinking they were immature or passé, this is the year to shake off all the stiffness that has set in from your important career, demanding family, and never-ending to-do list and release your inner Cleopatra! Or Antony—hell, it's Halloween, you can be him, too! That is the beauty.

Are you that zany, classic cartoon character you worshipped growing up, a parody of a political celebrity who has been in the news lately that you can re-create using your old business suit, or an abstract creation from things in the garage that your husband just can't throw away? It is your choice. Unlike the dressy holidays to come later in the year, use this fun, inexpensive holiday to show another facet of your style skills. Just remember, once in character, you have to live it for it to be believable. So choose wisely. I suggest steering away from anything that requires too much physical energy and charade acting to get people to recognize who you have become. Sometimes a repurposed old bridesmaid's dress can be the perfect start of a tooth fairy or good witch that actually looks kind of sexy.

OCTOBER 29 | A PERFECT WEEKEND BAG THAT WILL HOLD EVERYTHING YOU'LL NEED FOR THE TRIP.

Autumn is such a wonderful time to get away. Especially if you are near foliage and the countryside where every day the change of season bursts in color like unexpected fireworks.

There is nothing better than packing a single weekend bag that efficiently holds the basic style essentials in a snap. Your companion, if you are going the date route, will be thrilled that you can be spontaneous enough to be out the door in no time flat, and you will be amazed at how little you actually need when it is time to kick back and enjoy the view. Here is the checklist of the fashion "musts" for the perfect weekend bag.

TOPS

- ❑ A cozy, zip-front sweatshirt for traveling in velour, merino wool, or cashmere
- ❑ A crisp white button-down shirt
- ❑ A lightweight sweater set that can be worn together or apart for layering
- ❑ A black tank and a nude tank for layering

BOTTOMS/DRESSES

- ❑ A cozy pair of sweatpants for traveling in velour, merino wool, or cashmere
- ❑ Dark-rinse jeans for sneakers by day and heels by night
- ❑ A solid-colored knit jersey dress that wraps and can be easily steamed near the shower

OUTERWEAR

- ❑ A blazer in colorful corduroy, cotton velvet, or suede for long daytime walks or hot nights

FOOTWEAR

- ❑ Slip-on flat shoes with active/athletic soles for traveling and sightseeing
- ❑ Slim mules with a touch of shine or color for quick evening glamour
- ❑ Leather or suede knee boots with a dressy heel and toe

ACCESSORIES

- ❑ Simple diamond or faux studs for maximum versatility
- ❑ An array of bracelets, drop earrings, and necklaces to add flair to basics
- ❑ A wrap/scarf in cashmere or soft wool for neck by day and shoulders at night

OCTOBER 30 | DON'T LET TAGS SPOIL YOUR LOOK.

You've seen it countless times. Along the back collar of a woman in a gorgeous, sheer silk blouse. Near the chest of that woman who took so much time to artfully tie her printed Hermès silk neckerchief. Or—horror!—along the seam of a slinky dress. It's the dreaded, rectangular manufacturer's tag, materializing like a fashion apparition. And suddenly, that is *all* you can focus on.

What is it about those darned tags that make them so hard to part with? Do you really need to be constantly reminded of where your garment was made and the exact fabric content? I know, tags have important care instructions. I also know that some of you simply relish seeing that high-end designer name. But is holding on to these tags and labels worth a substandard look? I think not. Plus, you can always catalog the severed tags and refer back to them for cleaning care, or moments of designer pride.

Not taking the time to remove any visible interior manufacturer's tags is an absolute no-no. So today take a good look at your delicate wearables—those items that are sheer, revealing, or feather light—and carefully detach those obtrusive tags.

Did you know that it is a manufacturing requirement that tags be sewn onto clothes? Most designers would probably never even attach them if they didn't absolutely have to. Be they high-end designers or discount chains, most clothing makers want their wares to look their best on anyone who invests in them. Sporting tags inappropriately just isn't part of a high style equation. So take this as your permit to subtract anything with potential to detract from your best style.

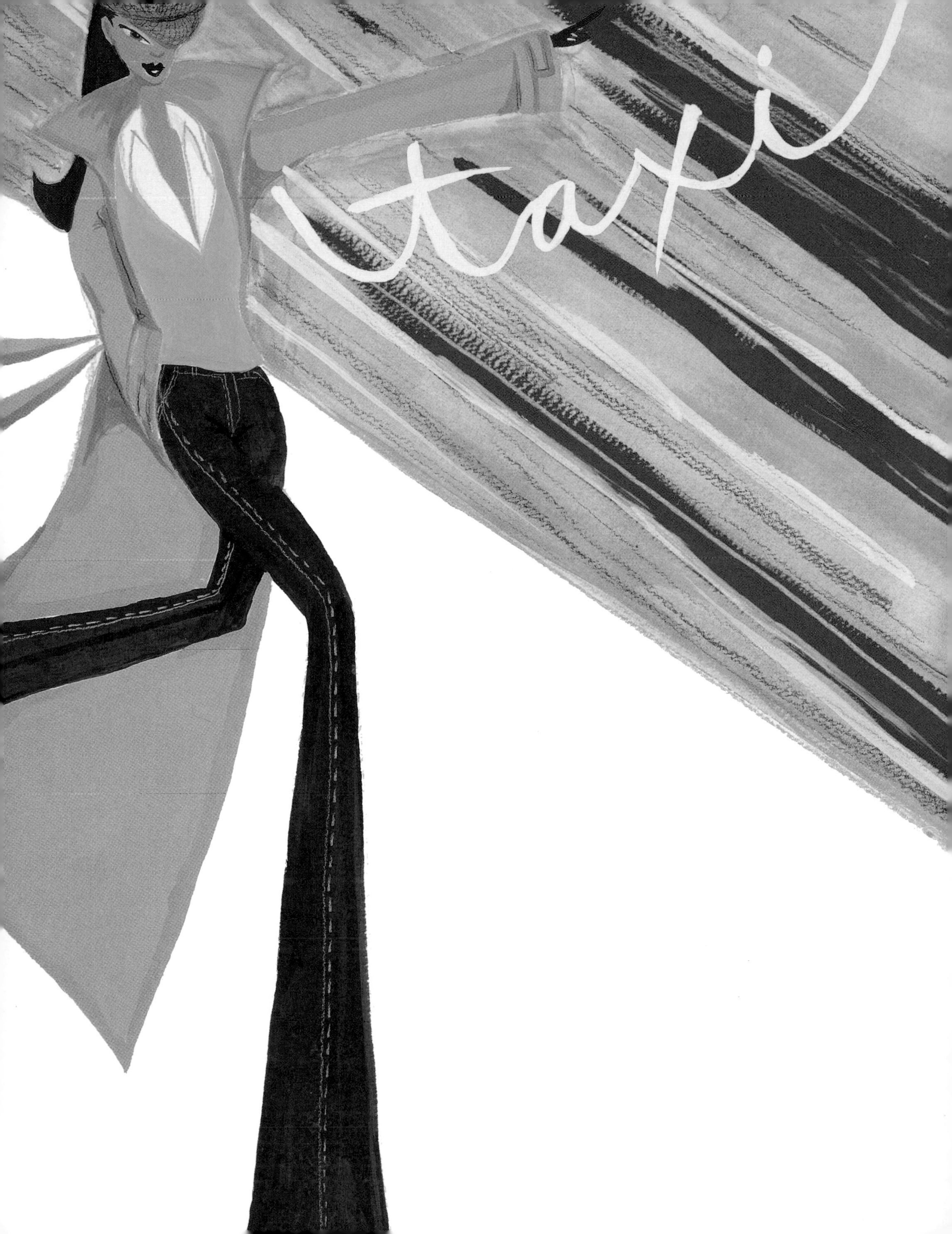
taxi

OCTOBER 31 | CREATE YOUR OWN VERSION OF THIS SUREFIRE, STYLISH OUTFIT COMBINATION.

Layer up your look to avoid the burgeoning autumn frost, but do it with thin layers that still flatter, not fatten. A fall trench is a great place to start. I say classic tan is fine, but why not go bright?

Top: A thin cotton V-neck sweater; even thinner solid cotton button-down shirt; a classic trench, belted with attitude
Bottom: Dark jeans in good condition
Shoes: Peep-toe heel in suede or leather
Accessories: Thin leather gloves
Flex piece: A wool newsboy cap

NOVEMBER

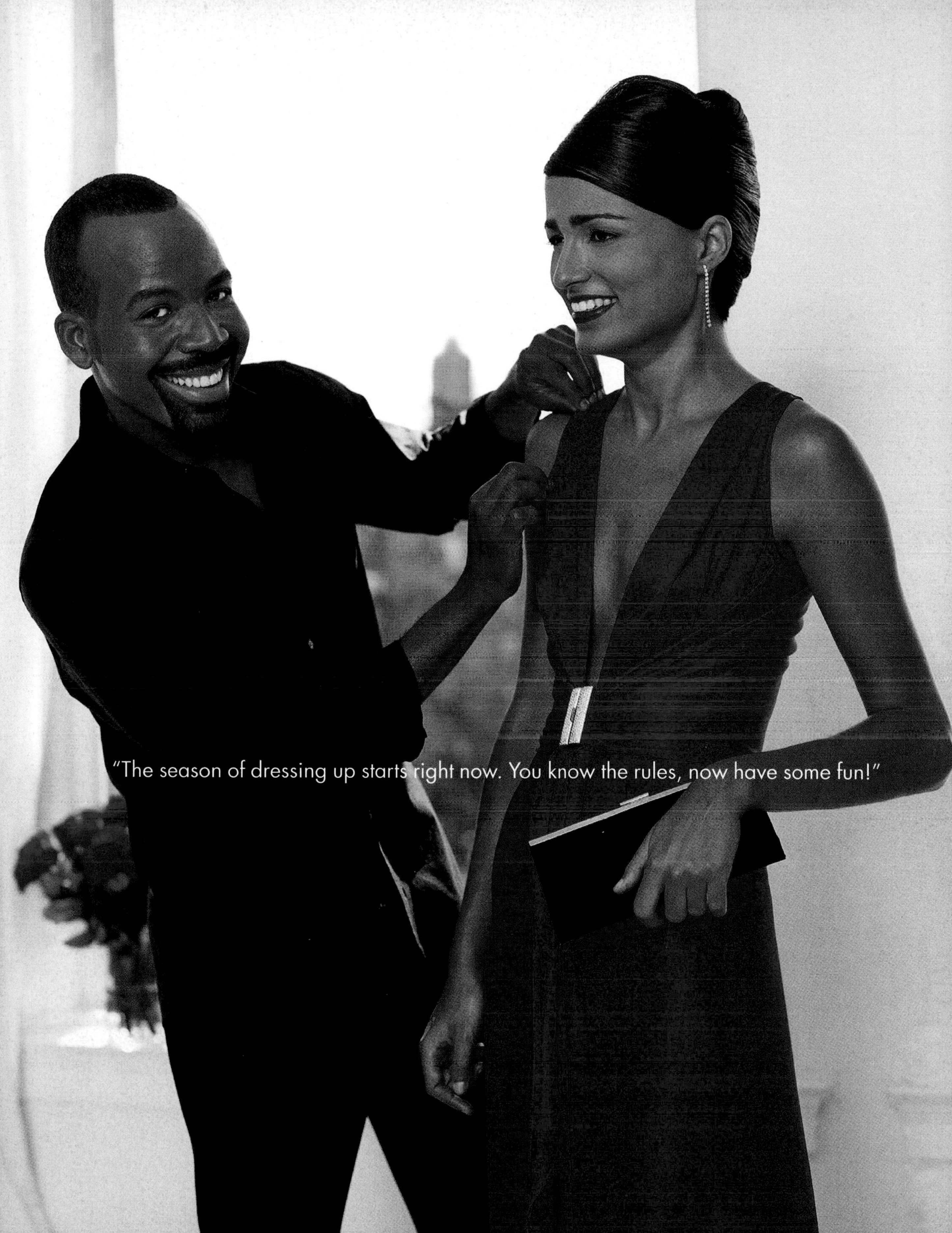
"The season of dressing up starts right now. You know the rules, now have some fun!"

NOVEMBER 1 | GIVE YOUR JEWELRY A BATH.

Jewelry, especially fine jewelry, is usually a precious possession, high in monetary or emotional value, and crafted to last a lifetime.

Before the glimmering rush of the holidays, when your jewels are front and center, make sure that your rings, diamonds, gemstones, pearls, and watches are properly maintained by taking them to a professional jeweler. It costs so much less than you think, and will help your pieces retain their value. Have your jewelry checked for loose prongs, tattered mountings, and general wear and tear. Use this day as an anniversary date to remind you to visit your jeweler at least once a year to have your jewelry professionally cleaned.

Just as you would do for your finest of dry-cleaned silk blouses, once you get all your jewelry back, keep it safe, secure, and out of harm's way with the following precious pointers:

• Always keep your jewelry in a clean area away from moisture.

• Invest in a jewelry case with a cloth interior, or in a simple box with divided sections, or you can swaddle each piece of your jewelry in basic tissue paper.

• To avoid permanent scratches, try not to tangle your jewelry pieces all together.

• When washing your hands, be careful not to place jewelry on the edge of a basin where it can quickly slip down the drain.

NOVEMBER 2 | TAKE AN EXPERT STYLE CUE FROM CYNTHIA ROWLEY, A TOP AMERICAN DESIGNER.

What is your best-kept personal style secret?

Pick out your outfit the night before. People are more inclined to experiment when they have more time and aren't in a panic because they're late.

What are the three fashion essentials every well-dressed woman should own?

1. Heels, because they make you feel confident and sexy.
2. Sunglasses so you can go out without makeup.
3. A great belt because it can fix many fashion mistakes.

What are the biggest mistakes women make when getting dressed?

1. Overaccessorizing.
2. Wearing clothes that are too tight.
3. Wearing looks that are too "matchy." Many women put together outfits exactly as they saw them on the mannequin and don't trust themselves to mix it up.

Who is the most stylish woman in existence, in your opinion? And what do you appreciate about her look?

The most stylish woman in existence is Scarlett Johansson because she manages to be sexy, sophisticated, and playful all at the same time.

If you could whisper a fail-safe style tip into the ears of women everywhere, without them feeling bad by hearing it, what would it be?

I would tell women to stand up straight. The right posture makes everything look better.

NOVEMBER 3 | UPGRADE YOUR UNDIES.

Think of how brides usually do this for their special day. Many women do it before a vacation. There is a private power in the newness.

Know that the same clean and new feeling that comes from stepping into the freshest of new underwear for a special event can be had all year long when you simply need an inexpensive lift. Keep a fresh set (tags still intact) in your dressing area at all times. And so you'll never be caught unprepared, when you pull off the tags, use it as a mental reminder to replenish your secret weapons with another set.

NOVEMBER 4 | WHAT'S YOUR SIGNATURE SCENT?

There are so many beautiful scents available these days, but likely only a few that really reflect your spirit. Know what they are. Here's a guide for finding out:

GIVE A HOOT

You're a woman who takes the spirit of the outdoors with her to dinner, dancing, and even to work! Woodsy, warm scents with notes of spicy sandalwood, oak, patchouli, a hint of cinnamon, and vanilla musk make you feel like you are communing with nature even in the heart of a big city.

SEA PRINCESS

Fresh and wet, you're a gal who dives right into life like a pool of possibility. Oceanic scents, like rain, sea grass, unexpected melon, cucumber, honeysuckle, and even a touch of sea salt take you right back to your last time on the surf and sand.

QUEEN OF CLEAN

You'd rather wear no signature scent at all, but if you must it is never musk. Just the opposite—succulent, fruity aromas with top notes of berry, florals like peony or sweet magnolia, and citruses like lime are a tropical scent sound track. You want others to hear you first, not smell anything artificial.

ACTIVATE ME!

Although a three-mile run releases the real you, the sweat is not the scent that matches your persona. You run to sporty scents like green tea, lemon, freesia, and a smidge of tuberose. Always ever so lightly applied, they match your endurance level and femininity equally.

GREEN THUMB

Nature girl, yes. Natural body odor, no! Though you live green, you know that grooming and flirty scents are where the crunchy lifestyle ends. Your fragrance garden is full of natural scents conjuring up leaves, lush flowering plants, touches of woody tones, and even bluegrass. Barefoot on a wet lawn is the mood—with a boost!

CANDY GIRL

Your sweet-sixteen party never stopped. The inner girl still loves all things pink and sugary and the smells of such bring you right back to high school. Scents with sweet cola, chocolate, mild vanilla, caramel, and even brown sugar are what you know to avoid but simply cannot resist.

A ROSE BY ANY OTHER NAME

A true romantic, the age of innocence is alive on your pulse points, and maybe even in your closet. You swoon over distinct floral scents like orchid, pure tuberose, lush violet, and wild country flowers. Jane Seymour has nothing on you.

NOVEMBER 5 | SMALL TIPS, BIG RETURNS.

Models usually have great posture.

This is no surprise since it's their job, a role originally designed to make a product look the best it can, and hopefully sell it. As a result, they are aware how anything they are dressed in looks at all times. Their posture never looks forced or self-conscious, just attuned to the fit and drape of their clothes. Real women can take a cue or two from them that has nothing to do with being skinny.

You may be sitting in an office all day, a far cry from strutting down an international catwalk, yet the tips can still help you preserve your look and sell the best you.

Post these two tips on a sticky note to remind you. This basic duo has been around for decades. Many real women may have seen their mothers applying it but never knew why. You'll never question them again, once you see how they can save an entire outfit.

(CONTINUED)

NO MORE KNEE-BAGGING

Lifting your pants a few inches when sitting to avoid knee bags is a simple trick to keep casual or dress trousers looking crisp. Be sure that the area of fabric that usually hits you at the knee when standing is hiked well above your knee when seated, especially when under a table, you have the leeway to lift them high for added knee-bagging prevention. Also, choosing skirts with slits is another way to avoid this frumpy look that results from sitting.

BYE-BYE SOCK GRABS

Remove casual, elastic leg socks at least an hour before dressing up in skirts to avoid "sock grabs." Most women have seen these gripping impressions caused by a day of long sock wear. The evening approaches and you opt for bare legs or sheer hose, and there lies the impression of a day of play in tube socks. Not a good look. Set an alarm, if only in your head, to remove your socks early enough before changing into leg-baring clothes.

NOVEMBER 6 | BAREFACED BY BEDTIME.

Top New York dermatologist Dr. Deborah A. Simmons says, "Women should never sleep in their makeup if they can help it." According to her, "going to bed in a full face of makeup can do damage to your skin over time, and not just temporarily. By thoroughly washing your face, you are not just removing cosmetics that can clog your pores overnight, you are first ridding the skin of pollutants that build up over the day, and oils, too—so the cleaning is threefold."

Cleansing the skin is easier and faster than ever. "From designer skin-care lines to trusted and inexpensive drugstore brands, women have options that make the messy facecloth and bar of soap a thing of the past," says Simmons. "There are several brands of face-cleansing cloths, both premoistened and 'just add water' that make it so simple to remove your makeup properly and fast at night. Always begin with a cleansing cloth made for sensitive skin, even if you think your skin is not, to prevent damage from an ingredient that may be too harsh." And the best news is that you don't have to spend a lot of money on department-store brands to get the best results. The good doctor feels that drugstore versions are just as capable.

A quick practical tip from Simmons for all skin types is to create your own quick-cleansing solution using equal parts basic antiseptic mouthwash and water—and cleanse with a cotton swab. Basic witch hazel and toners are mild enough to work on normal skin as well. She adds, "Pollutants plus daily build-up, plus oils and your day's makeup equals acne. These things clog your pores and, if slept on, you are basically *grinding* and packing them further into the pores, which could cause a lot of damage."

NOVEMBER 7 | WEARING HOSE.

Hosiery, at its best, should virtually disappear on the leg or be overtly dark enough to intentionally stand out and complement an ensemble.

THE SHOE-IN

Try and match the shade of your shoe color. Simply put, dark shoes look best with dark hose. This can get tricky if your shoes are dark and your bottoms are not. In this case, I suggest choosing hose in the color of your skin. Be careful of the old-fashioned, suntanned legs identified with weary flight attendants.

GO DEEP

In cooler months, complement your bottom. Again, dark skirts or pants call for dark hose. Go with navy, solid black, or even charcoal.

NOVEMBER 8 | TAKE AN EXPERT BEAUTY CUE FROM BJ GILLIAN, A TOP COVER GIRL MAKEUP ARTIST.

What is your best-kept personal beauty secret?

Let your true beauty shine through. Apply a natural-looking foundation just where you need it instead of applying a heavy mask that hides your skin tones and features. Concentrate on playing up one feature that you love with vibrant color or a great finish that makes it the focus of your look, then leave the rest of your face natural.

What are the three beauty essentials every woman should own?

Every woman should have a foundation or concealer they feel comfortable with. Today's best products don't just cover, they enhance. If you can't say that about the products in your makeup bag, it's time to invest in new ones that really create a natural, luminous look for you. A perfect canvas is key.

For a second product, blondes should pick separating mascara that delivers volume and darkens lashes. Blondes tend to have light eyelashes and mascara can help enhance their overall look. For brunettes, lip color is a must-have because it adds dimension to the face and provides the perfect accent.

(CONTINUED)

Finally, every woman should own an all-over face color that can be used on cheeks and eyes. Today's best blushes—like Cheekers from Cover Girl—provide a translucent, luminous shot of color that bronzes cheeks and adds a natural flush to the face. It can also be used on eyes to accent bone structure.

What are the biggest mistakes women make when applying makeup?

One of the biggest mistakes women tend to make when applying makeup is not embracing change. Women tend to find one look and stay with it year after year. Makeup gets better and better and women should look for new cosmetics that meet their changing needs. Not just with color, but also with technology. A great example is now we have lip color that feels and looks as good as traditional lip color but lasts eight to ten hours like CoverGirl Outlast Smoothwear lip color. Cosmetics offer so many possibilities on both the technology and color fronts that it's easy to look your best at any age.

Who is the most stylish woman in existence, in your opinion? And what do you appreciate about her look?

I work with women from every walk of life, from glamorous stars who are preparing to appear on national television to everyday women at mall makeovers. The most beautiful women share confidence in their own personal beauty and continually reinvent themselves to avoid staying frozen in time.

If you could whisper a fail-safe beauty tip into the ears of women everywhere, without them feeling bad by hearing it, what would it be?

Please don't sleep in your makeup. If it were made to sleep in it would be called night cream. Teach your children about sunscreen. Beauty is forever if you keep your skin out of the sun.

Keep it simple. The best approaches to beauty are those that are simple and easy. The more confusing it is the more confused you'll be. Beauty products should be used as tools to enhance what's unique and beautiful about you.

Finally, it's not how people judge you or see you that makes you beautiful, it's how you feel about yourself and how you portray that to the world.

NOVEMBER 9 | LEARN A NEW FASHION TERM.

***Batik** (bah-teek) • 1. Designs, usually in dark blue, rust, black, or yellow, made by using an Indonesian technique of painting with wax before dyeing. 2. Method of dyeing fabric by drawing the design on silk or cotton, then covering with hot wax all areas that are to remain white, dyeing, removing wax, resulting in a pattern with a crackle effect; process originated in Indonesia.*

Tuck this definition away for warmer months, but don't be afraid to feature chic batiks even this time of year. As I always say, the unexpected look is what sets you apart.

Batiks conjure up the festive prints of the East, but done simply in two colors so they still have a sort of minimal quality. Caftans, dashikis, tunics, and djellabas from Africa and Indonesia sometimes feature batik prints. The look is casual and celebratory all at once, giving you the option of pairing a batik top with dressy, satin pants and heels, or well-worn jeans and flats. Both are valid fashion combinations and total entrance makers.

The beauty of batik is the fact that you don't have to be of a specific ethnicity to flaunt its majesty. Sometimes the look stands out even stronger when you don't look as if you were raised in prints from the East. There is a sexy and interesting juxtaposition that happens when your visual identity meets that of a foreign locale, head-on. The visual conflict looks more than peaceful. Like a woman who had a ticket to see the world, used it, and relives her journey every time she slips into her batik top. Only she has to know that she grabbed it at a local yard sale.

NOVEMBER 10 | THREE WINTER LOOKS IN ONE.

Busy women, with or without a confident sense of personal style, know what it is like to have to change in a flash, in a moving taxi, in a ladies' room, or even in the backseat of a parked car. Space is limited, accommodations aren't ideal, and you just hope for the best outcome.

Fully loaded: Tan wool overcoat + white dress shirt + red V-neck sweater + black dress pants + black heels
Completely chic: White dress shirt + red V-neck sweater (over shoulders) + black dress pants + black heels
Simply fab: Tan wool overcoat + red V-neck sweater + black dress pants + black heels

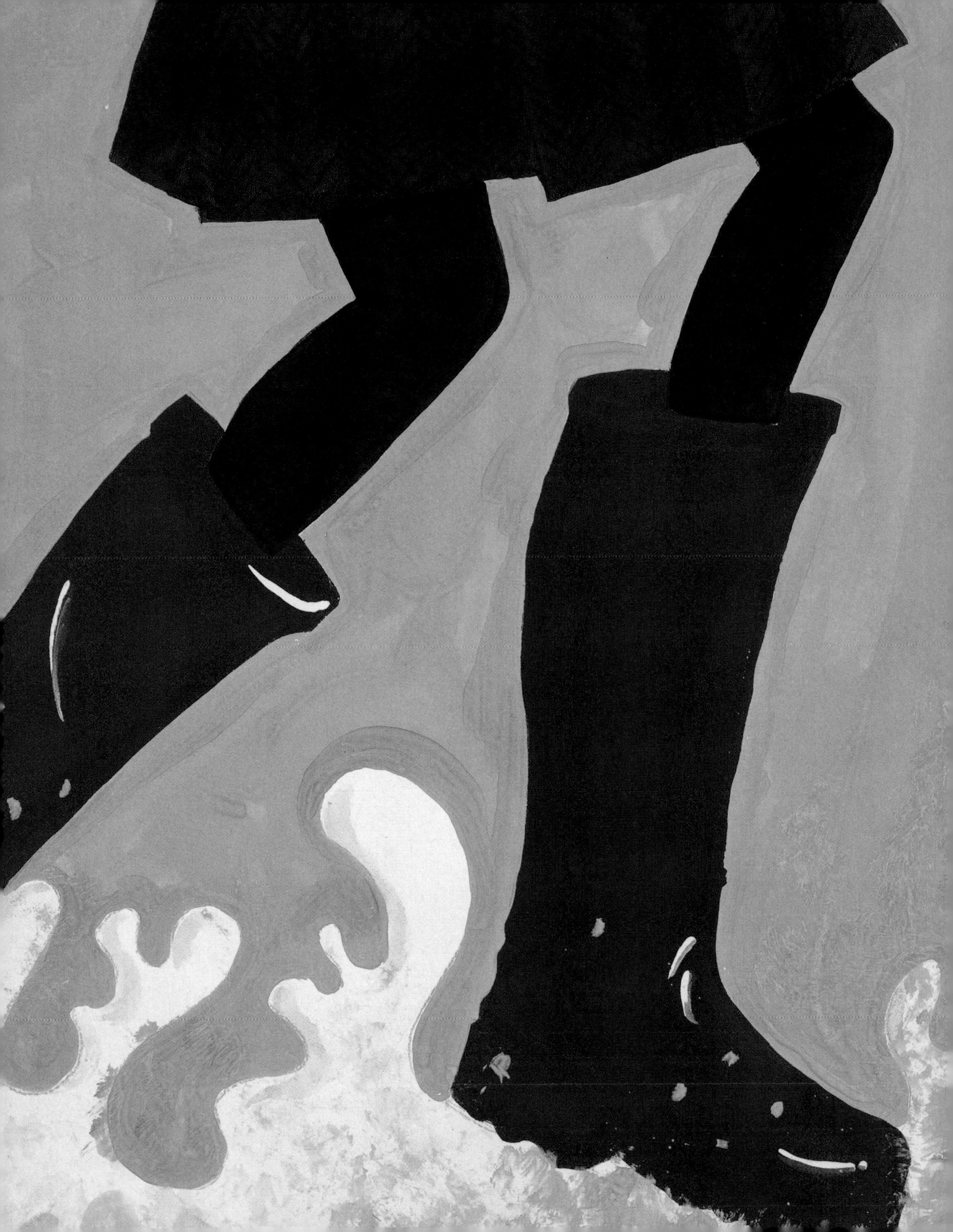

NOVEMBER 11 | JUMP INTO A PAIR OF WELLIES.

According to Hunter Boots, one of Scotland's most venerable boot manufacturers for over 150 years, the origins of Wellington boot making in Scotland date back to 1817. Arthur Wellesley, the first Duke of Wellington, instructed his shoemaker, Hoby of St. James Street, London, to modify a basic eighteenth-century boot, resulting in a new boot design cut closer around the leg, which was hard wearing for battle yet comfortable for the evening. The Iron Duke didn't know what he was starting, for the boot was dubbed the "Wellington" and the name has stuck ever since.

American manufacturers modified the concept in the mid-1800s by experimenting with the same design but using rubber to better brave the elements.

If you search, you'll find Wellies in the traditional hunter green, as well as more feminine colors like red and hot pink.

Pair them with opaque tights and a shorter skirt, or toss them on with jeans or khaki pants cuffed really high. The rubber will literally put a bit of bounce in your step as you make your way down the wet streets, and the youthful look will allow a woman of any age to splash around freely like a girl puddle-hopping her way to school even if you are heading to another boring day on the job.

NOVEMBER 12 | TRY ADDING AN ABSTRACT PRINT.

Abstract prints are very stylized designs of a non-naturalistic type, usually of the geometric print family yet a bit more "out of order" to the more conservative set. This is indicative of the roots of such prints, for before they trickled across to fashion, they became popular after a 1964 exhibit of Op Art paintings at the Museum of Modern Art in New York City set the conservative art world aflame—just like our "unapologetic" woman does today in a room of conventional fashion types.

And just like Op Art's signature bent lines—warped shapes that create an optical illusion (think checkerboards that look as if you've had a cocktail or two [or four] before sitting down to play)—prints of the abstract persuasion can do wonders to a figure that needs attention, or painterly distraction. The choice is yours. Hey, might you even be a bit unapologetic today?

THREE WAYS TO ALWAYS LOOK STYLISH IN ABSTRACT PRINTS

•Infuse fun into the cooler months when most women are running to safe tweeds and Donegal plaids. Set yourself apart with an abstract printed blouse, worn beneath a more serious solid-color suit—a great way to take on the night by just taking off your jacket.

•Abstract doesn't have to mean getting crazy. Consider incorporating a dynamic, abstract print in a tonal pattern—so all the elements in the design are in varied shades and weights of the same color.

•When in doubt, choose an abstract print top that you can pull back on in an instant by layering it beneath a solid sweater, jacket, or trench.

NOVEMBER 13 | DEFINE YOUR WAIST.

Bow-tied ribbons and superthick or ultrathin belts are great ways to mind your middle. The waistline is an overlooked area of a woman's body, which can really add interest to an otherwise boring outfit on any given day—why not right now? Look down at your waistline—at a very different place for each and every woman—and hold it. Are you high-waisted, have a long torso, or maybe even thick-waisted? Guess what, the waist is still there. It is probably just time to give it some attention.

Do what so many high-fashion designers do from season to season: play with your waist area to create drama and add shape to a shapeless top, skirt, or dress. Using anything from hand-crafted leather belts to a yard of $5 grosgrain ribbon from your local fabric and notions shop can have equally amazing results. Here are some ways to pull it off, or in, for that matter:

HIGH-WAIST GALS

The goal is to add more vertical balance to your frame when dressing. Reach for thick belts (four inches and up) that sling lower and close to your hips. The cinching action of a wide belt will add more length to your torso and even out your shape. Try one atop a tank and jeans, or even over a blousy peasant top.

LONG-TORSO GALS

You have it made, according to many women. Your best belts are slimmer and those that have excess dangle: handcrafted leather fringe, metal chain links and loops, or anything ornate that starts slim and keeps the eye going down. You can even create your own bow-tied ribbon belt with a strip of grosgrain ribbon.

THICK-WAIST GALS

Never despair, your waist is in there. It may just need a bit of unearthing or illusionist tactics. Many women with thick waists have to go higher than normal when adding attention to an area that has little shape. Just beneath your bustline is as high as you should go. Empire-waist dresses and tops are key. Funky Bohemian silhouettes that gather and tie up above the navel, and then blouse out can do the trick as well.

NOVEMBER 14 | POP STYLE QUIZ.

1. As designer hemlines change, which length is always timelessly elegant and appropriate?

A. Well above the knee
B. Just around the knee
C. Just around the ankles
D. Midcalf

2. Which American singing legend was made famous in Paris by wearing a skirt fashioned of artificial bananas?

A. Lena Horne
B. Nina Simone
C. Josephine Baker
D. Dorothy Dandridge

3. Which luxury knit fabric is created from the belly hairs of goats found in the most remote regions of the Himalayas?

A. Boiled wool
B. Cashmere
C. Alpaca
D. None of the above

4. To most women's surprise, which is the most flattering place to store a small cell phone?

A. In a compartment within a tote or purse
B. Tucked in the center of your bra
C. Attached to either side of your waistband or belt
D. In one outer breast pocket of a jacket

(Answers: 1-B, 2-C, 3-B, 4-A)

NOVEMBER 15 | GET TEN-MINUTE STYLE CHIC FOR TAILGATE EVENTS.

Here is a great ten-minute style solution for any outdoor tailgating party:

Minutes 1:00–2:00:
Cut the fuss! Heels and skirts are no good. Grab a fun pair of cargo pants—maybe even a pair of his if you can roll them up and pull it off believably.

Minutes 3:00–4:00:
Soften up your top by choosing ultrafeminine colors. Layer a pink short-sleeve T-shirt over a yellow long-sleeve T-shirt or similar contrasting colors.

Minutes 5:00–6:00:
Opt for cute, colorful sneakers that look active but are really just for styling. And toss on a classic denim jacket, the more worn the better!

Minutes 7:00–8:00:
Keep the woman in you present by going for sexy hair that is still easy to do. Something about a fun, high ponytail does both. Think cheerleader sassy!

Minutes 9:00–10:00:
Makeup is where you lose time and arguments! Take care of the under eye area, a little powder, mascara—and pack a lip gloss with you for the car. Go, girl, go!

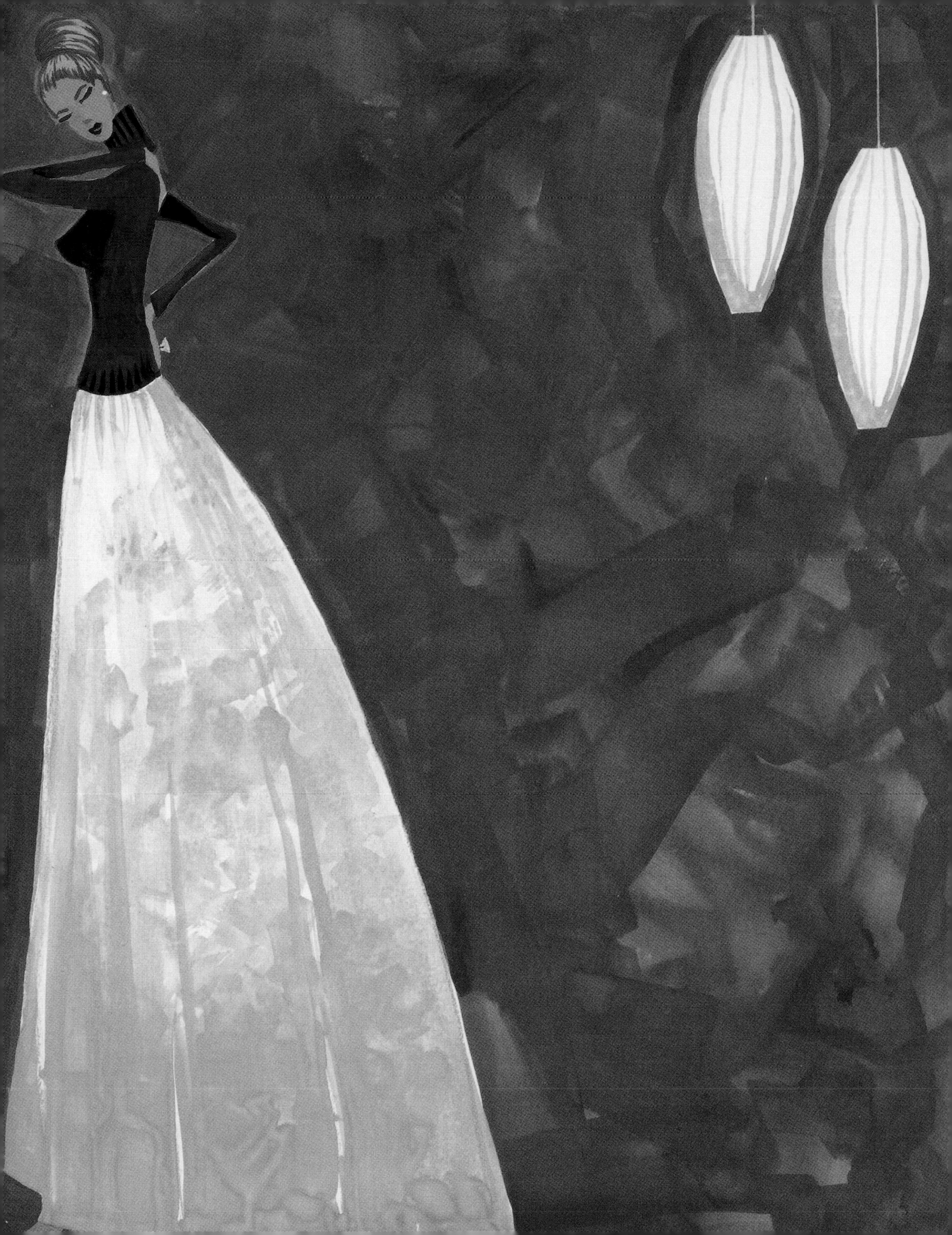

NOVEMBER 16

SIMPLIFY AND "SEXIFY" YOUR LOOK. WEAR YOUR MOST FLATTERING, FITTED BLACK TURTLENECK.

This garment may, in fact, be the only cool-weather top a woman needs—taking her from ultracasual to formal if the fabric is versatile enough. Imagine an ultrathin cashmere turtleneck that skims close to the body and hugs the neck high and snug.

Pair it untucked with flat-front tan chinos that flare at the leg and a sweet pair of magenta ballet flats in suede, creating a weekend brunch look that rivals any of Audrey Hepburn's finest moments off-camera. Conversely, you could take the same top right into the night for a gala evening affair by coupling it tucked with a solid black or pale, floor-length satin ball gown skirt and sparkly evening mule. Add an ornate vintage clutch and you are out the door with a sporty take for the red carpet that will look personal and unique.

Shake out your best turtleneck and allow it to breathe today.

NOVEMBER 17 | INVITE A PEACEFUL ELEGANCE INTO YOUR DAY BY WORKING THE COLOR LAVENDER.

Find a place in your look today for the color lavender. Why? Because this color will put the world around you at ease. Lavender is the one color that speaks of total relaxation and the nurturing spirit of femininity without being stereotypical, like baby pink.

Historically, lighter shades of purple suggest refinement along with grace, elegance, and that indescribable something that eases tension. I call it the color of meditation. And nature follows right behind with the lavender plant, orchids, lilacs, and violets, which are often superdelicate and considered the most precious of flowers.

Dash it into your ensemble in a dose that won't alarm or make you feel too powdery. Sometimes it is just a *hint* of something new that makes the most impact.

NOVEMBER 18 | THROW OUT THE MOST UNFASHIONABLE ACCESSORY OF ALL, THE CIGARETTE.

Every year around this week, across the nation, smokers seeking to quit participate in the American Cancer Society's popular Great American Smokeout by either smoking less or quitting just for the day (the actual day is the third Thursday of November). The event challenges people to cease tobacco use and raises consciousness of the many diseases that come from smoking.

The concept was hatched out of a 1974 event created by Lynn R. Smith, editor of the *Monticello Times* in Minnesota, who spearheaded the state's first "D-Day," or "Don't Smoke Day." The idea caught fire, and on November 18, 1976, the California division of the American Cancer Society successfully prompted nearly one million smokers to quit just for the day. The California event marked the first Smokeout, and the Society took it nationwide in 1977.

The Smokeout has helped bring about dramatic changes in Americans' attitudes about smoking, which have led to community programs and smoke-free laws that are now saving lives in many states, and making women look more stylish—at least in my view.

Seriously, though, research shows that smokers are most successful in kicking the habit when they have some means of support and the encouragement of friends and family.

Use this reminder to put down your habit if only for twenty-four hours, or if you know someone who is still puffing away, let him or her know that you care and are there to help.

Those around you may be too shy to tell you, but I am not. Nothing can ruin the look of a gorgeous woman with notable style faster than a burning cigarette smack in the center of the picture. The days of glamorous smoking became passé with the passing of black-and-white films. Your life in living color is real and precious, so honor it by respecting your body and keeping it smoke free!

NOVEMBER 19 | ALWAYS REQUEST A FRESHLY UNPACKAGED ITEM OF ANYTHING YOU'VE TRIED ON IN A CLOTHING STORE.

Garments are continually flowing in and out of boutique and department store doors each day. Many of them have been tried on by one, if not several, customers. Count yourself among this number. The idea is a simple one. You see it. You like it. You try it. You buy it. Yet somewhere between steps three and four, additional parties get involved and can leave their presence behind.

Trying on garments in the privacy of a dressing room allows people to be themselves. Some people take care of their clothes. Others do not. Some people take care of their bodies. Others do not. This list could get long and sordid.

You can always request what I call a "fresh" version from the stockroom, hopefully bagged and in a manufacturer's packaging, or just hanging untried by the masses. By making this small request, hopefully you won't experience the impressions of the hips from the person before you, traces of the deodorant from the girl in a hurry, or makeup from the more dolled-up shoppers before you.

NOVEMBER 20 | SILVER-SCREEN INSPIRATION.

I have a personal "top three" list of movies from three very different decades that knock me off my feet every time I watch them. It is not about the story lines, the romantic crescendos, or even the big-name stars—it is all about the clothes. The spectacular clothes! Use this autumn night to curl up with a movie that will do more than entertain. Let it inform your style. Allow it to inspire your clothing choices the following day and beyond. And most of all, look at the characters' ability to fearlessly embrace looks that are unique and signature without hesitation—or seemingly so. Let's count 'em!

#1 *BREAKFAST AT TIFFANY'S* (1961)

One of the silver screen's most fashionable female characters of all time, Holly Golightly. Audrey Hepburn's defining style role is summed up in the very first scene, when she is on New York's Fifth Avenue at daybreak, dressed to perfection in her black dress and tiara, sipping basic New York coffee and nibbling a pastry while window-shopping at Tiffany's—all beneath the film's illustrious score and opening credits. Genius! ***Take away:*** Wear what you like, whenever you like, and they will follow.

#2 *MAHOGANY* (1975)

Many would argue with me from a cinematic standpoint, but few would disagree with the story of a struggling fashion design student who makes her way from Chicago to the high life of Milan's fashion world, both as a top designer *and* supermodel—all in less than two hours. And the star, an in-her-prime Diana Ross, designed the drop-dead costumes herself, or at least the credits say so. ***Scene to beat all scenes:*** Diana swaps one of her own designs on a big-budget film shoot, gets reprimanded by the director (Anthony Perkins), and fires off the face-slap heard 'round the world.

#3 *THE WOMEN* (1939)

This film can be summed up in one word: glamour. A groundbreaking all-female cast of legends from Joan Crawford to Rosalind Russell being catty, gorgeous, dolled-up, fabulous girls—from the first scene to the last. The story is not so important. It is all about the lines and the delivery. ***Reason to buy instead of rent:*** Although billed as a black-and-white feature, there is a small portion of the movie, midway, filmed in color; a glorious "fashion show" scene that you will want to watch again and again!

NOVEMBER 21 | HOW DO I WANT TO BE REMEMBERED?

Ask yourself, "How do I want to be remembered, even for just today?" And try to answer with one word. Strong. Sweet. Hip. And the word can change weekly.

Use the answer to plot out your day's best look and what you reach for regularly. Here are some general guidelines for style choices and their meanings to discerning onlookers—and I would know, as I am one with a watchful eye on women.

STRONG

Clean, bold, classic lines

Avoid excessive amounts of embellishments and froufrou

Suits (pant or skirt), solid colors, and as few separates as possible

SWEET

Softer shapes and lines, more traditionally feminine color palette

Embrace pattern, texture, and whimsy

Select a sweater over structured, tailored jackets and tops

HIP

Mix the unexpected (linear shapes with romantic detailed garments)

Pair colors that speak to your exact mood every time and never question it

Trends are accents, whether vintage, hot-off-the-runway, or big bargains

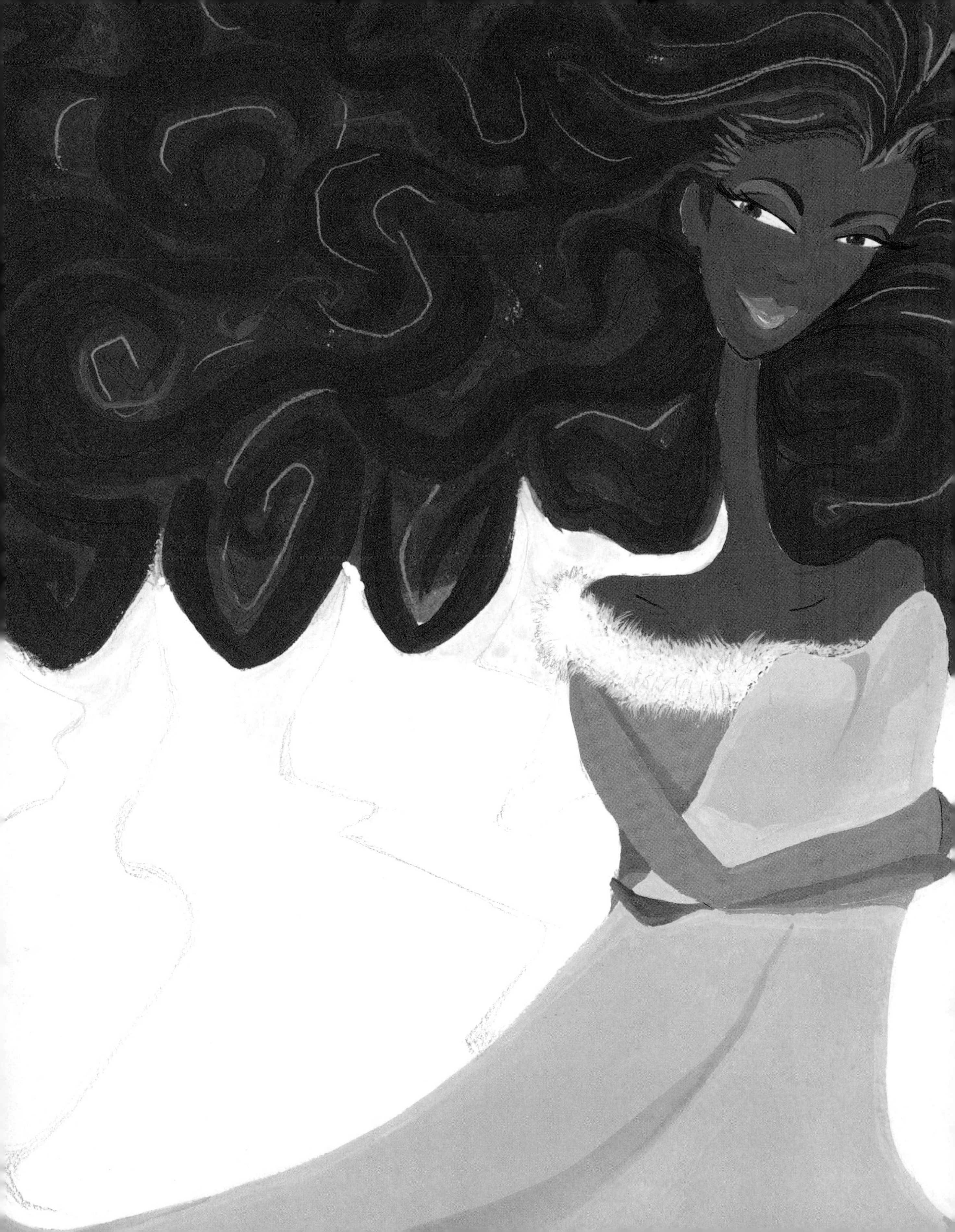

NOVEMBER 22 | HAPPY BIRTHDAY, SAGITTARIUS GIRL.

You are bohemian at heart and like to keep your wardrobe stylishly close to mother earth.

Talk about easy, you take life at your pace with the fluidity of a water sign even though you are a true fire sign. For you, the fire within actually allows you to stay cool on the outside. Your attire, or lack thereof, follows you organically and allows you remain cozy but never corny.

A natural style sensibility can take shape for the lively Sag in many creative ways that can fool others. You like to have fun on the go. Weekend getaways mean bringing loose-fitting skirts that sweep the earth and hint toward sassy (versus sexy) flats that lounge or take you hiking—leaving behind fussy hair products and pore-clogging makeup. Your glamour can happen from a simple lip balm. The fresh air makes you feel alive. You usually want your clothes to simply be a conduit to that feeling!

Daryl Hannah and Tyra Banks share your birth sign, and when not dolled up for the camera they are known for kicking back in easy, relaxed elegance. Just like you, they know when to turn up the artifice and glamour, but they reserve that power for when it really matters. This would be never, if the free-spirited archer were to always have her way.

NOVEMBER 23 | GO, HILLARY, GO!

November 23, 1999: Hillary Rodham Clinton announced her intention to seek a seat in the U.S. Senate from New York, an unprecedented move for the wife of a U.S. president.

Most women have the standard picture of what an American first lady should be etched in their minds. Appropriately dressed, platform ready to be shared at a podium, and full of the good "wifely" social graces. Think Jacqueline Kennedy—pillbox hat and all.

Well, Hillary Rodham Clinton had all of those things in place and more important ones just beneath the surface. My, how appearances can tell the world exactly what you *want* them to know.

On this very day, months before the new millennium, Clinton announced her intention to seek a seat in the U.S. Senate from New York. Many were shocked and curiously impressed. She dusted off any naysayers and kept her eyes on winning the election, which she in fact did.

Take a cue from her fire within when getting dressed, and don't put all your cards on the table. Keep in mind that certain clothes reveal too much way too soon. Choose an ensemble that peels away to reveal your many moods as the day passes. For work, tailored suits can conceal shimmery party tanks without anyone at the watercooler ever knowing, while saving you time going from day to night. Or, a casual black velour sweat suit can also become evening pants by just adding a white dress shirt, black patent leather flats, and a brooch, all of which can happen in your car if in a pinch. Very Hillary. Next stop, the White House maybe?

NOVEMBER 24

AVOID TRYING TO PASS OFF YOUR WORKHORSE OF AN OVER-COAT FOR SOMETHING SPECIAL ENOUGH TO GO ATOP GOWNS AND THE LIKE.

If your evening coat is special enough, it sometimes lets you ease back on your outfit's level of formality. The right evening coat can add that extra dose of glamour and help to balance out your entire look. Make sure you have one standing ready in your style arsenal, even if you only wear it once. You don't have to break the bank either. Unlined, solid satin trench coats can be perfect and cost less than a basic cashmere evening wrap. Floor-length wool coats with fur or faux fur collars have been around for decades; why not dig for one at a secondhand store and have it altered and refreshed for next to nothing. Or, simply go without and just don your best shoulder wrap or shrug—if you're just hopping from your door to a warm car—and back into another door. Just fake them out!

NOVEMBER 25 | GIVE THANKS.

According to the Women's Alliance (www.thewomensalliance.org), a national organization of independent, community-based individuals who provide professional attire, career skills training, and related services to more than fifty thousand women in transition from welfare and poverty, many American women you face daily are in crisis. And this very day may be one of the most difficult for them to face.

How can you help? The same closet that you see as a virtual wasteland could be a life-changing treasure trove for a woman in need. You can lend a sister a hand today by reaching in for both you and her. Choose something celebratory to wear for Thanksgiving Day, and while you're in the trenches, grab another gently used career suit or separate that you haven't worn since last bird-day. I'm sure you can think of the item before ever reaching in for a hanger.

The feeling will instantly lighten your day and layer a sense of calm over you before the joyously perfect time with family. Well, at least it *should* be a joyously perfect time. Either way, you'll be covered and so will another genuinely thankful woman.

Check out these great organizations as well:

www.dressforsuccess.org
www.wardrobe.org
www.suitedforchange.org

NOVEMBER 26 | BUILD YOUR OUTFIT WITH AN ABSOLUTE FAVORITE ITEM.

Pull a fast one on yourself and save minutes by making the first thing you pull out of your closet a tried-and-true favorite piece of clothing. You know the one. That suit, the one that makes you feel instantly skinny. The skirt covers you enough, yet has that hot back slit for amazing "exit strategy" from any meeting. Or it might just be your most comfortable shoes that make everything else feel a whole lot better. Whatever you decide to wear, if it's a favorite, you know that you'll feel better and ultimately look better. Those around you will let you know it, and what better way for a compliment to take the sting off any busy day.

Think about it, by using this simple style strategy, the first four minutes of getting dressed can really be given back to you and your day by reaching straight for what you know will never let you down, and structuring the rest of the look from there

NOVEMBER 27 | REAL STYLE BEGINS WHERE THE RULES END.

My mother once told me, "Real style begins where the rules end."

Your personal style can only be fully realized when you build upon what is standard, adding your own unique twists. Just step out far enough onto the ledge to experience the exhilarating thrill of the fall—without ever plunging to real harm. Each time you do, you instill character and a signature that acts as an identifiable extension of your personality.

Maybe you'll choose to wear white after Labor Day, when the women in your Southern town wouldn't dare. You may decide to mix your best navy blouse with a chic pair of black trousers to go to work in Denver, just like European women do. Or, today might be the day your husband's old tuxedo jacket goes off to the tailor to become your new evening jacket.

The trick is to own your nontraditional choices with as much confidence as you can muster and walk into any room with total confidence. If you happen to see another woman taking a similar chance, give her that nod of approval.

NOVEMBER 28 | GET A LITTLE MORE MILEAGE OUT OF YOUR FAVORITE LITTLE BLACK DRESS.

The little black dress is a staple for every woman, but don't let yourself and others get bored with it. Shake it up a bit, retro style. Take that classic sheath or spaghetti-strapped black dress and pair it with not one strand of pearls but six, or even eight, stacked as high and low as you can stand. Let them hang to your waist, fall just atop your bustline, and simply entwine as they may—for an edgy, Prohibition-chic look that just says fun and carefree. Keep the rest of the look simple and sophisticated, choosing a matching pair of black sling-backs or pumps, quiet diamond studs, and a cocktail ring at the most on your hands. If you don't need your watch, ditch it—and let your date lead you like a retro society lady heading out of the Cotton Club into a balmy night.

A few other great little black dress style solutions:

•Add knee boots in black or nude to give a Mod 1960s feel to a knee-length dress. Keep your makeup sheer and your lips nude to maximize the look. Opt for a square clutch with razor-sharp lines.

•Ignite your dress with attitude by pairing it with your longest, brightest trench coat, highest heels, and stacks of metallic necklaces stopping just *there*.

•If you dare to make it sporty, wear it with a lightweight matching leather jacket that hits you just at the waist, opaque tights in a bold color, and motorcycle boots.

NOVEMBER 29 | LOOK YOUR BEST BY MAKING THE MOST OF HOTEL AMENITIES WHEN TRAVELING.

My work takes me to about fifty different destinations each year. Some trips are longer than others, but the simple fact is that when you have to step out of your home routine by packing a bag, two days or twelve days really doesn't make too much of a difference. And taking your style along with you in a carry-on can be a challenge. What's the best way to look good coming and going?

Lean on the services provided by your hotel. Whether it's shining your shoes, pressing your shirts, or sending your dry cleaning out, it is a part of their business to provide you with the perks. It is your business to make the best use of the resources available to you.

There are three platinum style rules that you should follow upon check-in:

GIVE YOUR CLOTHES SOME MUCH NEEDED LEGROOM

Unpack as soon as you arrive. Hang and fold your clothes as necessary. Doing so allows fabrics to breathe after being compressed in a suitcase, and saves you time from having to iron them. If you find that you still need to smooth some wrinkles, use the bathroom to steam your clothes. Hang them on the shower rod spaced evenly apart, and run the hottest shower possible with the bathroom door closed for fifteen to twenty minutes. The steam will relax the wrinkles and have you ready to go in no time flat. If time allows, many hotels offer a twenty-four-hour valet who will arrange that your clothes be steamed or pressed for a fee. I recommend arranging this before you leave the lobby for your room.

HAVE YOUR SHOES SHINED

Most women know that footwear can make or break an ensemble. Traveling can add even more stress to our most stylish street soldiers. Many hotels have shoe-shine services set aside for business travelers. And for a few dollars and a small tip, your shoes can be polished professionally (and there is a difference), making even the most traveled suit look a touch better. If such a service is not available, you may want to inquire if the hotel has an automatic shoe polisher behind the scenes for employee use—better hotels always want their staff looking spiffy from head to toe. If so, a meager palm greasing and a smile will usually get your tootsies backstage for a quick hit of shine.

TOUCH UP YOUR LOOK WITH YOUR PILLOWCASE

Most of today's hotels have an iron and ironing board waiting for you in your room's closet. But often times these irons are not top of the line, nor are they intended to be. So, when giving a quick press to any of your clothing, simply remove one pillowcase from the bed's pillows to shield your clothes from potential scorching, snagging, or water that may leak from the iron.

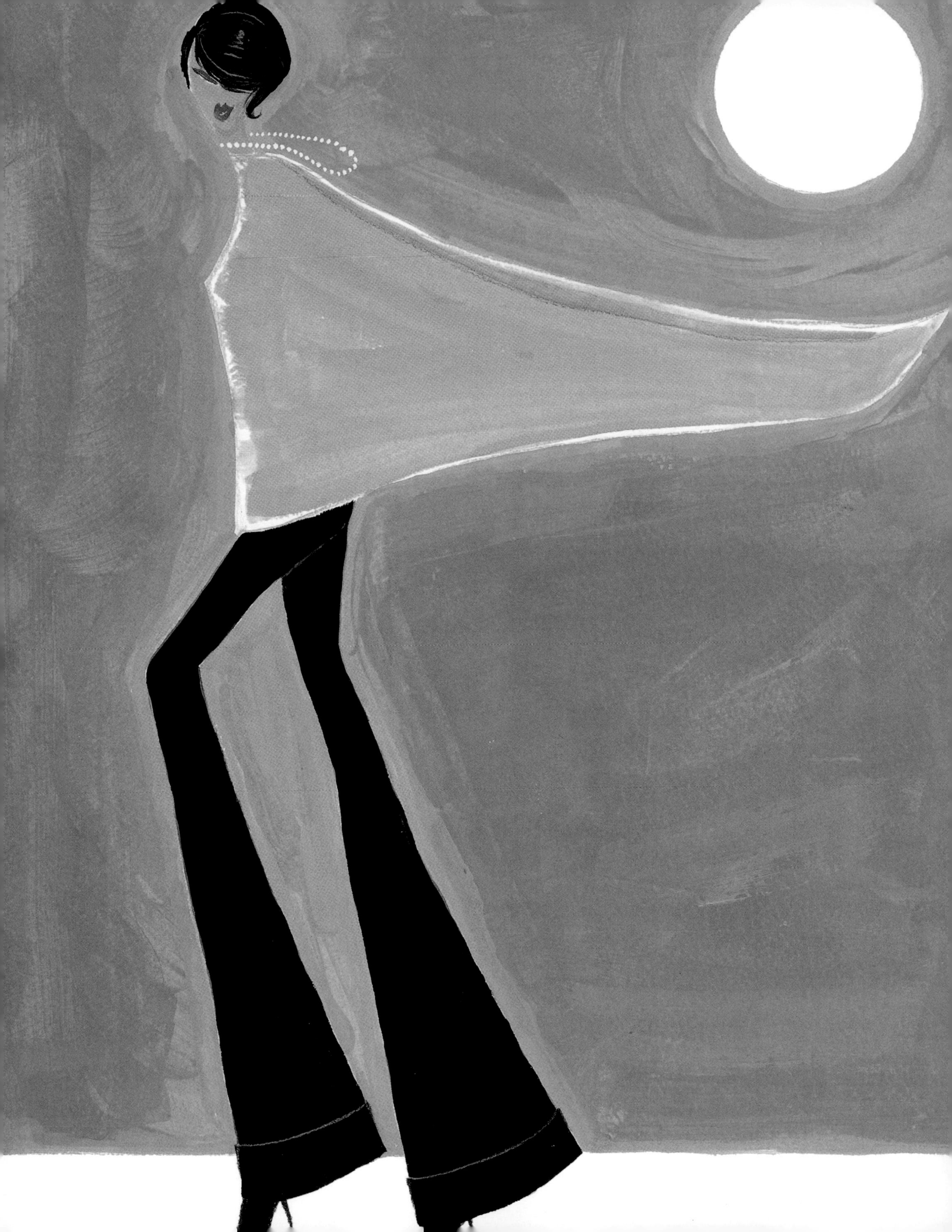

NOVEMBER 30 | CREATE YOUR OWN VERSION OF THIS SUREFIRE STYLISH OUTFIT COMBINATION.

Head straight for your power suit, stat! You know the one; it fits and flatters in the most important places. It always makes you feel like the woman in charge.

Juxtapose it with ultrafeminine underpinnings and accessories to create a sexiness that is irresistibly modern far and away from the predictable button-down blouse. (Snore!)

Make time right now to look in your closet and match this style equation as best you can with what you have. Don't worry if the items you own aren't an exact match. Within this template, choose your own colors and details. Getting the look not so letter perfect gives it your hint of personal style, which is always better than a carbon copy.

Top: Power suit jacket and sexy lace top
Bottom: Power suit skirt or pants
Shoes: Three-quarter boot with a sexy heel
Accessories: Single strand of pearls; the smallest of stud earrings
Flex piece: An oversized wrap in cashmere or merino wool (drape it over your chest with the loose ends dangling behind you for maximum chic)

DECEMBER

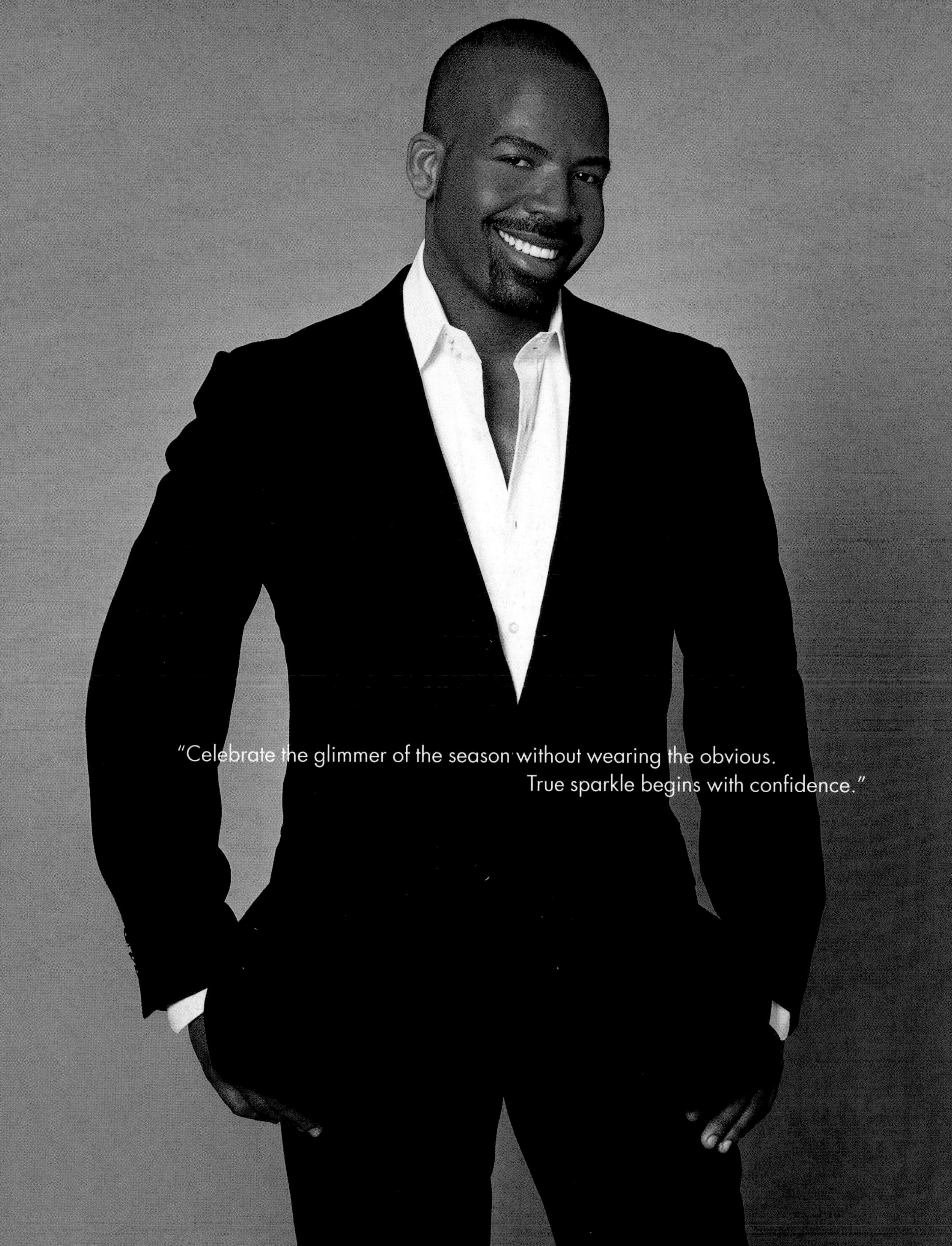
"Celebrate the glimmer of the season without wearing the obvious.
True sparkle begins with confidence."

DECEMBER 1 | RECHARGE AND DRESS DOWN, SO THAT YOU CAN REALLY GET DRESSED UP FOR THE HOLIDAY SEASON AHEAD.

Can you believe that an entire year is almost gone? From pretty spring outfits that hopefully brought out your ultragirly side, to summer swimsuits that made you feel a little more proportionate while poolside, to the perfect pair of jeans for the autumn months, we've almost covered it all. Tons of style information that will hopefully make getting dressed a bit more fun, flattering, and fulfilling.

As you look toward your final thirty days of style, take this one off. No cute skirts for the day, no pop of lip gloss before heading out, nothing. Relax (if circumstances allow).

Getting dressed up each and every day can be a mistake. Reason being, you begin to wear down your excitement and creativity trying to invent something special all the time. No one is capable of this, not even your biggest red carpet celebrities. (They have people like me to do it for them.)

Especially with the month ahead that boasts holiday parties, year-end office gatherings, making the rounds, and celebrating in special outfit after special outfit. Save your energy and creative looks for when it *really* matters. Take a personal day to plot your triumphant return!

DECEMBER 2 | TAKE AN EXPERT BEAUTY CUE FROM CYNDE WATSON-RICHMOND, A TOP CELEBRITY MAKEUP ARTIST AND BEAUTY INDUSTRY EXECUTIVE.

What is your best-kept personal beauty secret?

I keep my eyebrows groomed and shaped. It gives me a monthly eye lift.

What are the three beauty essentials every well-dressed woman should own? Why?

- A proper-fitting bra in three basic colors (black, white, and nude) and they should be convertible with a choice of clear straps, low back, or halter
- Classic accessories (diamond studs, diamond pendant, pearls, etc.)
- A basic black suit and a little black dress

What are the biggest mistakes women make when applying makeup?

- Not using enough concealer
- Using a foundation in the wrong formula

- Not shaping their eyebrows
- Wearing a lip liner that's too dark
- Not having the proper tools (brushes, sponges, Q-tips, powder puff)
- Trying to look exactly like a celebrity or a picture they see in a magazine

Who is the most stylish woman around, in your opinion? And what do you appreciate about her look?
Actress Michael Michele (today) and Diana Ross (back in the day).

If you could whisper a fail-safe beauty tip into the ears of women everywhere, without them feeling bad by hearing it, what would it be?
Wax.

DECEMBER 3 | GIVE YOURSELF A HAND AND ZIP UP YOUR OWN DRESS.

Sorry, Joan Crawford. A few wire hangers around the house can save you in a pinch (just don't use them to hang your clothes). They're great to zip up your dress and any other garment that challenges your reach.

Avid yogis can strike poses the average woman can't, and crane one arm behind them to zip up a cocktail dress from the lower back to the neck. All I can say to that is "Namaste!"

I learned a trick from my very unyoga aunt Linda. She a stylish fiftysomething gal who is single and quite resourceful, and besides making a mean vegetarian meal, she hipped me to the art of zipping yourself up!

Hold the hanger upside down behind you so that the base is inverted. Using the head, poke the slim pointer into the catch on the dress's zipper. Once locked in place, place your hand on the base and slowly pull up until the zipper is fully zipped. The hanger acts as an extension to your arm (you can always add more length by bending the hanger open as far as you need to), causing you less strain and saving you precious seconds to focus on something more important, like selecting the perfect earrings to wear.

Linda, you have liberated women everywhere, with the help of something they have been tossing out for years. For them, I thank you!

DECEMBER 4 | NAIL IT EVERY TIME.

In a month filled with outfit changes, your nails should be as versatile as possible. Around the holiday season, real women get a taste of what a starlet's life must be like. Going from day to night, casual to festive, and basic to sparkly sometimes all in one day.

With this in mind, the most stylish nail color choice is as close to natural as possible. This doesn't have to mean boring either. Sheer, natural nail colors create an elegant look that will keep you well suited for anything. Choose pale flesh tones that have undertones of shimmer or blushed hues so you can go from khakis to crystal earrings and never think twice about your hands looking commensurately elegant. This look does today what the French manicure did for stylish women in the 1980s. Hint. Hint.

Here are some surefire natural-inspired nail treatments you can request by name:

The American: A color that matches the flesh of your nailbed and skin followed by a topcoat.
Ballet Slipper: The palest of sheer pinks, followed by a topcoat.
Classic Clear: If you've got great, healthy nails, flaunt them by simply adding two strong, clear topcoats. This look speaks of youth and fresh clean hands.

DECEMBER 5 | STRIKE YOUR BEST POSE.

If last year's photos make you cringe, here are some ideas for how to prepare for your close-up:

KEEP YOUR SHOULDERS BACK AND AWAY

By positioning your shoulders slightly behind you and away from your side, you create the illusion of thinner arms since they are not pressed to your flesh, which makes them visually expand. Remember, the camera can add a visual ten pounds without warning. Don't help it out.

ALWAYS LOOK OVER THE SHOOTER'S SHOULDER

Never look dead on into the lens. Looking over the photographer's shoulder, or just above the lens, forces you to gently lift your chin and add a posture boost.

BEST FOOT FORWARD

Simply placing one foot in front of the other, and shifting your weight onto one hip, can give a leaner, more feminine look that speaks of poise and elegance. Think beauty pageant stance, only softer and more realistic.

DECEMBER 6 | FISHNETS MAKE YOU FLIRTY.

Rev up the sex appeal of a conservative knee-length skirt by highlighting your gams with a nuance of attitude. The classic fishnet stocking is one of my favorite ways for women to achieve this.

There are so many more tasteful options available today. No, the look doesn't have to speak of burlesque or the working girls depicted in the hit Broadway musical *Sweet Charity*. This era's fishnets are anything but trampy! From patterned mesh and warm fashion colors to flesh-toned microfishnets that virtually disappear on the leg yet offer an understated texture in the right light.

Fishnets work gorgeously with skirts in soft, ladylike fabrics like silk and chiffon. They add interest and elegance, and offer up more skin to the eye—a youthful touch that keeps lighter dresses looking as they should—fresh.

Another trick is keeping fishnets handy for a fast way to add nighttime glamour to a basic, skirted work suit. With the switch from sensible shoe to sling-back, the right fishnet can add another layer of drama without having to change your entire outfit. We're talking three minutes to marvelous!

DECEMBER 7 | TAKE AN EXPERT STYLE CUE FROM BETSEY JOHNSON, A LEGENDARY NEW YORK DESIGNER AND STYLE ICON.

What is your best-kept personal style secret?
I don't care what's "in" or "out," I wear that I want.

What are the three fashion essentials every well-dressed woman should own?

1. Lipstick for life! Red!
2. Rock 'n' roll T-shirts for comfortable "cool."
3. A leopard straight skirt to keep it simple.

What are the biggest mistakes women make when getting dressed?
If they worry about it, it usually fails. If women don't feel good, they won't look good. And nothing good happens.

Who is the most stylish woman in existence, in your opinion? And what do you appreciate about her look?
Gwen Stefani. Everything about her! Her daring, glamorous, punk, rock 'n' rollness, and she's so beautiful inside and out.

If you could whisper a fail-safe style tip into the ears of women everywhere, without them feeling bad by hearing it, what would it be?
Pretend you're in love or be in love!

DECEMBER 8 | LEARN A NEW FASHION TERM.

Houndstooth/hound's-tooth check • *Irregular colored one-half- to two-inch check like a square with points at two corners. Consists of colored checks alternating with white, produced by a yarn-dyed twill weave. Derived from resemblance to a dog's pointed tooth.*

In this season of layering up, bundling up, and wrapping up, bold, chunky woolens and tweeds abound. Glen plaids, argyles, tattersalls, tartans, and windowpane plaids are everywhere you look. You may not be sure which is which but you love the look.

Nonetheless, houndstooth scarves, overcoats, opaque hosiery, handbags, hats, jackets, pants—you name it—will always resurface each and every fall/winter season. Without fail, whether fashion magazines deem it "in" or "out," you can confidently don your houndstooth-check clothing and accessories with style.

The look of exploded houndstooth, where the pattern is enlarged to great proportions, almost distorting it, gives off a very high-fashion vibe. Smaller, more traditionally sized houndstooth patterns are a bit more classic and conservative. Either way, wear it with biting assurance all winter long.

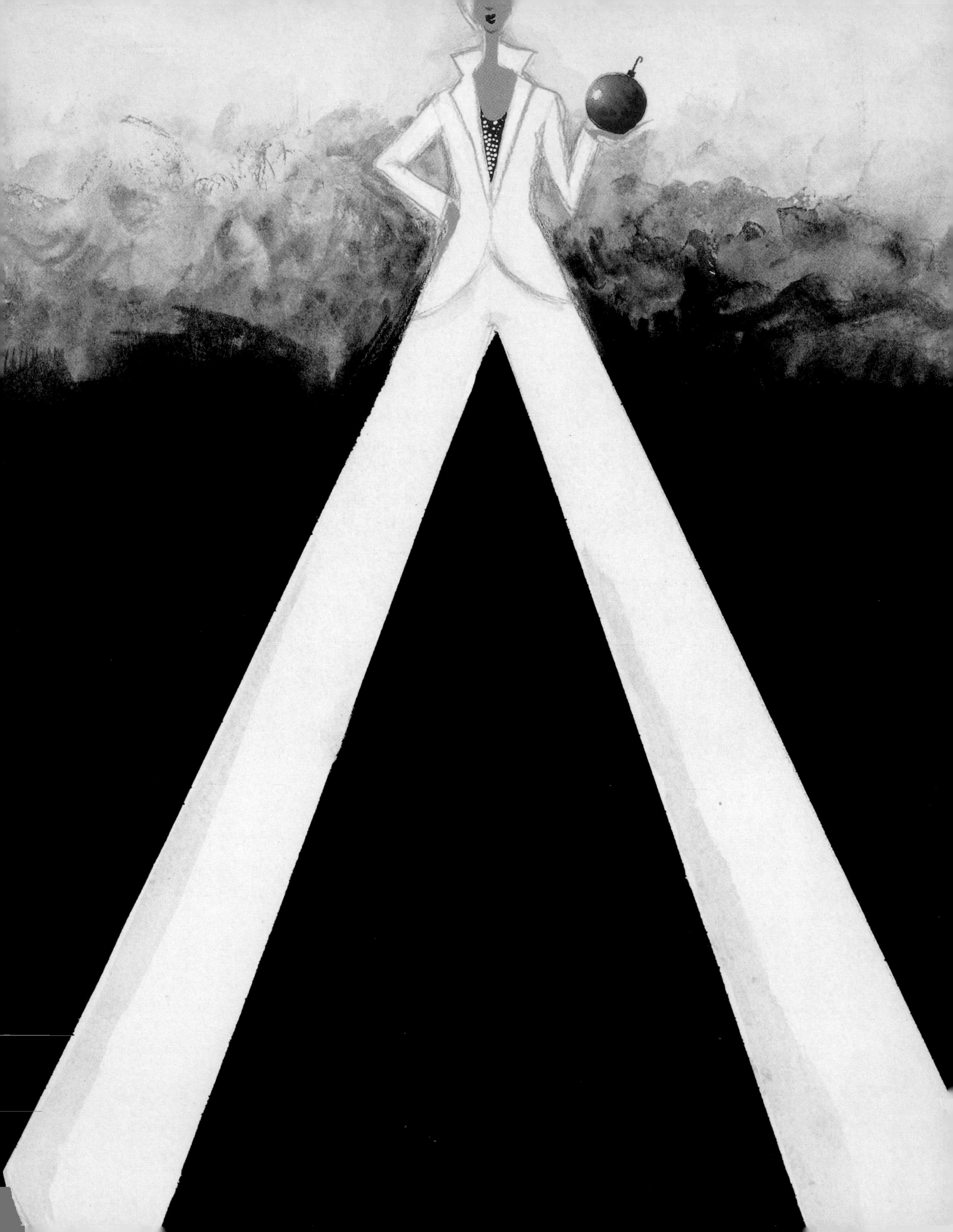

DECEMBER 9 | FLIP THE HOLIDAY DRESS SCRIPT AND RENT A MEN'S TUXEDO.

How many times have you walked into a holiday affair only to be yet another woman in some version of the "little black dress"? Or have you even noticed that you were?

Instead of jumping into your little black dress again, rent a men's tuxedo! The look speaks of classic elegance with a wink of menswear just like Coco Chanel or Marlene Dietrich may have worn. And unlike more conservative events (graduations, Easter, Passover, etc.), winter holiday season evening affairs are the perfect time to think out of the box a bit.

The average cost of a tuxedo rental these days is around $100, and you can get it fitted at a local rental store just like one of the guys. They will hem your pants just as you like, so bring heels.

The trick is renting only the jacket and pants. No need for anything else. You can add your own sparkly shell or tank, or even just a low-cut camisole for a sexier look. And work the jacket or pants as separates.

Rent a tuxedo in black or even white to add more femininity, and if you get it for a week, use it for your busiest block of nights and mix up the underpinnings, shoes, and evening bags. You will be amazed how modern you look, and how many compliments you get on your gorgeous tuxedo, for most women would have never thought to do the same.

DECEMBER 10 | SURPRISES AS CHIC.

Challenge yourself to put fashion before function with an accessory—namely the classic, printed neckerchief.

Most stylish women own at least one, or have almost bought one and were thwarted for not knowing how to wear it. Their images of women in neckerchiefs are ones of the not-so-distant past. That sharp, triangularly folded scarf worn by women (and some men) in the late 1960s and early 1970s. Or worn by cowboys in place of a traditional necktie, and Boy Scouts—not sexy or stylish images. If you continue to only toss it on around your neck, the look (or your perception of the look), will remain back there as well.

CONSIDER WEARING THIS

Printed neckerchiefs are fun accents in many unexpected places. Try it tied once onto the strap of a medium-sized handbag.

or

If you can wrap it around your waist (with excess at the knot), choose it over a belt when wearing solid pants.

or

Simply use a smaller, lightweight neckerchief as a dandy-inspired pocket square—by stuffing it into a blazer pocket from its center—and letting the tails dangle out with flair.

=

Mary Tyler "No" More!

DECEMBER 11 | KISSING SANTA IS BETTER THAN WEARING HIM ON A SWEATER.

BEFORE WEARING THIS

The Santa sweater: Give it up for a more modern look. (If you have one of these in your closet, there is no need to toss it. Just wear it for an audience of those twelve and under for maximum compliments.)

CONSIDER WEARING THIS

The solid velour sweat suit is queen this time of year! Choose a zip-front hooded version with loose, drawstring pants that flare a bit at the bottom. Go with classic red if you are really in the spirit, black for a day-to-night event, even cream or sky blue for a feeling that speaks to Hanukah!

+

Add that extra holiday flair with the help of fun accessories (not ornament earrings, or battery-operated Rudolph pins) like a stack of bangles or bracelets in a contrasting holiday color—or festive silver or gold.

+

Feature a lightweight solid T-shirt beneath your "Santa" suit in another identifiable color of the season, like pine green or snowy white. A fun candy-stripe T-shirt would dazzle just as brightly!

=

And to all a good night!
(Especially those who thought you'd never retire that sweater. Guess who has that last laugh!)

DECEMBER 12

ACCENT WITH HIP FAUX FUR—A CHUBBY, STOLE, OR SCARF. THE IDEA IS KIND TO ANIMALS AND YOUR POCKET.

The retro elegance of real fur adds instant cachet to the most basic pieces of dress attire. Women in the 1940s and 1950s viewed a fur coat as the ultimate signifier of affection, wealth, and luxury, next to diamonds, of course. As our society has become more aware of wildlife preservation, many women have begun to think differently, opting to leave real fur where it belongs—on the backs of unharmed animals. The choice is yours. Either way, something warm and fuzzy can give you high style.

Embracing faux fur might very well be the best solution for several reasons: The price is usually a fraction of what real fur will cost, the temporary and trendy look of any season can be captured without a load of financial guilt, and no animals lose their lives in the process.

A great way to incorporate faux fur in a classic way is by investing in a chubby (waist-length jacket) with a traditional button-front closure, a fun faux fur scarf for evening (instead of rushing to a fabric wrap time after time), or a stole that's popped on over the shoulders of a solid dress or your dressy jeans and a satin top.

Caution: A fur can add years if worn too seriously. Always try to look younger and more modern by going for the *un*fur look, both in the unexpected clothes you pair it with and in the type of fur you choose to buy. I say avoid the real thing fur sure!

DECEMBER 13 | RESERVE YOUR NEWEST CLOTHING FOR YOUR MOST IMPORTANT OCCASIONS.

How do women on television and in films always manage to look so sharp on camera? They are usually wearing new, or nearly new, clothing that is reserved only for wear in front of the camera.

The feeling of a new garment on one's body is like no other. Similar to that of a new second skin after an intense exfoliating spa treatment, a cleaner, fresher you seems to come shining through when an unfamiliar fabric makes contact with your skin. Not only is this an inward sensation, but there is an outward glow that radiates just as brightly, especially on the very first wear.

Don't ever waste this glimmering moment of the first wear. It could be a new silk blouse, a perfectly fitted pantsuit and sling-back combination, or simply a natty little hat that raises the visual value of your warm winter coat. Know that the very first time you decide to don that piece of clothing or accessory is the only time it will have 100 percent of its visual impact, so choose this event wisely.

Push your new clothes back into the closet for when they really need to work for you.

DECEMBER 14

LET YOUR HANDBAG BE YOUR "STATEMENT PIECE" BY TONING DOWN YOUR OUTFIT. SELECT A BAG THAT PEOPLE WOULD NEVER EXPECT TO SEE ON YOU, AND ALLOW IT TO TICKLE YOUR WILD SIDE.

Let your handbag stand out. You might choose a glimmery metallic mesh evening clutch and decide to feature it with something as simple as your black pencil skirt, a bleached-white T-shirt, and flat sandals. The French fashionista may want to come out of you today. This means you run to your swankiest designer bags with massive logos, or the sweet little exotic pastel sachet that is topped with feathers and slim ribbons, only to wear it with your strongest business suit—the one that gives you masculine authority atop your ultrafeminine wiles.

The trick is to pair your signature bag of the day with something subtle or opposite that will allow it to shine on its own stage. Think about outfits that are monochromatic from tip to toe, simple dresses that are one clean line, or supercasual separates like your "leggy" jeans and casual tops. Let all eyes go to your bag first today—whatever one you choose—and watch them rise to your eyes with looks of complete entrancement. This is the kind of "baggage" you should be happy to take along into any relationship.

DECEMBER 15

TAKE INVENTORY WITH AN EYE TOWARD PASSING THE GOOD THINGS ON.

Does your line of work or social life entitle you to fashion freebies? Giveaway totes, tops, hats, and mugs? If so, pile up your perks and see what really reflects your taste and image, and determine what you can use and what you can share. Be honest with yourself and maybe just rid yourself of one ball cap to start.

Giving away many of your giveaways might just give way to some room in your closet for clothes and accessories that really give off way more style!

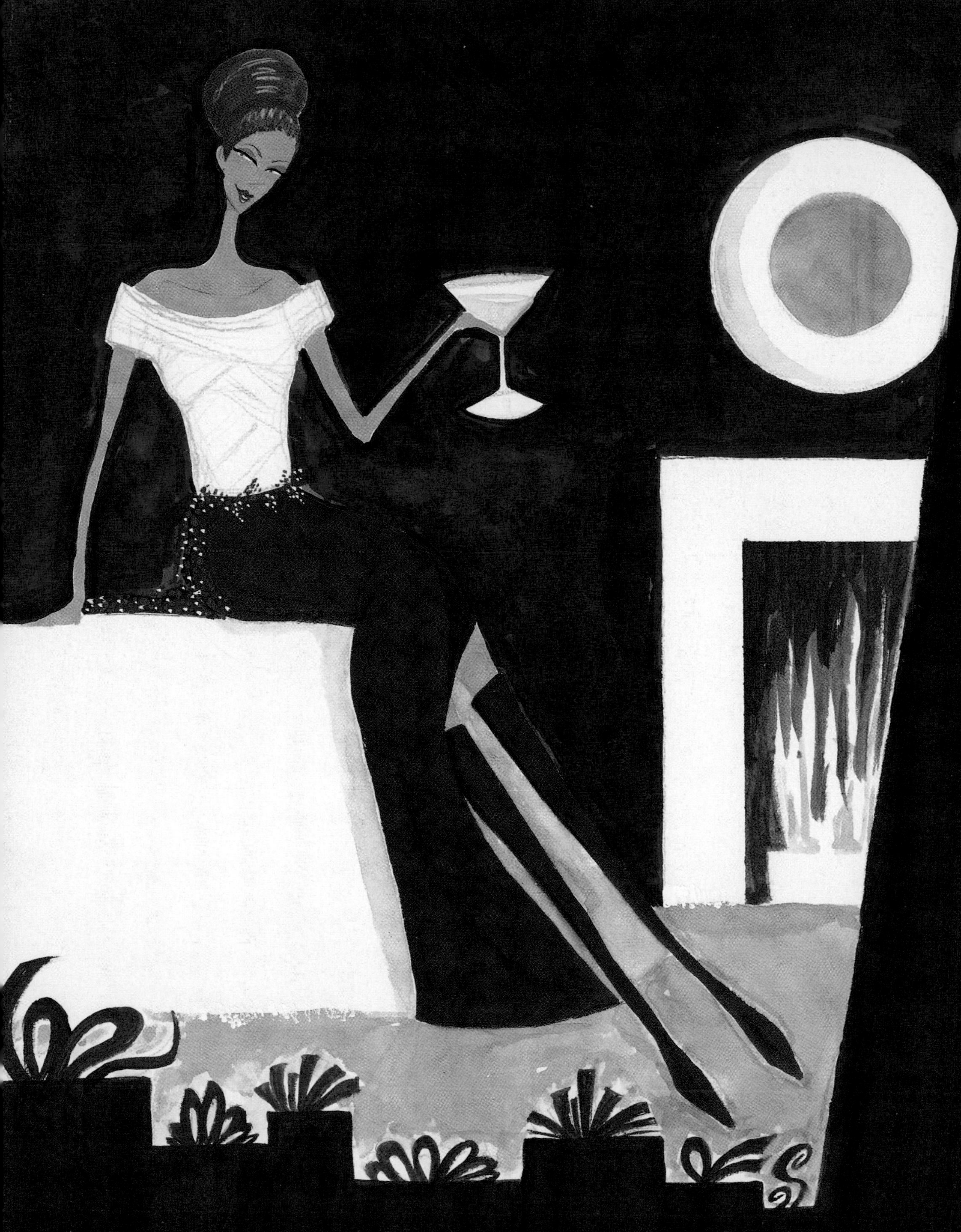

DECEMBER 16 | GET TEN-MINUTE STYLE FOR ANY CASUAL HOLIDAY PARTY.

You are stacking events like a true, high-society socialite, even if it is just about making the holiday rounds to see family, attending middle school concerts, and chatting up your better half's tipsy boss at the annual holiday soiree. Wearing the right clothes helps to make all of these functions a bit less taxing, and a whole lot less burdensome.

Guess what? Here is your first holiday gift from me, a ten-minute style stunner for any casual holiday party that will keep you sane and on schedule:

Minutes 1:00–2:00:
Snatch a pale solid sweater that has just a little sex appeal—like an off-the-shoulder white or camel cashmere or a merino wool sleeveless turtleneck.

Minutes 3:00–4:00:
Jump into a dark tailored bottom to ground it. A black pencil or A-line skirt, black suit trousers, or even a fun wool wrap skirt that hits the floor.

Minutes 5:00–6:00:
Keep warm in stylish boots that hit the knee and go with any of the above. Black leather pointed-toe boots, or even a black equestrian riding boot for a twist!

Minutes 7:00–8:00:
Select just one over-the-top accessory that says *"bling!"* A metallic belt that dangles low, a pair of oversized chandelier earrings, or a chunky vintage brooch.

Minutes 9:00–10:00:
Go for flawless skin by using an all-in-one foundation/powder. Add shimmer to your eyes but nowhere else. A holiday lip (for many it's classic red) and mascara, and hit the starry night like you just fell from on high!

DECEMBER 17 | CHOOSE YOUR OUTFIT BEFORE YOUR INTIMATES.

Oftentimes you get dressed on automatic pilot. You jump out of the shower or bath and toss away your towel. You crunch outfit ideas in your head while brushing your teeth or blow-drying your hair. But you pick out panty and bra without thinking. Hours later, you happen to pass a mirror and notice that you have the dreaded V.P.L.: visible panty line. And you are miles away from your closet.

If you are among the many women who choose their undergarments or intimates before choosing their outfit, reverse the process.

It is most important to think about your "inners" before your "outers."

There may be nothing worse than a fabulous A-line or pencil skirt that is diminished by a panty that has more seam than support. The end-all solution for today's smart woman: embracing the thong or smooth seamless panties.

As for tops, the undergarment options are limitless when it comes to ample support or further enhancement. So the more important issue here is the brassiere color choice, which ideally should be chosen *after* your top is selected. Case in point: the dreaded mistake of wearing the white bra beneath the white top. For years, women in the know felt that a black bra was the answer, when, in fact, the champion nude-to-match-your-skin bra is the overall winner. For it truly will disappear—along with the awkward stares.

DECEMBER 18 | USE YOUR CONSUMER RIGHTS.

Much of the pomp and circumstance that surrounds your purchase in clothing stores can intimidate you from returning what you have second thoughts about. Don't allow it. Stores are trying to move goods and make money, not be a revolving door of debits, credits, returned products, and dissatisfied customers.

Never be afraid to return or exchange unworn clothes or accessories (with tags attached) to the place of purchase, as long as it happens within the time stated on their return policy, which should be clearly posted near the register, if not clearly printed on the back of your receipt.

If the prospect of questioning as to why you are returning or exchanging intimidates you, simply have the golden answer ready and diffuse all fear. If asked why you are returning, look the salesperson straight in the eye and calmly yet firmly state, "I changed my mind." Enough said.

Believe me, there is no arguing with that, for the customer is always right, at least in upstanding businesses. If that fails, keep these few rights in mind, and feel free to mention them if the transaction gets the least bit uncomfortable:

WHEN CONSIDERING MAKING A RETURN OR AN EXCHANGE, ALWAYS REMEMBER

• Although consumer rights vary from state to state with respect to product returns, generally speaking a store can set up any return policy it wants, whether it is "all sales final," "merchandise credit only," or "all returns in thirty days." Most states require the policy to be clearly disclosed to the buyer prior to purchase, usually by means of a sign. If the customer is returning or exchanging within said policy, there should never be a problem.

• Select chain stores, such as Target, don't accept returns without a receipt but will search their system for a copy if you cannot locate the original.

• When holiday shopping, note that some retailers relax their regular return deadlines at holiday time by extending the return period into January.

DECEMBER 19 | POP STYLE QUIZ.

1. Which brand of women's hosiery revolutionized the market in 2000 by offering unique, "footless" panty hose that offered support and a bare-leg look?

A. Wolford
B. Spanx
C. Footloose
D. Hue

2. How often should tailored business suits be dry-cleaned?

A. After every wear
B. Once a month
C. Once a season
D. Once or twice a year

3. Which pant shape/detail provides visual balance to larger hips?

A. Slightly flared leg
B. Slightly larger waist
C. Permanently stitched creasing
D. None of the above

4. Shorts can be tricky to wear, especially with a tummy that takes center stage. Which shorts style will help to dim the stage lights best?

A. Flat-front shorts with slit pockets
B. Flat-front shorts with front cargo pockets
C. Pleated-front shorts without pockets
D. Short-shorts with a drawstring waist

(Answers: 1-B, 2-D, 3-A, 4-A)

DECEMBER 20 | BE CERTAIN THAT YOU HAVE AN EVENING CLUTCH ON STANDBY.

With the many evening bag silhouettes available today—from feminine pouches that will dangle from your wrist like a twentieth-century Gibson girl, to oversized coin-purse shapes with girly, jeweled handles that stand to attention even while you're off dancing across the candlelit room—there is none more versatile and sophisticated than the small, sleek clutch.

Stealthy in its shape, the cleanest of lines, and as discreet as a midnight flight to Paris with the man who makes your spine tingle, the clutch handbag speaks of timeless elegance and pared-down function.

The solid black satin version with a slim metal clasp, shaped like an envelope, might very well be the pièce de résistance of your clutch options. And you can find a great one new or secondhand with character and history. There may be a shoulder strap hidden inside for the forgetful gal, or a near-invisible strap on the bag's back through which one hand can be secured for a much better look. Even mini-clutch versions are chic options, which look amazing in overly ornate beading, crystal designs, and embroidery.

Always keep a few important things in mind when reaching for your evening clutch. Know that it will usually remain on an elegant table when you are not mobile. This means that it is on display as openly as the fine china, crystal, flowers, and silverware at any special evening event. Be sure the look of your bag is commensurate. Make it just as special and be sure it's in good condition. Don't overpack it. A lipstick, a credit card, a couple of dollars to tip the ladies' room attendant, and a small fragrance atomizer should get you through a few hours. With this in mind, you can actually keep an evening clutch packed and ready to go in your office desk drawer, work tote bag, or even your glove compartment if you are in a pinch to transition into an evening affair. Why not? Today's stylish woman can add it to a pantsuit and make it look like an intentional combo for nighttime. It is all in how you carry it. Which will hopefully be like you really meant it.

DECEMBER 21 | WELCOME THE WINTER SOLSTICE.

Winter dressing has a way of getting heavy, not only in the layers on your body, with the repetitive task of staying warm in the increasingly cold month, but simply beating the doldrums that invade your spirit when the sun is being blocked out by gray skies and snow. Themes help more than ever this time of year. It may sound silly, but it really works to keep you inspired and playful when peering at yet another pair of tights, chunky sweater, and snow boots. Think classic ice princess sweetness, or call on the look of Julie Christie as Lara Antipova in *Dr. Zhivago*—whatever it takes to give you a fresh point of departure for your outfit to battle the elements. Use today as scene one of your winter style statements. Here are a few fun season openers:

Black Leather Pants + Red Silk Blouse + Black Ankle Boots + Silver Clutch
= Winter Wonder Woman

Ice Blue Blazer + Ice Blue Turtleneck + Winter White Trousers + Nude Loafers
= The Tasty Freeze

Camel Wool Kilt + Black Cashmere Wrap Top + Gold Cuff + Black Knee Boots
= Known for the Holidays

DECEMBER 22

HAPPY BIRTHDAY, CAPRICORN GIRL. LOOK TO YOUR STARS AND DRESS ACCORDING TO YOUR COSMIC STYLE TRAITS.

The well-suited, sensibly high-heeled Capricorn is business first and foremost. Stately style is paramount to the way you structure your wardrobe. This is not to say that you are frigid or detached from your ladylike wiles.

Dressing the part for you is just that—a part of you whether it's the side that's a pragmatic thinker or a self-starter and do-er. One part has assured friends, and acquaintances are known to rely on you to get it done, whatever "it" may be. She's all about business, owning the tailored suits, classic separates, and eight-hour heels to prove it. The other part can turn off that PDA and, wearing silky pajamas that hold you better than any man could, curl up with a book set in a romantic time gone by.

All in all, style is about function before fashion for you. What can an item do for me in the workplace? Will this skirt help me seal the deal at a client dinner? Even in sweats, you want to know if they perform to the level of comfort you need in order to unwind. Accessories are your weak point, turning you into the mushy type who swoons at sight of the perfect accessory and pays the high price to shine—for you know the results of wearing the real thing.

Analyze supermodel Christy Turlington and ageless rocker Annie Lennox for a glimpse at how a Capricorn's style prowess can hypnotize anyone who stares too long. You know this deep inside, but keep your cards close to your chest, as any smart businessperson should. Or you might be covering that diamond pendant that will show your vulnerability. Only you know the real deal.

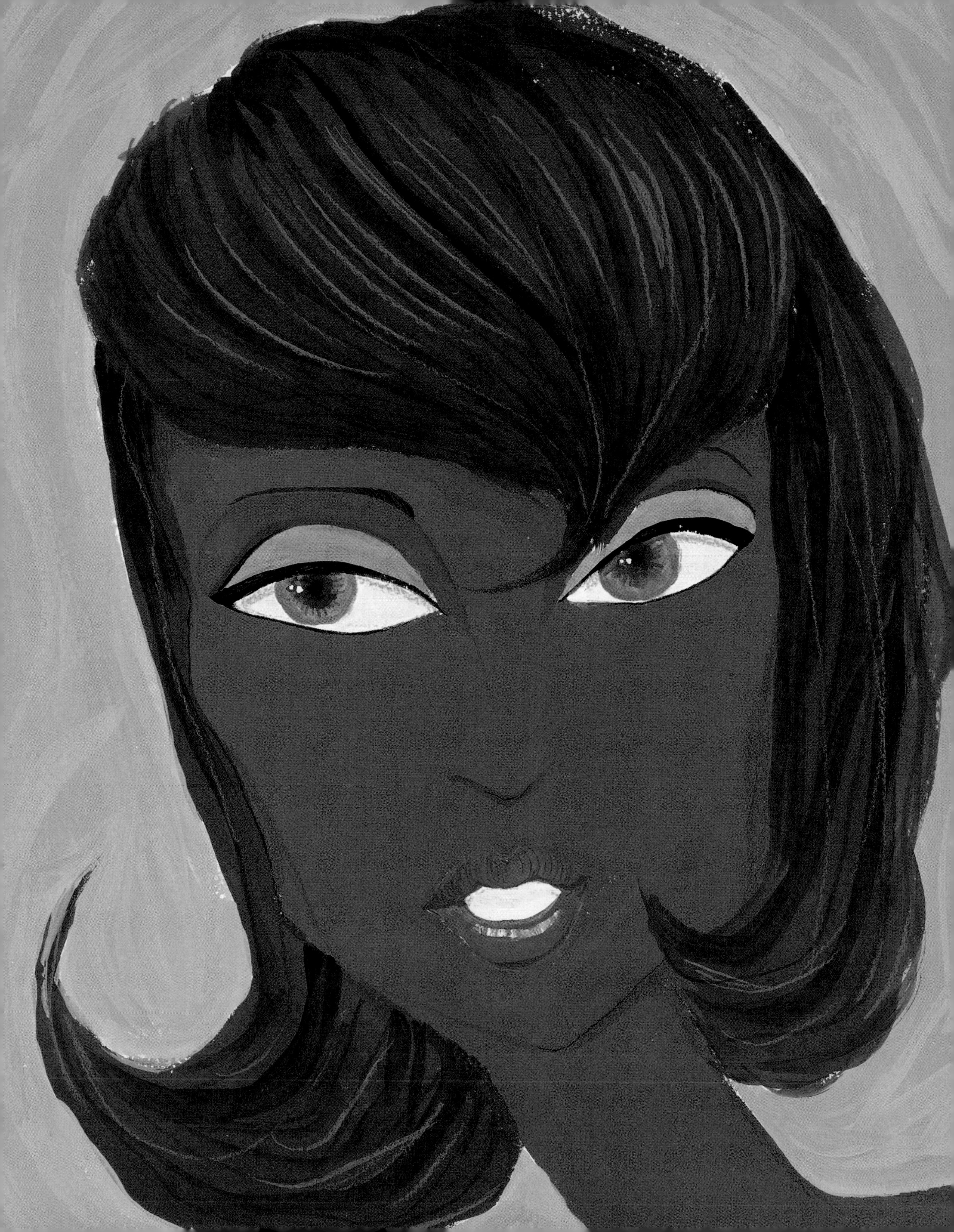

DECEMBER 23 | ADD A WIG TO YOUR WARDROBE JUST FOR FUN!

Before you even turn the page and decide that this tip is not for you, hear me out. Today's quality wigs are no longer worn out of necessity; they are sported for style and a shot of glamour. They are on high-fashion runways, movie screens, and Hollywood red carpets, but you'd never know it!

One thing about celebrity hairstyle trends that most women probably don't even realize when they exclaim how much they love it, is the *volume* of the star's hair. You think you just love the color, or adore the cut, but it is the healthy, full, rich volume that creates such a statement on film and in photographs. And guess what, sometimes it's a wig—and a very expensive one at that. These stars shall remain nameless.

The next time you are in search of a new hairstyle and would rather test the waters slowly before going under the scissors or getting a dye job, check out a wig store. Sport it when you're at home hosting a party in an outfit that could use a lift, or simply skipping town with your best girlfriends for some fun in Las Vegas. Try doing it in a super-cool, so-not-like-you style. Buy it on sale so no guilt ensues. Choose a hot new color that you've always wanted to try. And wear it like it is your own, natural hair. Wear it with confidence among friends first; in other words, throw it like you actually *did* grow it!

DECEMBER 24 | WHY NOT EVENING GLAMOUR, ALL DAY LONG?

Before heading off to your job, or day's activity, steal a little extra time to apply your makeup and style your hair as if you are headed right out for a night on the town. I know it is easier said than done, but here is why it is worth stealing the time.

Big-name celebrities lead lives that appear pretty glamorous from the outside, and mind you, they are quite privileged in their day-to-day rigors. They are usually driven from place to place, served the exact food they have a yen for, and ushered like royalty into whatever place they want to go. Those red velvet ropes are nothing but a big green light in their minds.

Within this dream also lives the reality of being "on" at a moment's notice. Meeting your fans in person, speaking with the press (who can kill your career with one wrong quote), and appearing on live television shows and stages all while being calm, articulate, and, most of all, nice.

Almost every celebrity who has to face a day of publicity does it with the help of a professional hairstylist and makeup artist hired expressly to create the best-looking person they can. Beautifully finished makeup and hair that speaks of time and styling send a message of polish, but also puts the star in his or her best comfort zone. It allows them to feel almost bulletproof.

You can get a sliver of this without an expensive beauty team knocking at your door at five in the morning. Just take the essence of the idea to boost your confidence and visual security today. Don't go overboard with a superdressy updo and dramatic eye shadow, only to look like you didn't go home last night. Simply eke out some extra time to go beyond your basic quick lipstick and comb-out. You'd be amazed at how tall you feel, even if you are petite in person, like most of our big-screen idols. Doesn't that just astonish you every time! Now you know why.

DECEMBER 25 | GIVE A GIFT TO YOURSELF FIRST—THE GIFT OF STYLE.

If you are like many of the women I see on this day, you start the morning serving everyone but yourself and end the day putting away the last dish from a day of doing the same.

You would never complain, but it sure would be nice if the gift-giving spirit of the day would come your way first, and alleviate just a portion of the pressure to shine as bright as the twinkling holiday lights.

If you'd accept this little style prescription gift from me, you may just have one sliver of stress shaved off your plate way before it is time to carve the holiday bird! Think of it as a high/low ensemble that is ultracomfortable when it is time to bounce around with the tiniest of holiday guests, and so versatile that you can clink glasses with the gals by night without a last-minute holiday fashion overhaul. Give it a try, and if it works, pass the formula on to another busy woman you love today, because you know you'll see plenty of them:

Breakfast with the Family: Solid velour or cashmere sweat suit + boatneck T-shirt + cozy slippers
Making Holiday Rounds: Solid velour or cashmere sweatpants + solid turtleneck + comfy flats
Local Volunteering: Solid velour or cashmere sweat suit + solid turtleneck + sneakers
Dinner with the Family: Solid velour or cashmere sweatpants + boatneck T-shirt + chunky necklace + festive sparkly flats
Fireside Cocktails with Friends: Solid velour or cashmere sweat suit + solid turtleneck + festive sparkly flats

DECEMBER 26 | FEATURE A LONG SKIRT THAT ARTFULLY DANCES AROUND YOUR LEGS.

Did you know that there are still countless women who will never wear a skirt? They would rather wear pants then show any leg whatsoever. This baffles me since unlike in past decades, there are so many amazing long-skirt options today that can cover a woman's legs and flaws yet still be amazingly feminine, flirty, and authoritative. And anything longer than just below the knee would fit right into this category.

There are three rules to keep in mind when going for the long-skirt look. So pull out your old long skirts and see if they get past the rules, or peek at a new one on your next shopping trip and try challenging what people expect to see you in. This is where the more stylish you begins—by varying your usual silhouettes. Here is a short list of rules for going long:

RULE #1 AVOID THE STRAIGHT AND NARROW

Choose an A-line, go for a trumpet-flare bottom, fun kick pleats—just keep it interesting, romantic, feminine, and anything but simple straight and narrow. The fit of your skirt around your hips is always the most important area, so make sure it hugs your hips firmly without squeezing.

(CONTINUED)

RULE #2 THE FULLER THE SKIRT, THE MORE FITTED THE TOP

Long skirts make you seem a bit taller to those checking you out. The trick is to wear long skirts that are usually a bit fuller with fitted tops that reveal some skin. I love cap-sleeved fitted stretch tops, tanks with thin straps, and body-skimming shells.

RULE #3 FOR ONCE, HITTING THE FLOOR IS A GOOD THING

Take the length to the floor to avoid the no-man's-land of lengths—midcalf—which actually makes you appear heavier than you are.

DECEMBER 27 | HAPPY BIRTHDAY, MARLENE DIETRICH.

Before you jump so confidently into a pair of pants today, remember that women didn't always have the option of doing so. So give a nod of recognition to style pioneer Marlene Dietrich.

Noted English drama critic and author Kenneth Tynan said it best when he described such a complex historical figure as an icon of independence for real women everywhere. "She has the bearing of a man; the characters she plays love power and wear trousers. Marlene's masculinity appeals to women and her sexuality to men."

Dietrich actually began her career playing the role of nightclub performer in several of her first German films. Her breakout role, *The Blue Angel,* where she portrayed Lola, a heartbreaking woman who confidently donned a men's top hat, is the one that began the style murmurs. Unheard of!

She arrived in America and struck gold with notable dramatic performances, the most famous of which is the 1930 classic *Morocco*, where she scandalously featured a men's tuxedo and kissed another woman. Even more of a shock to audiences!

Some feel her acting prowess paled at times to her personal style, off-screen and on. But Dietrich always wore the pants, literally and figuratively, being the highest paid woman in the world in 1936.

If you choose to go with pants over a skirt for the day, give a wink to Marlene when you zip up and secure the final button in honor of her birthday. Walk a little taller and free with legions of women doing the same, knowing she'd see it as a very clever birthday gift. Top hats off!

DECEMBER 28 | ARRIVE AT YOUR HOLIDAY EVENT LOOKING FESTIVE AND FRESH.

'Tis the season to look very carefully at how you express yourself at festive events. And we are not just talking about light banter over the cheese log, or tasteful fireside chats with friends old and new. This is about examining your clothing expressions and the messages it sends.

Sometimes we get so caught up in the season that we forget that the fun-themed decorations, lights, artful ornaments, and classic "frosty" icons were designed to enhance one's home and tree. The party invites arrive and out come the sweaters, with images of Santa popping up where Mrs. Claus would never have allowed his face. Faux candy canes adorn earrings and necklaces, and my favorites, the miniature Christmas tree ornament earrings.

Send a similar celebratory message, more chic by far than the Santa sweater or the ornaments as earrings:

REPLACE	WITH
Holiday icon earrings (e.g.: Frosty, Rudolf, Santa)	Vintage crystal cluster earrings à la icy snowflakes
Holiday-themed necklaces	Chunky red coral necklaces with a black or white top
Merry holiday hair ornaments	Black lacquered chopsticks
Holiday character/seasonal scene sweaters	Metallic solid sweaters in silver or gold

DECEMBER 29 | A TEN-MINUTE MAKEOVER.

Here are some quick ways to look like a celebrity hostess who spent all day getting ready—and only you'll know that you did it in a flash.

HAIR WE GO AGAIN

Never forget the power of the classic chignon! Whether you place it high (slimming) or low (sleek), it looks neat and elegant. Add an ornate chopstick à la Auntie Mame, a jewel-encrusted clip in the vein of Grace Kelly, or a whimsical winterberry to make it youthful and quirky.

SHAKE UP YOUR MAKEUP

Less is so much more. Many makeup lines offer all-in-one shimmery powders that can enhance cheeks, eyes—and even bare shoulders in seconds. Tis the season to stand out, effortlessly: Choose a beautiful lip color you wouldn't ordinarily wear; dot a touch of concealer under your eyes; stroke on a coat of rich black mascara, and you are done!

MAKE THEM ALL PANT

Velour sweats can look relaxed and sophisticated when paired with the right top. Look for drawstring versions (so that the waist is adjustable should you overindulge) that flare at the leg. Choose ink black, bright white, classic camel, cream, or even soft pink to add a plush look to a basic white blouse. Pair them with satin flats inspired by ballet slippers or very low kitten heels, and smile through the whole night.

GO OVER THE TOP!

Go for glitter, glimmer, and glitz! Buy that one shiny top with beaded or sequin embellishments—you know, the type your flashier friend wears with abandon. It's the perfect topper for nights like this. Don't spend too much on it, though. Just be sure it brings out your joyful, celebratory side. Wear it in the safety of your own home, with your closest friends, and feel more glamorous.

THE NO-REGRET DRESS

Look for a one-piece wonder that speaks of holiday charm yet allows you to eat, drink, dance—and not worry about bulge. Let it drape the body in a sumptuous fabric that makes you feel like a lady! Try a wrap dress that ties at the waist. If the price is right, invest in a few, ranging from classic black to berry reds. Add festive, colored accessories to make your look really pop.

DECEMBER 30 | DRESS TO WIN! SCORE MORE ON YOUR CLOTHES-SHOPPING TRIP BY DRESSING ACCORDINGLY.

Post-holiday sales are abundant right now. Here is a checklist of the best "clothes-shopping clothes":

Tops: Quick on and off, zip-front sweaters and sweatshirts; easy to remove, wide boatneck pullovers
Bottoms: Drawstring waist pants with open bottom hems; loose or stovepipe elastic-waist pants
Footwear: Slip-on flat shoes with active/athletic soles; slip-on sneakers; pack a pair of average-height heels for try-ons with pants/skirts
Hosiery: Wear or pack along a pair of knee-high stockings for shoe try-ons; cotton booties/anklets to reveal your leg when trying on skirts
Underwear: Wear or pack along a strapless bra for dress try-ons; wear or pack along a thong for a true V.P.L. (visible panty lines) test during try-ons
Accessories: A large canvas tote to consolidate small purchases and house any excess clothing layers while shopping

Happy shopping!

...that's my song!

DECEMBER 31

BEFORE YOU RAISE YOUR GLASS AT THE MINUTES TICKING TO MIDNIGHT, RAISE YOUR GLASS TO A YEAR OF STYLE BUILDING.

Look in the mirror before you get dressed and know that whatever you choose to wear, the final night of the year will be perfectly appointed to you.

ACKNOWLEDGMENTS

God, thank you for allowing me to see yet another dream come to life.

Naima Turner, for "Joking" up the best book title ever, and being the perfect right hand at all times. Glad you found me. Your humor is brillant! Your style is even better.

Stephanie Scott, my left hand, for handling any task tossed your way, and the stellar interviews, with grace and total professionalism.

Faith Childs, for never letting me down and being the consummate literary agent with such style to boot!

Malaika Adero, for seeing the value of my words, and editing all 365 tips with time and care as if each were the first. Stylish women everywhere now have you to thank.

Judith Curr, Karen Mender, Justin Loeber, Angela Stamnes, Krishan Trotman, Linda Dingler, Isolde Sauer, Dana Sloan, Jim Thiel, Monica Hopkins and everyone at dix!, Julian Peploe, and all the stylish executives at Atria Books, thanks for rolling out the red carpet for me.

My entire family, especially my mother and rock, Lynell Kollar, for always having my back.

Craig Rose, Cynde Watson, and Sean Allison for giving constant love and support to this only child as only blood siblings could. And for Steve Barr, truly man at his best.

Armstead Edwards, my manager and friend, who'll get up at four AM to check on my car and driver. Thanks, "Pa!"

Archie Dixon, my power rep at the William Morris Agency, strong men keep a comin' on!

Jeff Google, your time, vision, and support of my television work makes me feel like my star is rising, thanks, and stay close.

Julia Chance, for taking the time to be the first set of 20/20 eyes over all my words, I thank you.

The entire NBC *Today* show family, for allowing me to help millions of women look their absolute best. It is an honor.

My Jones New York family—Mark Mendelson, Stacy Lastrina, Amy Rapawy, Shirley Imig, and Frank Belfatto—for choosing me to represent your brand to your loyal audience, and supporting the book from day one. Thanks a million purchases over!

My LensCrafters family—Kathy Clark and Seth McClaughlin—and the power team at Ogilvy—Shari Kurzrok and Bethany Eppner. I love being the "chief" face behind your stylish frames. It is a joy.

Tommy Hilfiger and the entire Tommy family, for love and support as if I'd never left.

Keith Major, for always making me look a little thinner, taller, and rested in your extraordinary photos. And hopefully I won't be single forever!

Liz Dewey and my entire *Full Frontal Fashion* family, for allowing me to do what I love every day.

Phil Shung, for helping me create a cover concept that I will always be proud of, and Erica Kennedy for "allowing" me to borrow him. Thank you, makeup assistant Loran Alvator. You rock!

Carmen Marc Valvo, for creating the perfect little black dress that defines the name and ignites the book cover. And to each and every designer, retail executive, makeup artist, hairstylist, skin-care specialist, and fashion editor who lent their voices. We can add style to a nation if we stick together.

Jacqueline Hackett, for saving the day at the last minute. I thank you.

Dana Hibbard, my intern during one of the busiest times of my career. I really appreciate your hard work and good attitude.

To my growing TV and book fan base of women and men seeking more stylish lives, you've had it all along! Thanks again and again for choosing me to show you the best way to allow it to shine.

SOURCES

Alumni information page. 6 April 2005 www.oberlin.edu

Appearance quotes page. 15 February 2005 http://www.quotableonline.com/quotesubjectcss.php?subject=Appearance&page=2

Bathing study page. 5 January 2005 http://www.psu.edu/

Biography page. 2 February 2005 http://www.ameliaearhart.com/about/biography.html *and* 22 February 2005 http://www.marlene.com/

Buying pearls page. 19 February 2005 http://www.pearlinfo.com/consumer/buying.html

Calasibetta, Charlotte Mankey. *Fairchild's Dictionary of Fashion*. New York: Fairchild Books, 2000.

Care and cleaning page. 7 February 2005 http://www.jewelers.org:8080/3.consumers/info/wysk_care.shtml

Celebrity tattoo page. 14 March 2005 http://www.vanishingtattoo.com/celebrity_tattoos.htm

Census information page. 20 March 2005 http://www.forbes.com/

Civil War information page. 18 March 2005 http://www.civilwarhome.com/

Color meaning page. 17 February 2005 http://www.color-wheel-pro.com/color-meaning.html

Cromie, William J., "Why Women Live Longer Than Men." 9 March 2005 http://www.harvard.edu/

Deaths: Preliminary Data for 2002 page. 7 April 2005 http://www.cdc.gov/

Drinking water page. 18 January 2005 http://www.weightlossforall.com/

Editors of Phaidon Press. *The Fashion Book*. London: Phaidon, 1998.

Fox, Patty. *Star Style: Hollywood Legends as Fashion Icons*. Santa Monica, Calif.: Angel City Press, 1995.

Gardner, Jody Kozlow, and Cherie Serota. *Pregnancy Chic: The Fashion Survival Guide*. New York: Villard, 1998.

Joyce, Linda. *The Day You Were Born: A Journey to Wholeness Through Astrology and Numerology*. New York, Citadel Press, 1998.

Ludot, Didier. *The Little Black Dress: Vintage Treasure*. New York: Assouline, 2001.

Martin, Richard, *The Boutonniere: Style in One's Lapel*. New York: Universe, 2000.

Mizrahi, Isaac. "Isaac Mizrahi." Behind the Label. Ultra HD. New York, 9 March 2005.

Moore, Donnica, M.D. 5 January 2005 Drdonnica.com home page. http://www.drdonnica.com/today/00007230.htm

O'Hara Callan, Georgina. *The Thames and Hudson Dictionary of Fashion and Fashion Designers*. London: Thames and Hudson Ltd., 1986.

Pedergast, Sara, and Tom Pedergast. *St. James Encyclopedia of Pop Culture*. Stamford: Gale Group, 1999.

Poitier, Sidney. *The Measure of a Man: A Spiritual Autobiography*. New York: HarperCollins, 2000.

Smoke-Out information page. 29 February 2005 http://www.cancer.org/docroot/home/index.asp

The diamond information page. 22 March 2005 http://www.jckgroup.com/

"The shelf life of cosmetics: when should you ditch that product?" 12 January 2005, www.findarticles.com/p/articles/mi_m1264/is_5_33/ai_90989876

Women's voices page. 3 March 2005 http://womenshistory.about.com/library/qu/blqulist.htm